Obstetrics and Gynaecology:

A PROBLEM-SOLVING APPROACH

Illustrations by

Peter Cox

For W. B. Saunders

Publisher Ellen Green
Project Editor Jane Shanks
Project Controller Frances Affleck
Design Direction Erik Bigland

Obstetrics and Gynaecology

A PROBLEM-SOLVING APPROACH

Mark James
MBChB MRCOG

Research Fellow in Urogynaecology,
Southmead Hospital, Bristol Urological Institute, Westbury on Trim, UK

Tim Draycott
MRCOG

Research Registrar,
Gloucestershire Royal Hospital, Gloucester, UK

Robert Fox
MD MRCOG DChE

Consultant Gynaecologist,
Directorate of Obstetrics & Gynaecology,
Taunton & Somerset Hospital, Taunton, UK

Michael Read
MD FRCOG FRCS

Consultant Obstetrician and Gynaecologist,
Gloucestershire Royal Hospital, Gloucester, UK

W.B. SAUNDERS

EDINBURGH • LONDON • PHILADELPHIA • TORONTO • SYDNEY • TOKYO • 1999

W. B. Saunders   24–28 Oval Road
                  London NW1 7DX

                  The Curtis Center
                  Independence Square West
                  Philadelphia, PA 19106–3399, USA

                  Harcourt Brace & Company
                  55 Horner Avenue
                  Toronto, Ontario M8Z 4X6, Canada

                  Harcourt Brace & Company, Australia
                  30–52 Smidmore Street
                  Marrickville, NSW 2204, Australia

                  Harcourt Brace & Company, Japan
                  Ichibancho Central Building, 22–1 Ichibancho
                  Chiyoda-ku, Tokyo 102, Japan

An imprint of Harcourt Brace & Company Limited

First published 1999

ISBN 0 7020 22519

British Library Cataloguing in Publication Data
A catalogue record for this book is available from the British
Library.

Library of Congress Cataloging in Publication Data
A catalog of record for this book is available from the Library of
Congress.

Medical knowledge is constantly changing. As new information
becomes available, changes in treatment, procedures,
equipment and the use of drugs become necessary. The
authors and the publishers have, as far as it is possible, taken
care to ensure that the information given in this text is
accurate and up to date. However, readers are strongly advised
to confirm that the information, especially with regard to drug
usage, complies with current legislation and standards of
practice.

Printed in China
NPCC/01

Preface

For the medical student starting an obstetric and gynaecology attachment, the diverse array of medical conditions, the multidisciplinary team approach, the dogged ethical issues, and the extreme psychological distress pose a bewildering set of new problems. In our clinical teaching, we have often been impressed by the endeavour of students in coping with these issues and yet frequently disappointed by the inability of many to deal with the simplest of clinical problems in a logical fashion. It was of course not their fault. We were providing too many facts and not enough stucture. Memorising a list of 20 causes of sperm dysfunction does not help a student to sit down with a childless couple and guide them through the investigation and treatment of infertility. Helping the student to think as a mature clinician and not as a contestant on a quiz show is the challenge. To meet that challenge, we have attempted to present common clinical problems in a coherent manner and at the same time outline some of the attitudes which make for excellence in women's health care.

Obstetrics and gynaecology is a difficult specialty, but ultimately the rewards received are greater than the efforts needed to become a skilled practitioner.

Robert Fox
Mark James
Tim Draycott
Mike Read

Contents

Introduction

ORGANISATION OF THOUGHT

Most doctors will have a very clear image of their arrival on duty for the first time just a few weeks after passing final MB. Despite being told that we had enough factual knowledge to pass MRCP, those first days seemed full of feelings of chaos and inadequacy. Facts were not enough. Organisation and structure were equally important. On the ward and in health centres, doctors are not set the task of writing essays about abstract concepts, nor of answering multiple choice questions, but of organising care and dealing with clinical problems.

We are concerned to help students develop a structured approach to medical care. Within the text of the book, we have attempted to present the management of the commonest clinical problems in a consistent format. Within each chapter we have given statistical information, but this is provided more to illustrate clinical points. A good knowledge base is important to a practising obstetrician, of course, but only a very small proportion of medical students will enter our speciality. Our wish is to give students a taste of 'OBGYN', avoiding information overload if possible, but also importantly to use obstetrics and gynaecology as a model for teaching general aspects of clinical practice which ultimately will benefit most doctors.

ATTITUDES TO PATIENTS

Most senior doctors will be able to recall, too, instances of causing great upset to patients, quite inadvertently, by making assumptions about their needs and emotions. Most medical students are caring and sympathetic, but few have learnt to be empathic by the time of qualification. Sympathy arises out of one's own previous emotional experience; empathy is an attempt to observe the emotions of others and respond to their needs, to see what emotion they are experiencing and not impose some emotion we have experienced in our past. As part of this, it is important for us all to learn that individuals behave very differently in response to physical disease, and that it can be disadvantageous to assume the nature of the emotional response. To ignore

or override the woman's response to physical symptoms can only lead to discord. One example is that of the complaint of heavy periods. Studies measuring blood loss have shown that many such women seem to have a menstrual loss within normal limits. However, to inform a woman who has taken the courage to report her symptoms to her GP that her menstrual loss is normal does not solve her problem (as she sees it) and only serves to creates barriers within the professional relationship. It is all too easy for us to forget that visiting a doctor per se is a frightening experience for many people. Simple questions become difficult to answer, advice given quickly by the doctor is misinterpreted for the worse. If the doctor shows disapproval because the patient is slow to react to questions or vague about giving historical details, or if the doctor reveals prejudice about some behaviour such as cigarette smoking or drug abuse, anxiety and anger intervene between doctor and patient. Care cannot then be delivered effectively.

The quality of health care should not only be measured by the expertise of the staff and the sophistication of the technical equipment but must also include the way people are dealt with at a human level. For a patient, the attitude of the doctors and nurses may be all that she remembers of her consultation. It is not an issue of which is better: a skilful surgeon or a thoughtful surgeon. The aim has to be a skilful and thoughtful surgeon.

It is difficult to help students to learn about attitudes. Much of this only comes with maturity and watching others in practice. Nevertheless, we have included small passages on the social and psychological aspects of obstetrics and gynaecology without, we hope, appearing to be self-righteous. Healthcare cannot be delivered effectively without concern for the dignity and comfort of our patients. Similarly, clinical medicine cannot be learnt properly without attention to the ethics of delivery of care.

THE STRUCTURE OF THE BOOK

Section 1 gives some basic knowledge of the speciality to enable the reader to understand the contents of the problem-based chapters in Sections 2 and 3. Each of these chapters is structured according to a standard format.

- On the first page, the clinical significance of the symptom is briefly outlined. This includes public health issues as well as details of the impact on the individual.
- The causes of the clinical symptom are given as a list together with a small section detailing the most frequently seen conditions.
- The next section of the chapter explains how care is organised, particularly if this is unusual in any way, and the methods used for clinical assessment. The clinical history aims to explain the importance of the symptoms so that the student can understand why the questions are being asked. Similarly, the description of physical examination tries to explain which parts need to be examined and why. This section continues with the relevant investigations that should be performed and the value of the information that is obtained.
- The commonest conditions are explained in some length, with particular attention being paid to the method of diagnosis of each and the treatment options. Of course, some conditions cause a variety of clinical symptoms, and cross-references are then used to avoid duplication.
- Finally, each chapter ends with a 'Golden points' box of important issues to be emphasised. The small amount of blank page that follows gives room for personal notes to be made. A template showing the structure of these chapters follows.

Clinical symptom

CLINICAL SIGNIFICANCE

Public health impact and effect on individual woman.

DIFFERENTIAL DIAGNOSIS

MAIN CATEGORY	DIAGNOSIS
Physiological causes	
Physiological	
Pathological causes	
1. *Congenital*	Malformation
	Single gene disorder
	Chromosomal rearrangement
2. *Neoplastic*	Benign
	Borderline
	Premalignant
	Primary malignancy
	Secondary malignancy
3. *Infective*	Bacterial
	Intracellular bacteria
	Viral
	Protozoal
	Fungal
4. *Degenerative*	Vascular
	Neurological

General information on frequency or other important diagnostic points.

CLINICAL ASSESSMENT

Rapid emergency assessment

Immediate measures to be taken if presentation is a severe emergency. Includes details of resuscitation.

Organisation of care

Any special points about how care is delivered, including screening, specialist clinics and inter-specialty referral.

Relevant history

Presenting complaint

MAIN SYMPTOM – Description of main symptom and questions to ask about it.

COMMONLY ASSOCIATED SYMPTOMS – Symptoms aiding assessment, which the woman may not mention spontaneously.

EFFECT ON PATIENT – Any deleterious effect on the woman's lifestyle, family, occupation, etc. Helps to gauge seriousness of complaint.

Gynaecological history

GYNAECOLOGICAL DISEASE – Ask of details such as previous PID or endometriosis, and of previous gynae surgery including complications.

MENSTRUAL HISTORY – Are there symptoms of the menstrual cycle not mentioned above?

CERVICAL CYTOLOGY – Is a smear due now? Any previous abnormalities or treatment?

CONTRACEPTION – Anything being used now? What was used in the past? Methods may be cause of symptoms or influence management.

FERTILITY REQUIREMENTS – May influence management. For example, should the gynaecologist offer conservative surgery (myomectomy) or hysterectomy for fibroids?

Obstetric history

DELIVERY – Number of babies and timing of recent delivery. Gynaecological symptoms may arise out of recent pregnancy.

OBSTETRIC COMPLICATIONS

Medical history

MEDICAL CONDITIONS – Any medical conditions that may be the cause of symptoms, e.g. antiphospholipid syndrome increases chance of miscarriage. Alternatively, medical disease may influence treatment, e.g. OCP is contraindicated in women with history of thrombosis.

SURGERY – Previous surgery may be the cause of symptoms or make repeat surgery more difficult.

PSYCHOLOGICAL DISORDERS – May be cause of symptoms or influence their interpretation by the woman.

ALLERGIES

Drug history

MEDICATIONS – Medical therapy may cause gynaecological symptoms, e.g. warfarin may lead to menorrhagia. Any gynaecological therapy might interact with concurrent medical therapy.

SMOKING AND ALCOHOL – May be a cause of problems; e.g. smoking is associated with higher chance of fetal growth delay.

ILLEGAL DRUGS – Again may be a cause of disease, including pregnancy complications.

Social history

AGE – Disease frequency changes with age.

OCCUPATION – Few occupational diseases, but stress may play a part in presentation, e.g. premenstrual syndrome.

LIFESTYLE – Excessive exercise is a cause of amenorrhoea.

Relevant clinical examination

General examination

GENERAL CONDITION – Any stigmata of anaemia, thyroid disease.

BODY-MASS INDEX – May influence disease, e.g. low BMI is a cause of amenorrhoea. Also may influence therapy, e.g. surgery more difficult with morbid obesity.

BREASTS – Not routinely examined by most obstetricians/ gynaecologists but should be in suspected breast disease or if going to prescribe drugs which influence the breast, e.g. OCP or HRT.

Cardiorespiratory system

Most important for pre-operative assessment.

Abdomen

CONTOUR – Any evidence of tumour or pulsation.

OLD SCARS – Woman may have forgotten an operation she had in past.

PALPATION – For masses, tenderness, etc.

BOWEL SOUNDS – If obstruction suspected.

Pelvic

VULVA – Evidence of skin disease or excoriation.

VAGINA – Evidence of tumour, discharge, prolapse, etc.

CERVIX – Evidence of tumour, discharge, excitation tenderness, etc.

BIMANUAL EXAMINATION – Evidence of tumour, tenderness etc.

RECTAL EXAMINATION – Only if suspect bowel disease.

Relevant clinical investigations

Haematology

HAEMOGLOBIN – For anaemia.

WHITE CELL COUNT – If suspect infection but not an accurate indicator.

PLATELET COUNT – To look for evidence of thrombocytopaenia, e.g. in menorrhagia or pre-eclampsia.

CLOTTING STUDIES – To look for congenital or acquired disorders. Includes both tendency to bleeding and thrombosis. Examples include screen for thrombophilia in recurrent miscarriage and screen for DIC in placental abruption.

Biochemistry

SERUM UREA AND ELECTROLYTES – Most often as part of preoperative screen to check renal function but also used in pre-eclampsia.

SERUM LIVER FUNCTION TESTS – Similar to U+Es.

RANDOM BLOOD SUGAR OR GLUCOSE TOLERANCE TEST – Screening for diabetes mellitus.

Endocrine tests

OESTRADIOL

β-hCG AND ALPHA-FETOPROTEIN – Pregnancy testing or tumour markers.

THYROID-STIMULATING HORMONE – Screen for thyroid disease, e.g. menorrhagia.

LUTEINISING HORMONE / FOLLICLE-STIMULATING HORMONE – Used mostly to investigate women with ovulatory disorders.

Microbiology

URINE – For microscopy and culture to look for evidence of infection or tumours.

Diagnostic imaging

ULTRASOUND – One of the most commonly used gynaecological investigations. Investigation of pain, pregnancy problems, etc.

PLAIN FILMS – Not often used but important if suspect urinary tract disease.

CONTRAST RADIOLOGY – IVU used if urinary tract disease suspected. GI enema studies if bowel disease suspected.

AXIAL IMAGING – Rarely used but assists gynaecological oncologists in the investigation of pelvic masses. Pituitary MRI used for women with hyper-prolactinaemia.

Cytology

CERVICAL – Part of screening for cervical cancer.

Histopathology

ENDOMETRIAL – Investigation of abnormal bleeding.

Direct visualisation

LAPAROSCOPY – Used in infertility, suspected ectopic pregnancy, and chronic pelvic pain.

HYSTEROSCOPY – Used mostly for abnormal bleeding but also recurrent miscarriage.

DETAILS OF COMMON CONDITIONS

1. Name of condition

Background

DEFINITION – A brief but precise statement of the nature of the condition.

AETIOLOGY – Causes of the condition.

ADDITIONAL TESTS – Investigations needed to clinch or refine diagnosis.

DIAGNOSIS – How to spot the clinical pattern and then confirm the diagnosis.

MAIN COMPLICATIONS – Consequences of the condition.

SCREENING/PREVENTION – Mention of any methods of screening and/or prevention before clinical presentation, e.g. cervical cytology screening. Also methods of secondary prevention to avoid complications, e.g. use of corticosteroids in preterm labour.

Treatment options

ADVICE – Combination of explanation and education. This may be all that some women wish for.

CHANGE OF LIFESTYLE/DIET – Methods of improving health by simple means, e.g. stopping smoking in subfertility.

DEVICES – Use of small device to control symptoms, e.g. vaginal ring pessaries for prolapse.

DRUG THERAPY – List of available drugs with side effects.

SURGERY – List of available operations with complications.

OVERVIEW – Brief resumé of the condition and a guide to the best treatment(s).

Follow-up

SHORT TERM

LONG TERM

GOLDEN POINTS

Pointers of things to remember.

Abbreviations

AC	Abdominal circumference	EPAC	Early pregnancy assessment clinic
ACA	Anticardiolipin antibodies	ERPC	Evaluation of retained products of conception
AFP	Alpha-fetoprotein		
AIP	Autoimmune profile	ESR	Erythrocyte sedimentation rate
ALT	Alanine transaminase	ET	Embryo transfer
ANC	Antenatal clinic	EUA	Examination under anaesthetic
APH	Antepartum haemorrhage	FBC	Full blood count
ARM	Artificial rupture of membranes	FL	Femur length
β-hCG	Beta unit of hCG	FMC	Fetal movement chart
BMI	Body-mass index	FSH	Follicle-stimulating hormone
BP	Blood pressure	FT3	Free tri-iodothyronine
BPD	Biparietal diameter	GDM	Gestational diabetes medicine
bpm	Beats per minute	GHb	Glycosylated haemoglobin (HbA$_1$)
BSO	Bilateral salpingo-oophorectomy	GI	Gastrointestinal
BSS	Blood sugar (glucose) series	GIFT	Gamete intrafallopian transfer
BV	Bacterial vaginosis	GnRH	Gonadotrophin-releasing hormone
Ca	Cancer	GnRHa	Gonadotrophin-releasing hormone analogue
CIN	Cervical intraepithelial neoplasia		
CMW	Community midwife	GP	General practitioner
COPP	Combined oestrogen/progestogen preparation	GSI	Genuine stress incontinence
		GTT	Glucose tolerance test
CPD	Cephalopelvic nisproportion	Hb	Haemoglobin
CPN	Chronic pyelonephritis	HC	Head circumference
CRP	C-reactive protein	hCG	Human chorionic gonadotrophin
CTG	Cardiotocogram/-graphy	HDL	High-density lipoprotein
CVP	Central venous pressure	HELLP	Haemolysis, elevated liver enzymes, low platelets
CVS	Chorionic villus sampling		
Cx	Cervix	HLA	Human lymphocyte antigen
D&C	Dilatation of cervix and curettage of uterus	HRT	Hormone replacement therapy
		HVS	High vaginal swab
DES	Diethyl-stilboestrol	IBS	Irritable bowel syndrome
DHEAS	Dehydroepiandrosterone sulphate	ICSI	Intracytoplasmic sperm injection
DI	Detrusor instability	IDDM	Insulin-dependent diabetes mellitus
DIC	Disseminated intravascular coagulation	IMB	Intermenstrual bleeding
DUB	Dysfunctional uterine bleeding	IoL	Induction of labour
DVT	Deep vein thrombosis	ISC	Intermittent self-catheterisation
E$_2$	Oestradiol	ITU	Intensive therapy unit
EA	Endometrial aspiration	IUCD	Intrauterine contraceptive device
ECV	External cephalic version	IUD	Intrauterine death
EDD	Expected date of delivery	IUGR	Intrauterine growth retardation
EDF	End diastolic flow	IUI	Intrauterine insemination
EFW	Estimation of fetal weight	IVF	In-vitro fertilisation
ELISA	Enzyme-linked immunosorbent assay	IVH	Intraventricular haemorrhage

IVP/IVU	Intravenous pyelogram/urogram	SFD	Small for dates
LAC	Lupus anticoagulant	SRM	Spontaneous rupture of membranes
LDL	Low-density lipoprotein	STD	Sexually transmitted disease
LFTs	Liver function tests	SVD	Spontaneous vaginal delivery
LH	Luteinising hormone	T4	Thyroxine
LLETZ	Large loop excision of the trans-formation zone	T21	Trisomy 21
		TAH	Total abdominal hysterectomy
LMP	Last menstrual period	TAS	Transabdominal ultrasound scan
LSCS	Lower segment caesarean section	TCI	To come in (be admitted)
Mane	Tomorrow	TCRE	Transcervical resection of endometrium
mcg	Microgram		
MI	Myocardial infarction	TFTs	Thyroid function tests
MRI	Magnetic resonance imaging	TOP	Termination of pregnancy
MSU	Midstream specimen of urine	ToRCH	Viral screen for toxoplasma, cyto-megalovirus and rubella
NIDDM	Non-insulin-dependent diabetes mellitus		
		TSH	Thyroid-stimulating hormone
NTD	Neural tube defect	TVS	Transvaginal ultrasound scan
OA	Occipitoanterior position	TZ	Transformation zone
OCP	Oral contraceptive pill	U+Es	Urea and electrolytes
OP	Occipitoposterior position	UAD	Umbilical artery Doppler
OPD	Outpatient department	UDS	Urodynamic studies
OT	Occipitotransverse position	USS	Ultrasound scan
P4	Progesterone	UTI	Urinary tract infection
PCB	Postcoital bleeding	VaIN	Vaginal intraepithelial neoplasia
PCOD	Polycystic ovarian disease	VH	Vaginal hysterectomy
PCT	Postcoital test	VIN	Vulval intraepithelial neoplasia
PE	Pulmonary embolism	WCC	White cell count
PET	Pre-eclampsia	X-match	Cross-match
PI	Pulsatility index	XPT	Crossed-penetration test
PID	Pelvic inflammatory disease	46XX	Normal female karyotype
PMB	Postmenopausal bleeding	46XY	Normal male karyotype
PMS	Premenstrual syndrome	47XX+21	Notation for female with trisomy 21
PoC	Products of conception	47XXX	Triple X syndrome
PoP	Progestogen-only pill	47XXY	Notation for male with Klinefelter's syndrome
PPH	Postpartum haemorrhage		
PRL	Prolactin	45XO	Notation for female with Turner's syndrome
RBS	Random blood sugar (glucose)		
RDS	Respiratory distress syndrome	/7	Number of days
Rh	Rhesus blood group	/12	Number of months
RIF	Right iliac fossa	/52	Number of weeks
RPoC	Retained products of conception	/40	Number of weeks of pregnancy
RUQ	Right upper quadrant	6/28	Notation of menstrual cycle; days of loss/length of cycle
SCBU	Special care baby unit		
SCJ	Squamo-columnar junction		

Outline of Clinical Practice

1 Obstetrics and gynaecology: requirements for professional care

PROFESSIONAL SKILL MIX

Women's Health is an enormous speciality involving a large variety of highly trained professionals, not just obstetrician/gynaecologists. Specialist gynaecology nurses, midwives, general practitioners, anaesthetists, family planning practitioners, breast surgeons and psychosexual counsellors all play important parts in the care of women in health and disease. The variety of skills needed to be a successful obstetrician/gynaecologist is also wide, ranging from microsurgical fertility techniques to non-directive counselling, from team management to ultrasound-guided invasive procedures, from endo-crinology to radical cancer surgery. Perhaps the most important of all is the ability to recognise the needs and wishes of the women we care for and to respect the differing skills of our colleagues.

EMOTIONAL RESPONSES

Perhaps more than any other speciality, extreme happiness and profound sadness are to be found side-by-side. In the morning an obstetrician may help comfort the mother whose baby was stillborn by emergency caesarean section for massive obstetric haemorrhage. Later the same day there may be news to break of successful fertility treatment or of a normal amniocentesis result.

The clinician may share in the emotional feelings of a patient, but it is not his/her role to decide or judge what the nature of those emotions should be. It is easy for a doctor to feel a patient's response is somehow in-adequate, misplaced or annoying, but such instincts have to be suppressed in order to maintain the patient's trust and deliver quality care. After all, we rarely know the full background to someone's life. A vaginal exam-ination may bring back memories of child sex abuse, and a blood test may remind a mother of her child's drug misuse.

2 Basic gynaecological care

HISTORY TAKING

Basic Skills

Everyone attending a hospital clinic tends to feel anxious – partly from fear of serious disease and concerns about pain during outpatient procedures, but also because of the thought of meeting a doctor. To make the woman feel as relaxed as possible and to make the clinic run smoothly, it is useful for all the members of the team to facilitate the arrival of the patient in the clinic. Simple things like a comfortable waiting area and keeping to appointment times help to lessen any apprehension and create a favourable impression of the unit. On first meeting, the doctor should greet the patient, introducing herself/himself and explain her/his position. Some doctors ask the woman what she wishes to be called, e.g. by Miss/Mrs and her surname or by her first name.

Surveys have shown that patients want their doctors to appear confident and sympathetic but without being too informal or overly assertive. It is difficult to get the balance right initially, but this comes with practice. Patients also like to feel that the consultation is not rushed, and yet the doctor may have a lot of other women to see at the clinic. The clinic therefore needs to run efficiently so that as much time can be given to the patient as possible. The taking of the history needs to progress reasonably quickly but it should be remembered that many patients do wish to tell their story. This should be encouraged, therefore, but within limits. Notes need to taken, and explaining that you will write as the interview continues often prevents the woman feeling that the consultation is impersonal. It is easy to forget certain questions in a busy clinic, and it may help to have formatted history sheets which act as prompts (see Figure 2.1). These sheets can be modified for different conditions such as subfertility, recurrent miscarriage and abnormal cytology. History sheets also cut down on some of the writing that is needed.

Functions of Gynaecological History

The primary reason of the interview is to enquire into the nature and severity of the woman's symptoms. This allows the gynaecologist to work toward a diagnosis and undertake an appropriate physical examination and set of investigations. The clinician can also gauge the effect the symptom is having on a woman's life.

The history is also used to assess the woman's fitness for anaesthesia and her thromboembolic risk if surgery seems likely.

Special Aspects of Gynaecological History

The gynaecological history should involve inquiry into the sexual and reproductive aspects of a woman's health. These may cause some embarrassment, but a gynaecological assessment is incomplete if details of problems with libido and intercourse are not known. Most women will speak freely if the questions are posed in a straightforward manner.

The possibility of pregnancy must be kept in mind all the time. X-rays, drugs and surgery are generally to be avoided in pregnancy. Details of the LMP were used to discount the possibility of pregnancy, but this is not accurate, and a high-sensitivity pregnancy test should be performed in all women with symptoms that might be accounted for by pregnancy, and in those who are admitted for surgery.

PHYSICAL EXAMINATION

General Gynaecological Examination

The gynaecological examination is in some ways very simple but it requires great care because of the intimate nature of the pelvic assessment. For the woman's comfort it is helpful if she can be made to feel as at ease and as confident as possible. Simply telling a woman to relax is counterproductive, but attention to small details (see Box 2.1) will make the examination easier for many individuals.

Breast Examination

In former times, many gynaecologists routinely undertook a breast examination at first consultation. This was considered to be a useful screening exercise, but it has not been shown to be of benefit, and many women found the combination of a pelvic and breast examination too much to tolerate. There has been a move over the last few years to leaving breast screening to general prac-

WOMAN'S DETAILS

Name   DOB   Ref No

PROBLEMS (list)

CURRENT HISTORY

Age   Parity   LMP

LAST SMEAR

Date

Normal/abnormal

Ever abnormal

CONTRACEPTION

Steri/IUD/OCP/Other

Sex active

Family complete

SYSTEMS

GI

GU

CVS/RESP

MEDICAL & SURGICAL HISTORY

DRUGS

Medications

Tobacco

Alcohol

Allergy

PHYSICAL EXAMINATION   Weight

                                             BP

                                             Urinalysis

ABDOMEN   CVS/RESP
                                             HS

                                             BS

PELVIS

Vulva   Vagina

Cervix

Uterus

Adnexa

IMPRESSION

ADVICE GIVEN & TREATMENT

Leaflet

INVESTIGATIONS

Fbc   USS

U+E/LFT   Smear

FSH/T4   Pipelle

Chlam serology   Urodynamics

Swabs   Other tests

MSU   Alert anaesthetist

ARRANGEMENTS

Follow-up: Operation/GOPD/By letter/Cross-referral to ....

SIGNED ....   **DATE** ....

Fig 2.1 *Formatted gynaecology history sheet.*

Box 2.1 Guidelines for vaginal examination

- Always ask permission to do a pelvic examination.
- Explain that she can stop the examination at any point.
- Allow the woman to empty her bladder before examination.
- Allow the woman to undress in private.
- Provide facilities for sanitary towels.
- Offer to let a companion attend.
- Always provide a chaperone (for benefit of both woman and doctor).
- Secure the room so that others cannot interrupt.
- Keep exposure of body parts to the minimum consistent with clinical needs.
- Keep medical instruments covered.
- Warm speculum before insertion.
- Explain procedure throughout.
- Avoid comments about personal details such as tattoos or suntans.

---

titioners using more satisfactory methods and to reserving breast examination for specific indications. These are relatively uncommon but include checking for occult breast primaries in women with apparent ovarian cancer and as a (medico-legal) check before commencing hormone therapy such as the oral contraceptive pill (OCP) or hormone replacement therapy (HRT).

SPECIAL GYNAECOLOGICAL INVESTIGATIONS

Cervical Cytology

Cervical cells are removed for staining and microscopy to look for cytological abnormalities (dyskaryosis) as part of the national screening programme for premalignant disease of the cervix. The test is performed by exposing the cervix with a Cusco speculum, and a spatula is used to gently remove the surface cells from the ectocervix and lower part of the endocervical canal. The cells are ideally taken from the transformation zone (TZ) around the area where the squamous and columnar tissues meet in the squamo-columnar junction or SCJ. This is confirmed at microscopy by the presence of both cell types. If either is present in insufficient numbers then the smear is reported as inadequate and a repeat test is taken. The ideal time to take a smear in premenopausal women is at midcycle, when the external cervical os is opening under the influence of oestrogen and the SCJ is exposed. The material removed

is then smeared over a glass slide and fixed with alcohol. The cytological stain is then added in the laboratory.

This is a screening test and is therefore used in asymptomatic women with an apparently normal cervix. It is not a diagnostic test and is of little value for the investigation of symptoms or an abnormal-looking cervix. If the cytology result is abnormal then further tests are undertaken to identify the cause. This involves microscopic examination of the cervix (colposcopy) (see Chapter 10).

Bacteriology

Vaginal and pelvic infections are a common source of problems, particularly in young women. Some infections such as candida, bacterial vaginosis and trichomonas are largely confined to the vagina and are best detected by taking a vaginal swab and performing immediate microscopy and culture. Other infections such as chlamydia and gonorrhoea involve the upper genital tract (cervix, uterus and adnexa), and these will not show up so frequently on a vaginal sample. To test for these it is important to take swabs from the endocervix. A general swab is sent for bacteriology and a special swab is sent for chlamydial ELISA. It is also important to consider taking urethral and rectal swabs.

Sampling of the Endometrium

Disease of the endometrium is common. Some lesions are focal, such as small cancers and benign polyps, while others, such as hyperplasia, are diffuse. Traditionally, a dilatation and curettage (D&C) was used to sample the endometrium for histology and to find polyps. This was a blind technique, however, and a significant proportion of pathological lesions were missed. Several groups developed hysteroscopy to allow inspection of the cavity and directed biopsy. This has practical problems, however, and so more recently there has been a move to

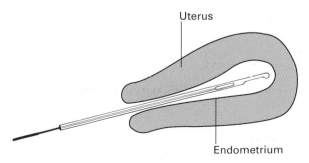

Fig 2.2 *Endometrial sampling.*

using endometrial aspiration (EA) with fine catheters (Figure 2.2). This is also a blind technique but, with the development of high-resolution transvaginal ultrasonography, the combination of EA and transvaginal scanning (TVS) gives a comprehensive assessment of the endometrium, myometrium and ovaries. Where any doubt exists, then a hysteroscopy can be performed.

Ultrasound Imaging

Ultrasound imaging has been a great advance in gynaecology. It has proved invaluable for the assessment of pain and bleeding in early pregnancy and for the investigation of pelvic pain and ovarian masses. Other specialities rely on transabdominal scanning but TVS is often more valuable for gynaecological problems because the image obtained is far superior. The probe is closer to the structures of interest and not separated from the transducer by layers of fat and muscle which attenuate sound energy and distort the image (Figures 2.3 and 2.4). Moreover, because the sound has less far to travel, higher-frequency sound can be used which provides better resolution of fine detail. Some women initially think that it is an odd way to scan, but the vast majority find it much easier than a standard bimanual examination, and many women who have previously had transabdominal scans comment that TVS is easier because there is no need for a full bladder. Others worry about safety in pregnancy, but there is no evidence that vaginal examination per se is dangerous, and the quantity of sound energy used is lower since the structures are closer and the examination is quicker. Disadvantages of

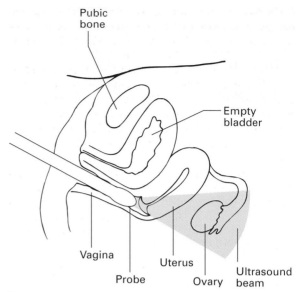

Fig 2.4 *Transvaginal ultrasound scanning.*

TVS are that it cannot be used to examine the urogenital tract and it may miss ovarian lesions high in the pelvis.

Urodynamic Studies

See Chapter 11.

PERIOPERATIVE CARE

It is not just the skill of the surgical team which influences the success or failure of an operation. Attention to medical care before and after surgery is equally important. This includes psychological and social preparation.

Preoperative Assessment and Perioperative Precautions

Medical assessment is important and should include a detailed history of current and previous medical and surgical problems and of current medications. It is easy for the patient to forget important issues, and the gynaecologist should ask questions such as, 'Are you under any other specialists?', 'Do you attend any other clinics?'. A general physical examination is performed, particularly looking for cardiovascular and respiratory problems. The assessment is mostly about cardiovascular and respiratory disease, but other issues such as chronic orthopaedic problems are very important because of positioning of the woman during surgery. The front of the notes should be clearly labelled if there is a history of spinal or hip conditions.

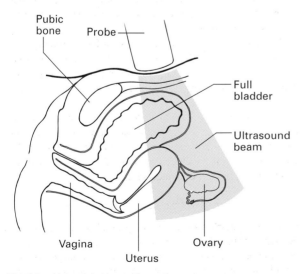

Fig 2.3 *Abdominal ultrasound scanning.*

For most women with gynaecological problems, few preoperative investigations are necessary. The common tests and the indications are given in Table 2.1. Not all tests are performed on all women.

If medical problems are identified, they should be optimised before surgery is undertaken, or special precautions should be taken. This includes use of an intravenous glucose/insulin/potassium regimen for women with established diabetes and the administration of corticosteroids for women who take oral steroids (see Table 2.2).

Blood grouping is used for two reasons. Rhesus grouping is necessary for pregnant women, to consider the need for anti-Rh(D) gammaglobulin. Grouping also allows for rapid cross-match if complications arise. For very major surgery such as radical hysterectomy, blood is cross-matched in advance.

Thromboprophylaxis

Thromboembolism is one of the commonest causes of postoperative mortality and thromboprophylaxis is thought to reduce that risk. The measures taken vary

Table 2.1	Preoperative investigations
Test	Indication
Pregnancy test	All women in reproductive years
Full blood count	Screen for anaemia
	Screen for thrombocytopaenia
Coagulation studies	History of bleeding tendency
	On anticoagulant therapy
U+Es/LFTs	Elderly (>70 years)
	Diabetes
	On diuretic therapy
	Renal/hepatic disease
	Severely ill
Serum calcium	Malignant disease
Serum lithium	On lithium therapy
ECG	Elderly (>70 years)
	Hypertension
	History of cardiovascular/ respiratory disease
Chest x-ray	Elderly (>70 years)
	Hypertension
	History of cardiovascular/ respiratory disease
Urine bacteriology	Urinary tract surgery

Table 2.2	Perioperative precautions
Bowel preparation	If bowel surgery possible (e.g. fixed pelvic mass)
Prophylactic antibiotics	Major surgery
	Valvular heart disease
Thromboprophylaxis	See Table 2.3
Sliding scale insulin regimen	Diabetes
Corticosteroids	Recent parenteral steroid therapy
Chest physiotherapy	Routine for major surgery
High-dependency monitoring	Radical surgery, e.g. Wertheim hysterectomy
	Severe intercurrent illness

with the estimate of risk, which depends on several factors (see Table 2.3).

The OCP is a risk factor for thromboembolism, and at one time the advice was that women discontinued the pill before surgery. The incidence of unwanted pregnancy was such that this advice has now been changed.

Psychological Preparation and Consent

Psychological preparation starts at the first consultation and includes giving information about the nature of the operation and what should be expected in the days and weeks after surgery. A clear explanation of the benefits and complications is mandatory. If a woman chooses not to have surgery after a detailed discussion, that should not necessarily be seen as a failure. She can always change her mind at a later date. Detailed leaflets can supplement the information given by mouth, and videos are now available for some operations.

The taking of consent the day before surgery is a medico-legal procedure, but the opportunity should be used for explanation and clarification. Always ask the woman if there is anything that she does not understand.

Social preparations include the timing of surgery to fit in with the woman's occupation and/or family life whenever possible. In addition, many women may need help with the care of an elderly relative during their stay in hospital and during convalescence.

Standard Postoperative Care

With the operation note, the surgeon should list instructions. Most units have a protocol for the type and timing of routine observations, which usually include pulse, blood pressure, temperature and urine output. This may be increased to incorporate pulse oximetry, central

Table 2.3 Thromboprophylaxis

	Low risk	Moderate risk	High risk
Assessment of risk	Minor surgery (< 30 min): no other risk factors Major surgery (< 30 min): age < 40 years and no other risk factors	Minor surgery (< 30 min): in women with a personal or family history of deep vein thrombosis (DVT), pulmonary embolism or thrombophilia Minor surgery (> 30 min) Laparoscopic extended surgery Obesity (> 80 kg) Gross varicose veins Current infection Immobility prior to surgery Major illness: cardiovascular, respiratory, renal or malignancy Heart failure or recent myocardial infarction Major surgery (> 30 min): in women with personal or family history of DVT, pulmonary embolism or thrombophilia Paralysis or immobilisation	Three or more of the above Major pelvic/abdominal surgery or gynaecological surgery
Options for prevention	Early mobilisation	Early mobilisation and **one** of the following specific methods of prophylaxis: Low-dose heparin Graduated elastic compression Intermittent pneumatic compression Dextran Low-dose aspirin	Early mobilisation **with both** low-dose heparin and leg stockings

venous pressure, and blood glucose if there are special indications.

On the first morning after surgery the gynaecologist reviews the woman's physical condition, and this is repeated daily until discharge. The assessment includes questions about symptoms such as pain, nausea and any cardio-respiratory problems. The observation chart is reviewed, and the woman's chest, abdomen and scar are examined. Her legs should also be examined for evidence of venous thrombosis. The drug chart should be reviewed regularly to see the analgesia requirement but also to decide whether any medications can be discontinued. The need for intravenous fluid therapy is also reassessed frequently, and this should be removed as

soon as possible. Patients become more mobile when lines are removed and generally feel as though progress is being made. While i.v. fluids are in progress a blood sample should be sent for urea and electrolyte (U+E) analysis daily to check for electrolyte disturbance such as hypokalaemia. A sample is usually sent for haemoglobin estimation on about the third day. If the sample is sent too early the level may be falsely lowered because of haemodilution by crystalloid infusion therapy.

At the first visit a reasonably detailed account of the surgery should be described. At each subsequent visit the woman should be told of her condition and congratulated on progress being made, however small. On the day of discharge, details of follow-up are given, and time should be taken to explain what can and cannot be done and things to report such as swelling of the leg and fever.

COMMON MEDICAL THERAPIES

Drugs Used to Control Menstruation

- **Mefenamic acid** is a prostaglandin synthetase inhibitor reducing both menstrual flow and pain. It is most commonly used in women with dysfunctional uterine bleeding (DUB) and fibroids who wish to avoid hormone therapy. It is started the day before menstruation, if the woman is able to predict the start, and continued until the bleeding has decreased or stopped. It is generally very safe but should be used with caution in women with peptic ulceration, asthma, renal disease or platelet disorders.

- **Tranexamic acid** is an antifibrinolytic agent which prevents clot lysis. Large studies in Scandinavia have shown it to be an extremely safe drug. It has been shown to be the most effective non-hormonal drug for DUB, reducing both blood loss by about 50% and menstrual pain scores. Its use is limited in some women by nausea and diarrhoea. It should be used with caution in women with arterial disease and a history of venous thrombosis.

- **Dicynene** is an unusual drug which has an effect on capillary fragility. It has been popular because of absence of serious side effects, but a recent trial showed it had no effect on the volume or duration of menstrual loss.

- **Combined hormonal contraceptive** is very effective both in regulating cycle length and reducing blood loss. It may cause venous thrombosis, and there are concerns about the chance of arterial disease and breast cancer. It is a very safe product for women, even over 40, who are slim, normotensive and who do not smoke, but many women prefer not to use it for therapy because of newspaper reports.

- **Progestogens** given orally are the most widely used medications for menstrual disorder, and yet there is no evidence to show that they are effective. They are valuable for acute episodes of severe menstrual haemorrhage but they do not appear to be useful for maintenance therapy.

- **Progestogen-containing IUCDs** do appear to be very effective and very safe. Bleeding is erratic initially, and some women get symptoms of progestogen in the first year.

- **Danazol** is a complex synthetic steroid with mixed oestrogenic, progestogenic and androgenic properties. It acts directly on the endometrium and it also suppresses ovarian activity by inhibiting release of follicle-stimulating hormone (FSH) and luteinising hormone (LH). It is very

effective but has many side effects, including weight gain, breast atrophy, hirsutism, acne, and mood depression. This can be limited by using low-dose therapy, but it remains unpopular because of early reports with high-dose treatment.

Analogues of GnRH

Native gonadotrophin-releasing hormone (GnRH) is a decapeptide which is released in pulses by the hypothalamus. It stimulates release of pituitary gonadotrophins (LH and FSH). Changes to the amino acid sequence produce changes in function with superagonist or antagonist effects. Agonists have been identified and paradoxically they inactivate the pituitary gonadotroph cells and induce ovarian quiescence and oestrogen deficiency (Figure 2.5). This effect is entirely reversible. Side effects include vasomotor flushes and vascular headaches. Prolonged use leads to loss of bone mass, but this can be prevented by giving tibolone (add-back therapy) which is a weak oestrogenic/progestogenic compound that prevents flushes and bone loss but without stimulating the endometrium.

In gynaecology, GnRH analogues are used to reduce fibroid volume and vascularity, and to treat endometriosis. In reproductive medicine, they are used in ovulation induction programmes and assisted conception. By preventing spontaneous surges of LH, they allow the reproductive physician to have greater control of folliculogenesis and the timing of ovulation/oocyte retrieval.

Drugs to Induce Ovulation

The ideal drug for ovulation should be simple to use, requiring minimal monitoring. It should have a low incidence of side effects and be associated with a normal miscarriage rate and a low chance of multiple pregnancy. It should also be inexpensive. The drug chosen depends mostly on the cause of the ovulatory failure (see Chapter 20). No drug is always effective, and, for each condition, an alternative agent is tried if the first proves unsuccessful.

- **Clomiphene** is an oestrogen receptor blocker (with partial agonist activity). It acts by fooling the hypothalamus/pituitary that there is insufficient oestrogen, which initiates release of GnRH and FSH. FSH then promotes folliculogenesis. It is given by mouth, and side effects such as flushing are well tolerated. Minimal monitoring is required (midluteal serum progesterone). It is moderately effective in polycystic ovarian disease. The

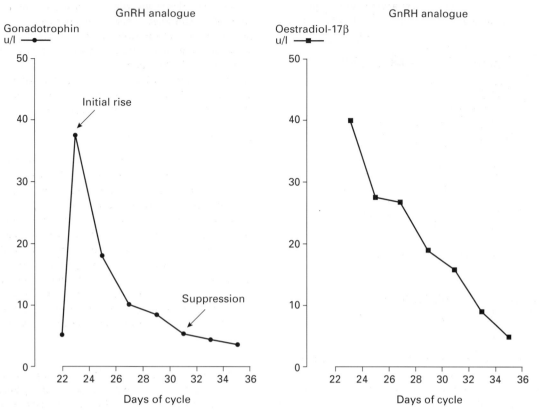

Fig 2.5 *The effect of gonadotrophin-releasing hormone analogues on gonadotrophin and oestradiol levels.*

twin rate is moderately high (10%) but high-order multiple pregnancy is rare. Miscarriage rates are high (30%). It may increase the chance of ovarian cancer, but this is unproven. If women with polycystic ovarian disease (PCOD) do not respond, the next step is to try laparoscopic ovarian surgery.

- **Pulsatile GnRH** is used for hypothalamic dysfunction (previous tumours, Kallmann syndrome). Native GnRH synthesised in a laboratory is given subcutaneously by pump. The pump delivers a dose every 90 min, mimicking the action of the hypothalamus. This activates the pituitary to produce FSH and LH, and ovarian function returns. Ovulation is confirmed by scan, after which the pump is removed and hCG is given to support the luteal phase. It is moderately effective with no drug-related side effects, and the multiple pregnancy and miscarriage rates are near-normal, but many women find it inconvenient to carry the pump for 2 weeks.
- **Exogenous gonadotrophin therapy** is the administration of human FSH (and sometimes LH) to

directly stimulate the ovary, overriding the control of hypothalamus and pituitary. It therefore requires close monitoring with serial oestradiol measurement and ultrasound assessment of ovarian follicular size in order to avoid an excessive ovarian response which may result in high-order multiple pregnancy and ovarian hyperstimulation syndrome. It is generally used as a second-line or third-line therapy for ovulation induction. It is also used as the main ovarian stimulant for assisted conception techniques (see Chapter 19).

- **Dopamine agonists** (bromocriptine and carbergoline) are used to induce ovulation in women with hyperprolactinaemia. They act directly on the pituitary to inhibit prolactin release. Normal ovular ovarian cycle resumes within about 6 weeks in most women. Side effects such as nausea and postural hypotension can be troublesome, but multiple pregnancy is very rare and the miscarriage rate is normal. They are discontinued when pregnancy is confirmed unless the tumour was known to be very large.

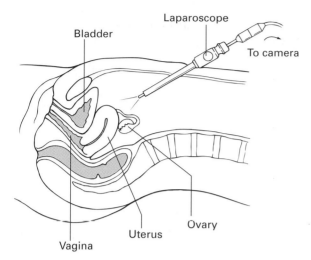

Fig 2.6 *Laparoscopic visualisation of the pelvic organs.*

COMMON GYNAECOLOGICAL OPERATIONS

Laparoscopy

Laparoscopy is a form of endoscopy allowing inspection of the peritoneal cavity (Figure 2.6). A rigid telescopic device is inserted through an incision at the umbilicus after the peritoneal cavity has been insufflated with carbon dioxide gas through a Verres needle. It is used for diagnosis and for a range of therapeutic procedures including clip sterilisation, ovarian cystectomy and hysterectomy. Side effects include bruising and pain, particularly subdiaphragmatic pain referred to the shoulders. Its main complication is trauma to bowel, urinary tract and major vessels. If the Verres is placed incorrectly into a major vein, gas embolism may occur.

Dilatation and Curettage

This is the technique of opening the cervix with a graduated dilator (dilatation) and removal of endometrial tissue (curettage). It is largely a diagnostic procedure for women with menstrual disorder or postmenopausal bleeding but may occasionally be used to stop acute haemorrhage in women with severe menorrhagia. Complications include uterine perforation and infection. It is now largely replaced by diagnostic hysteroscopy or endometrial aspiration and transvaginal scanning.

Hysteroscopy

This is a method of visualising the uterine cavity. It is used to investigate menstrual disorders, recurrent mis-

carriage and infertility. It is also used for minimal-access surgical techniques, including endometrial ablation, polypectomy and division of uterine septa. It involves insertion of a 5 mm rigid telescopic device into the cavity through the cervix. The cavity is opened out by infusion of carbon dioxide gas or liquid medium such as glycine or saline. Complications include uterine perforation, infection and gas embolism (very rare).

Endometrial Ablation

This is hysteroscopic removal or destruction of endometrium as treatment for menstrual disorders (Figure 2.7). Methods include laser, electrodiathermy coagulation, and electrodiathermy resection. It is a simple technique with more rapid recovery than for hysterectomy, but only 30% are amenorrhoeic and 10% have no relief at all. Complications include perforation with intra-abdominal trauma, haemorrhage (and emergency hysterectomy), and equipment failure (incomplete operation). It is not fully contraceptive, and sterilisation should be offered in conjunction. It is likely to be replaced by the levonorgestrel intrauterine contraceptive device (LNG-IUCD).

Simple Hysterectomy

Hysterectomy is removal of uterus. It is performed for menstrual disorder, endometriosis with pelvic pain, uterine prolapse, massive fibroids with pressure symptoms, and endometrial cancer. It is often combined with prophylactic oophorectomy. Complications include urinary tract trauma, vault haematoma, and dyspareunia.

It is performed in various ways. Routes include transabdominal, vaginal and laparoscopic. The vaginal route has the advantages of quicker recovery and absence of

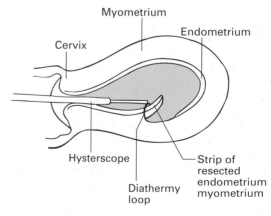

Fig 2.7 *Hysteroscopic resection of endometrium (TCRE).*

abdominal wound, and this is the preferred method for all but difficult cases or those with cancer. The vaginal route makes oophorectomy more difficult, which can be overcome by taking the ovaries laparoscopically.

Subtotal abdominal hysterectomy (conservation of the cervix) has been advocated by some gynaecologists, since the incidence of haematoma is lower and sexual function (orgasm) is said to be less affected. The evidence for better sexual function is poor, however, and the disadvantage of a subtotal procedure is that cervical smears are still required and the treatment of cancer of a cervical stump is difficult. Subtotal hysterectomy is used if removal of the cervix proves difficult because of a deep pelvis or endometriosis.

Prophylactic Oophorectomy

Prophylactic removal of (normal) ovaries is offered by many gynaecologists at the time of hysterectomy. There are many views on this, however, and there is a lot of debate. The advantage is that removal prevents trapped ovary syndrome (secondary to surgical adhesions), repeat surgery for benign ovarian cysts, and ovarian cancer. In order to prevent just one case of ovarian carcinoma, 250–400 pairs of ovaries would need to be removed. The average age for the menopause is 51 in this country, so if the woman is under 45 years of age it would mean she would be taking hormone replacement for nearly 10 years unnecessarily. In addition, HRT is not suitable for all women, and some are left with menopausal symptoms but no suitable therapy. The final decision should be made by the woman after careful explanation.

Radical (Wertheim) Hysterectomy and Pelvic Lymphadenectomy

This is the operation of choice for localised cancer of the cervix (Stages 1b and 2a). It involves removal of the uterus, Fallopian tubes, parametrial tissues and a large cuff of vagina. At least one ovary is usually preserved in young women. It is a radical operation and it should only be undertaken by specialist gynaecological oncologists. Morbidity is common, particularly when combined with postoperative radiotherapy.

There is disagreement about the role of the lymphadenectomy. It was initially proposed as a therapeutic procedure but it is unlikely to control spread and is probably more important as a prognostic test which determines the need for radiotherapy.

Myomectomy

This is the removal of one or more fibroids from the

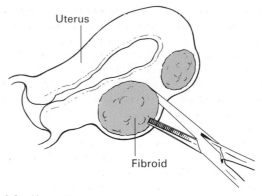

Fig 2.8 *Myomectomy.*

uterus in women who wish to retain their fertility (Figure 2.8). It can be performed as an open procedure or laparoscopically. Complications include emergency hysterectomy for massive haemorrhage, postoperative tubal adhesions and tubal infertility, and scar rupture in future pregnancies. The chance of hysterectomy is low, particularly if the size and vascularity of the fibroid(s) is reduced by preoperative GnRH analogue therapy.

Ovarian Cystectomy

This is removal of a simple ovarian cyst while conserving the body of the ovary.

Vaginal Repairs

This is surgery for vaginal prolapse. It is often combined with vaginal hysterectomy if there is uterine descent as well. It involves opening of vaginal mucosa over the area of prolapse, removal of redundant tissue and repair of underlying fascia. In addition to risks of urinary tract trauma, infection and haemorrhage, there is a chance of vaginal narrowing and dyspareunia.

Surgery for Tubal Pregnancy

The aims of tubal surgery are prevention or arrest of haemorrhage, retention of fertility when needed and the prevention of further ectopic pregnancies. There are a variety of operations including open and laparoscopic routes, and conservative and radical approaches. The radical approach is salpingectomy, and this is undertaken if the woman has had a previous ectopic in that tube or if haemostasis cannot be achieved. Conservative procedures include partial salpingectomy (removing a segment of the tube and ligating the ends for future reconstruction) and linear salpingostomy (opening of the tube along its axis over the site of the implantation and removal of the pregnancy). Conservative operations may help to preserve fertility, particularly in women with only one Fallopian tube, but the evidence that this is much superior to radical approaches in the majority of cases is lacking. Furthermore, conservative surgery for ectopic pregnancy is more likely to be complicated by recurrent haemorrhage, persistent trophoblast and recurrent ectopic pregnancy.

In the future we may resort to even more conservative methods such as systemic cytotoxic therapy with methotrexate, which eliminates surgery. As yet, these techniques have not achieved widespread popularity.

Tubal Microsurgery

Reconstructive surgery of the Fallopian tubes and ovaries is used to restore fertility in women with damage secondary to pelvic inflammatory disease (PID), appendicitis or endometriosis. The technique involves careful holding of tissues, accurate apposition of structures during reconstruction, careful attention to haemostasis, use of non-irritant suture materials, avoidance of tissue dehydration with saline lavage, and prevention of infection. Overall, the pregnancy rates are low. The success rates are best for pelvises damaged during previous surgery for ovarian cysts, because the ciliated tubal mucosa has not been damaged by infection.

As well as being used in reconstructive operations, these techniques can be employed to prevent fertility problems arising after surgery in young women.

Burch Colposuspension

This was initially designed to elevate the vagina for women with severe prolapse but is now used for the treatment of genuine stress incontinence. Through a transverse suprapubic incision the potential space behind the symphysis pubis is opened and the bladder mobilised to reveal the vagina. Sutures are then run from the vagina to the iliopectineal ligament on the superior pubic rami. As the sutures are tied, the bladder neck is elevated with the vagina. It has success rates of about 90% at 2 years, but morbidity is common. Complications include inability to pass urine, detrusor instability, pelvic pain and enterocoele formation.

3 Basic obstetric care

PRE-PREGNANCY CARE

Bevan, the founding father of the National Health Service, coined the phrase 'healthcare from the cradle to the grave'. With growing evidence that the intrauterine environment influences the wellbeing of the fetus and ultimately the child, this philosophy has been extended to before conception has even occurred. Pre-pregnancy care is intended to improve the outcome of pregnancy not only for the fetus but for the mother as well.

In addition to the many genetic influences, it is clear that environmental factors affect development and fetal maturation. Viruses, maternal disease and poor nutrition, drug therapy and abuse have all been shown to cause fetal disease. As with adult medicine, avoidance of adverse factors can prevent disease, and increasing numbers of healthy women and women with specific diseases seek advice and treatment before conception.

General Measures

General measures which should be discussed with all women include advice about healthy eating and cessation of smoking and moderation of alcohol intake. It is now known that folic acid supplements by tablet help prevent neural tube defects such as spina bifida and anencephaly. Vaccination against German measles helps to prevent the congenital rubella syndrome. Dietary modification may influence the incidence of adult disease such as Type II diabetes, hypertension and coronary artery atherosclerosis.

Pre-pregnancy Care for Specific Maternal Diseases

Not all chronic maternal diseases have an impact on pregnancy, but some, such as diabetes mellitus, phenylketonuria, epilepsy and antiphospholipid syndrome, may be associated with significant fetal risks. Advice about the nature and chance of known problems, together with methods of prenatal diagnosis, allows couples to make appropriate choices and prepare themselves emotionally. Optimisation of care is often associated with an improved outcome; there are good data to suggest that stabilisation of glycaemic control reduces the number of fetal malformations (Table 3.1). Adjustment of drug therapy to avoid teratogenic agents is an important part

Table 3.1 Fetal malformation rate in women with diabetes mellitus		
	Pre-conception care	
	Given	Not given
Age	27.5 years	25.2 years
HbA$_1$[a]	8.9%	10.9%
Anomalies	2/143 (1.4%)	10/96 (10.4%)

[a]HbA$_1$ is an indicator of glycaemic control.

of pre-pregnancy care. A good example is the substitution of another antihypertensive agent for angiotensin-converting enzyme inhibitors which cause fetal malformations and oligohydramnios.

For some women with chronic disease, pre-conception care is more about assessment of chance of poor maternal outcome. For women with severe medical disease such as severe diabetic nephropathy or Eisenmenger complex (ventricular septal defect and pulmonary hypertension), the chance of an adverse outcome in pregnancy may be so great that some choose to avoid conception. It is not the role of the doctor to say pregnancy must definitely not take place but simply to advise of the risks carefully and with compassion. Overly directive statements against pregnancy may be met with resistance rather than compliance and result in the opposite of the intended effect.

Pre-pregnancy Care in Families with Genetic Disease

For couples who have had a previously abnormal baby or in whom there is a family history of genetic disease, pre-conception care should focus on advice about the chance of recurrence in the next pregnancy and on prenatal diagnostic tests which can be offered. This work is undertaken by the clinical genetics team. Often tests on the couple and other relatives are needed to identify genetic markers before the availability of tests is known. It is better to arrange this before pregnancy so that time pressure does not force the couple into making a wrong decision for them. Advice is often given about single gene disorders such as cystic fibrosis and on chromosomal rearrangements (translocation). It is also entirely appropriate for couples with a history of pregnancies affected by sporadic genetic defects such as trisomy 21 (Down's syndrome) and syndromes with multifactorial aetiology such as spina bifida, to receive advice from clinical geneticists.

Psychological Care

Where there has been a previous stillbirth or neonatal death, there may be issues of guilt and blame of both themselves and of others. It is sometimes helpful to spend time simply listening to the couple's tale without interruption. Attention to psychological morbidity is often very important to prevent failed grieving, depression and marital disharmony. Referral to a perinatal bereavement counsellor may be justified many months or even years after such a loss.

It is important, when discussing issues about care in future pregnancies, that doctors and midwives outline the psychological support that will be given as well as describing more usual medical details. Particularly after a previous pregnancy loss, it is important to acknowledge that emotions may be very mixed even after delivery of a healthy baby. It may help to emphasise that it is quite appropriate for them to wish to discuss any sadness that they may be experiencing.

STANDARD ANTENATAL CARE

Pattern of Care

Most pregnant women are healthy and with normally formed fetuses. Antenatal care is therefore mostly about support and preparation for delivery and parenthood. The pattern of care for normal women varies widely across the United Kingdom and is currently changing in units. Many women still have one or more visits to see a specialist obstetrician but, increasingly, normal women are having all their care with the community team of midwives and general practitioners.

The first visit to the GP or midwife at 6 to 8 weeks is to establish the diagnosis of pregnancy and to set out a provisional plan; this includes an assessment of the need for a specialist opinion. At a second visit at 8–10 weeks a detailed personal and family history is taken to identify any important risk factors. Routine booking blood and urine tests are arranged. The tests performed and the reasons for undertaking them are explained in Table 3.2. Many of these tests are arranged routinely but, for some, the choice lies with the woman and her partner as to whether or not to have the tests performed, particularly those tests screening for fetal abnormality. It is important that any choice is based on good information, and leaflets may help to impart this.

A proportion of normal women will develop problems in pregnancy, many of which are asymptomatic, and so routine checks are carried out at each visit to screen for problems such as pre-eclampsia, anaemia and fetal growth delay. In doing so it is important not to undermine the confidence of women, many of whom feel anxious and vulnerable. Emphasis on the normality of any findings is in some ways just as important as identification of complications.

Table 3.2 Routine antenatal booking tests		
Test	Principal screening indications	Screening policy
FBC	For anaemia	All women
Hb electrophoresis	For sickle and thalassaemia	Certain racial groups
Blood group	Prepare for delivery	All women
	? Need for anti-Rh (D)	All women
Anti-red cell antibodies	For isoimmunisation	All women
Rubella	? Need for vaccination after delivery	All women
Hepatitis B	? Need for vaccination of neonate	All women
HIV	Alters antenatal care	? All women
MSU	For occult bacteriuria	All women
HVS	For bacterial vaginosis	High risk for preterm delivery
Serum markers	For trisomy 21	Woman's choice
	For neural tube defects	Woman's choice
Basic ultrasound scan	For twins and dating	Woman's choice
Detailed fetal scan	To detect fetal anomaly	Woman's choice

General Advice

At booking, the women are informed of the choices of schemes of care suitable for them, and advice is also given about available prenatal diagnostic tests.

The risks of exposure to toxoplasma, listeria and chlamydia organisms are explained to all women. These infective agents may cause severe maternal and/or fetal disease. For toxoplasma there is no method of prevention other than avoidance and hygiene, as no active or passive immunisation is possible. Serological screening for toxoplasmosis is currently advised against, as the results can be difficult to interpret or there is no effective treatment. Chlamydia is screened for using endocervical swabs in high-risk women, and treatment with antibiotics can be given. Listeria is extremely rare, and screening is not effective. The diagnosis of listeria should be considered in all women with a flu-like illness, and antibiotic therapy should be prescribed if there is reasonable suspicion.

Parentcraft Classes

Interspersed between the routine antenatal visits are classes that help to prepare both partners for labour, delivery and parenthood. Topics covered include relaxation exercises, analgesia in labour, and breast feeding. The meetings are generally run in health centres by community midwives. Some non-NHS organisations such as the National Childbirth Trust also run classes and meetings. Other activities for pregnant mothers include swimming sessions (aquaerobics) at local baths at which a midwife attends.

Second Trimester Ultrasonography

Most obstetricians and midwives believe that ultrasonography has transformed maternity care for the good. Cynics would say there is no evidence for this. Most women find it a thrilling social event (see Figure 3.1).

Ultrasound (high-frequency sound energy) is thought to be safe for the fetus, although this is impossible to prove with certainty. Obstetric ultrasonography is highly accurate but, like any medical test, has problems of false positive and negative results.

Scanning can be performed on two levels. A basic examination can be used to check the menstrual dating, identify the number of fetuses, check for fetal viability and look for evidence of adnexal pathology. Some units also use the basic scan to determine the placental site, but evidence from prospective studies suggests that this is a poor method of predicting placenta praevia. It should be remembered that accurate dating is also an essential

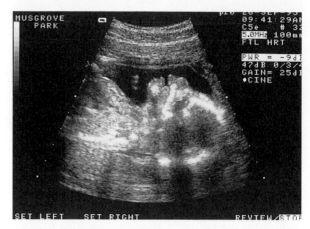

Fig 3.1 *Abdominal ultrasound of fetus.*

prerequisite of serum marker testing for trisomy 21 and neural tube defects.

More advanced scanning techniques allow detailed examination of the fetus (and placenta) to look for evidence of structural anomalies, markers of aneuploidy, and fetal infection. The features examined in a routine detailed fetal anatomy scan are given in Box 3.1. A study in Yorkshire showed sensitivity for structural abnormalities to be 75%, with a false positive (inappropriate termination) rate of 0.1%. The false negative rate is much higher. This is in part due to operator error but is more often because some problems do not become visible until late pregnancy, e.g. talipes equinovarus, and others are not generally identifiable at scan, e.g. trisomy 21.

Some units operate a selective policy, only offering a detailed scan to those women with a specific indication

---

Box 3.1 Detailed fetal scanning – anatomical parts examined

- Skull shape
- Cerebral ventricles, cerebellum and cisterna magna
- Face
- Eyes
- Chest, lungs and diaphragm
- Four chamber view of heart
- Spinal column
- Arms, hands, legs and feet
- Stomach and liver
- Kidneys and bladder
- Liquor volume and placental consistency
- Cord insertion
- Fetal behaviour
- Fetal growth

Table 3.3 Potential benefit(s) from fetal ultrasonography

Potential benefit	Example
Reassurance	Previously affected fetus
Preparation of parents	Any abnormality
Opportunity for termination of pregnancy	Anencephaly/spina bifida, etc.
Medical treatment of fetal disease	Cardiac arrhythmia
Surgical treatment of fetal disease	Insertion of chest drain
Early delivery	Cerebral ventriculomegaly
Delivery in tertiary centre	Gastroschisis
Delivery by caesarean section	Conjoined twins
Neonatal treatment of otherwise occult disease	Renal pelvis dilatation
Avoidance of maternal complications	Trisomies 13 and 18[a]
Avoidance of caesarean delivery of fetus with lethal problem	Trisomy 18/renal agenesis

[a]Greater chance of early, severe pre-eclampsia

such as a previously abnormal fetus or a family history of fetal malformation, but most units now offer scans routinely to all women. The benefits of undertaking detailed fetal scans are given in Table 3.3.

In addition to these uses, ultrasonography can be used to guide invasive procedures such as amniocentesis, chorionic villus sampling (CVS) and cordocentesis.

Finally, some workers have used Doppler assessment of fetal or maternal blood flow to predict the chance of pre-eclampsia and fetal growth retardation. The success of this has been variable, and currently it is not a routine practice in most units.

Communication

Communication is important as in all areas of medicine. Because women are being cared for jointly by the hospital and community team, and because they may transfer about the country, most units have a system of hand-held notes which the woman keeps with her. The experience of most units is that the women rarely lose the notes and that availability is generally better than that of conventional hospital notes.

ANTENATAL BOOKING HISTORY
General Principles

The obstetric history can be taken by a midwife or doctor. The details are usually entered onto a computer database as a permanent record which can be updated with each pregnancy.

The history is used to help the maternity team decide on the type of care to be provided. Questions should be directed at important issues which materially influence maternal and fetal care. Questions such as a family history of twins are now irrelevant because all women should be offered a scan to screen for multiple pregnancy.

Social History

The woman's age is important particularly with respect to prenatal diagnosis for trisomy 21. Details of her occupation and family life will indicate possible social problems which may need to be addressed.

Medical History

Details are taken of the woman's medical and surgical history. Most medical conditions have little effect on pregnancy, but some may directly affect the fetus (e.g. diabetes mellitus), whereas others carry serious implications for the mother (e.g. aortic stenosis). It is often necessary to liaise with consultant physicians to set out a clear plan for pregnancy and delivery. Remember too that the woman may need an emergency anaesthetic in labour and the obstetric anaesthetists should be informed of any potential serious problems.

Drug History

The vast majority of medications do not affect the fetus, but a proportion will cause serious problems including malformation (e.g. thalidomide), dental discoloration (e.g. tetracycline), spontaneous haemorrhage (e.g. warfarin) and renal dysfunction (e.g. indomethacin, angiotensin-converting enzyme inhibitors). A detailed history of medications is therefore essential, and this should include drugs supplied by alternative medicine practitioners. The general advice is to avoid all drugs in pregnancy unless they are necessary or considered very safe (such as paracetamol).

If any medicines have been taken, information should be researched either through the hospital Drug Information Bureau or by contacting the National Teratology Unit in Newcastle-upon-Tyne. It is usual to offer a detailed fetal ultrasound scan to screen for anomalies even if the drug is thought to be safe.

Doses of insulin, thyroxine and antiepileptic drugs should be carefully recorded, as these are often adjusted in pregnancy and returned to pre-pregnancy dose afterwards.

It is also important to ask about recreational drugs such as tobacco, alcohol and illegal substances. This needs to be done with sensitivity otherwise the woman will not offer information. Advice can be sympathetically given, and the pregnancy can be monitored more closely. If the woman has ever injected drugs, a screen should be offered for HIV and hepatitis B status so that the fetus can be given vaccination at birth.

Family History

Particular attention should be given to relatives being born with malformations or developing mental deficiency. This may result from a genetic defect, and prenatal diagnostic tests might be available. The clinical geneticists will be able to assist in the search for further details.

Previous Gynaecological History

Gynaecological disease such as pelvic infection increases the chance of ectopic pregnancy, and an ultrasound scan should be performed at about 6 weeks to site the pregnancy.

Cervical cytology is generally not undertaken in pregnancy, but the case notes can be marked for it to be offered sometime after delivery.

PHYSICAL EXAMINATION AT BOOKING VISIT

General Principles

Most women are fit and healthy, and the chance of finding a significant abnormality is small if there are no adverse features on the history.

General Examination

Weighing is undertaken at the first visit as a baseline and to use for the serum marker tests for trisomy 21 and neural tube defects. There is no evidence that serial weighing is of value, except for women with established medical disease such as the nephrotic syndrome. It is essential to measure blood pressure and preferable for the heart sounds to be auscultated for asymptomatic cardiac murmurs.

Breast Examination

Many obstetricians no longer undertake routine breast examination, as it is rarely helpful. It does not predict those who can lactate, and breast tumours are very rare. In addition, it is unpopular with women.

Abdominal Palpation

With the advent of routine ultrasonography abdominal palpation is virtually valueless for a woman with no symptoms.

Vaginal Examination

Before the introduction of ultrasonography, genital examination was undertaken in early pregnancy to help with the dating of pregnancy. This is clearly no longer relevant, but some clinicians advocate examination for asymptomatic lesions such as congenital malformation of the vagina, although these are extremely rare. A pelvic examination is still indicated if the woman has bleeding or an abnormal discharge.

PREGNANCY PLAN

When all the details of the maternal history, examination and booking tests have been reviewed, then a plan should be made for the rest of the pregnancy. Usually this is very simple, but for some women it needs to be very detailed and specific. A formatted pregnancy plan sheet (see Figure 3.2) may help the obstetrician to prepare this quickly and comprehensively.

FOLLOW-UP VISITS

Routine Care

Antenatal care needs to be tailored to the needs of the woman. Most units have a set plan of visits for healthy women with normal pregnancies (see Table 3.4), but even some of these visits may be cut out if all is well or the woman chooses against certain aspects.

Most of the visits in late pregnancy are undertaken to offer advice and support to the mother and to screen for asymptomatic conditions. The three most important conditions are pre-eclampsia, fetal growth retardation and maternal anaemia.

Maternal History and Physical Examination

There is a set routine for looking for problems, but this will need to be revised if specific problems do arise. Enquiry should be made into the woman's general wellbeing. The most common complaints are the side effects of pregnancy such as reflux oesophagitis, nausea, mild headaches, non-specific abdominal pain and urinary frequency. Although these are to be expected and gene-

PREGNANCY PLAN SHEET

RISK FACTORS (list)   Name etc.

PLAN FOR ANTENATAL CARE (tick or write comments)

Fetal surveillance 1st trimester (serial USS & see prog)

Detailed anomaly USS: Standard/Fetal echocardiogram

AFP/hCG testing

Amniocentesis/CVS

Fetal surveillance 3rd trimester

Diabetic screen (GTT @ 28 weeks)

Infection screen (Toxo, Hep B, Hep C or HIV)

Hb electrophoresis

Low-dose aspirin

Iron/folate therapy

REFERRAL (ring and give details)

Specialist care/low risk care/next visit @ ——————————— weeks

Medical/Anaesthetic/Neonatal/Social work consultation

PROVISIONAL PLAN FOR LABOUR/DELIVERY (ring and write on partogram)

Elective delivery at ——————————— weeks by induction/caesarean section

Decide at mode and timing of delivery at 36 weeks

Standard CDS protocol

Continuous fetal monitoring

Venflon/Group and Save/X-match

Please contact ——————————————— on admission

Other instructions _____

SIGNED ————————————————————————— **CONSULTANT/REGISTRAR/SHO**

DATE ———————————————————————

Fig 3.2 *Pregnancy plan sheet.*

Table 3.4	Routine antenatal visits	
Gestational age	Reason	Tests/action
6 weeks	Diagnose pregnancy	Discussion
8 weeks	Booking visit with midwife/GP	History General examination Routine bloods Discussion
12 weeks	Ultrasound scan	Dating and screen for twins Nuchal translucency
16 weeks	Serum markers	T21 and neural tube defects
18 weeks	Ultrasound scan	Fetal anomaly
24 weeks	Routine progress visit	
28 and 32 weeks	Routine progress visits	BP/urinalysis Fetal size on palpation FBC/rhesus status
36, 38, 40 weeks	Routine progress visits	BP/urinalysis Fetal activity charts Fetal size on palpation Fetal presentation
41 weeks	Postdates visit	Ditto Fetal assessment (CTG/USS) ? Induction of labour

rally do not signify serious disease, they can cause great anxiety and discomfort. It is, therefore, important to maintain a sympathetic approach.

Questions should be asked about fetal movements and instructions given about action to take if they reduce in number. Some units use a fetal kick-to-ten chart to improve maternal compliance.

At each visit the woman's **blood pressure** is measured and her urine is tested for **protein**, mostly to screen for pre-eclampsia. The urine is also tested for glucose and leucocytes to screen for gestational diabetes and urinary tract infection.

The woman's abdomen is palpated to assess the **fetal size**, the **presentation** and the **volume of liquor**. The fetal heart is listened to with an ultrasound device, largely for the mother's pleasure. Only very rarely will an abnormality be detected by this means.

Blood Tests

Blood is sent to **screen for maternal anaemia** at 28 and 36 weeks gestation. If anaemia is diagnosed it is important to identify the cause. Iron deficiency is relatively rare in the United Kingdom, and the most common cause of anaemia is physiological (dilutional) anaemia of pregnancy. This is a sign of a healthy pregnancy, and mothers can be reassured that the fetus is not starved of blood because the low viscosity allows rapid flow through the placental vascular tree. Indeed, there is evidence to show that women who maintain a high haemoglobin are more likely to develop pre-eclampsia.

Some units also routinely perform **screening tests for gestational diabetes** but the value of this has not been proven. There is clear evidence to show that gestational glucose intolerance is associated with larger babies, birth trauma, and neonatal hypoglycaemia, but the evidence that the perinatal mortality rate is worse is less good, and there are no definite data that unequivocally demonstrate that knowledge of the diagnosis improves pregnancy/neonatal outcome. Many units no longer undertake screening at all or run a selective policy for high-risk groups.

Rhesus isoimmunisation is sensitisation of a rhesus (D) negative mother to the Rh(D) antigen, usually by leakage of fetal cells into the maternal circulation. Isoimmunisation may cause a haemolytic anaemia in a Rh(D) positive fetus because of transplacental transfer of antibody into the fetal circulation. This can be prevented by the administration of pooled anti-Rh(D) gammaglobulin at the time of delivery, miscarriage, antepartum haemorrhage, or invasive procedures. Some maternity units are now giving routine anti-Rh(D) prophylaxis for all mothers at 28 and 34 weeks gestation to prevent sensitisation during the antenatal period. If the antibody screen becomes positive there is a risk of fetal anaemia and cardiac failure (hydrops fetalis). For women who are rhesus (D) negative without anti-Rh(D) antibodies, antibody screens are repeated at 28 and 36 weeks gestation. Detailed fetal surveillance is then undertaken using ultrasonography and/or invasive testing. If necessary, delivery is brought forward so that the fetus can be transfused. Other anti-red-cell antibodies can cause fetal anaemia, as gammaglobulin is not available, but sensitisation of the mother cannot be prevented.

Repeat Ultrasound Scans

Studies of the use of serial ultrasonography in normal pregnancy suggest that it is of no value. Further scans should be undertaken if there is suspicion of small for dates, polyhydramnios, abnormal presentation and reduced fetal movement, etc.

STANDARD INTRAPARTUM CARE

Place of Delivery

During the pregnancy the midwife and/or doctors will discuss place of delivery with the woman. Most women choose to deliver in hospital, largely because that is the current tradition, but some women wish to deliver at home. The woman's medical and obstetric details are then reviewed and advice given. For normal women with a healthy pregnancy, home delivery appears to be a safe option with some advantages over hospital birth: women tend to feel more relaxed. Disadvantages are that transfer to hospital in labour is quite common – about 30% of primigravidae labouring at home will deliver in hospital – and that entirely unforeseen maternal and neonatal problems may arise at delivery for which care would not be available. These are very rare, however.

Sometimes it is important to consider delivery in a regional centre, either because the fetus needs immediate specialist medical care (e.g. pacemaker insertion for congenital heart block) or neonatal surgery (e.g. gastroschisis).

Mode of Delivery

For normal women with apparently normal, well-grown fetuses, it is very difficult to predict who will labour well and who will require a caesarean delivery. Maternal height, estimated fetal size, head engagement and position, and x-ray pelvimetry all lack sufficient power to be used as clinical tests. The routine policy for primigravidae, therefore, is to attempt vaginal delivery unless there is a specific complication antenatally or during labour which is best dealt with by elective caesarean delivery.

Increasingly, some women are requesting elective caesarean section because of maternal anxiety, to protect the baby, or to avoid pelvic floor trauma. Such requests are best not dismissed out of hand but considered carefully and sympathetically. The risk to the fetus of severe respiratory problems after elective caesarean delivery must be taken into account, but overall the chances of maternal and neonatal problems after labour and elective abdominal delivery are similar. After explaining their anxieties, listening to the issues and being offered support, many women do choose to try for vaginal delivery. However, if the woman continues to request elective caesarean delivery, it should be borne in mind that the true reason for the request is sometimes not given by the woman who cannot bring herself to talk of previous rape or childhood sex abuse.

Support in Labour

Whenever possible it is important to create a safe, private and comfortable environment for the mother and her companions. Labour is a time of great anxiety, and it is important not to undermine confidence by undermining the woman's plans for delivery. Allowing choice may give a sense of control, which is important to many women. Control gives confidence, and confidence allays anxiety. This may not only increase the enjoyment of labour and delivery but actually improve the outcome. There is some evidence that women in South America accompanied by professional lay attendants (dumas) have a lower caesarean section rate than women who do not. Failure to give the appropriate support may not only influence the progress of labour but leave psychological damage which lasts for years and results in post-natal depression, sexual dysfunction, chronic pain syndromes, divorce and child neglect. Some authorities have likened the effect of labour on some women to post-traumatic stress disorder. It would be foolish to suggest that labour should always be a fulfilling experience, but care to empathise with the needs of women may prevent some of these problems.

Maternal and Fetal Monitoring in Normal Labour

Maternal and fetal problems can arise spontaneously in any labour. Maternal complications include failure to progress, infection, pre-eclampsia and intrapartum haemorrhage. The commonest fetal problems include hypoxia acidosis, cord prolapse and infection. Some of these conditions are often overt (massive abruption or amniotic fluid embolism), but others may be occult (pre-eclampsia and fetal hypoxia). Monitoring of the fetal and maternal condition is therefore potentially helpful but may also give rise to problems (Table 3.5).

All of this information is recorded graphically on an observation chart (partogram). If serious complications do arise, both maternal and fetal monitoring may be intensified to include fluid input/output, serial haematology and biochemistry, pulse oximetry, central venous pressure, fetal heart rate tracing, etc.

Table 3.5   Maternal and fetal monitoring

Test	Indication
Routine maternal monitoring	
Maternal blood pressure	Pre-eclampsia
Urinalysis	Pre-eclampsia
Temperature	Maternal infection
Cervical dilation	Progress of labour
Routine fetal monitoring	
Liquor colour	Infection
	Meconium aspiration
Intermittent auscultation	Hypoxia acidosis
	Chorio-amnionitis

The optimum policy for fetal monitoring has still to be defined. The difficulty is that the incidence of significant fetal hypoxia is very low at perhaps just 3 cases per 1000 normal labours, and some of these will be because of sudden acute events, such as a massive intrapartum haemorrhage, which are unpredictable. The test developed to detect occult hypoxia-acidosis, fetal heart rate pattern analysis (cardiotocography, CTG), is being asked to look for a needle in a haystack. Three additional problems with CTG monitoring are, first, that it is non-specific and most trace abnormalities do not result from fetal disease. Second, that it gives rise to maternal and fetal problems (Table 3.6) which numerically far outweigh the number of cases of neonatal hypoxic–ischaemic encephalopathy which lead on to cerebral palsy that could be prevented. And finally, a large majority of infants with cerebral palsy have not been subjected to intrapartum hypoxia at all, but the neurological state is the result of some other condition. This final issue may lead to medico-legal problems.

Other methods of routine electronic fetal monitoring have been tried, including fetal EEG and fetal ECG

Table 3.6   Disadvantages of electronic fetal monitoring

Problem	Reason
Maternal anxiety	Non-pathological CTG variants
Maternal immobilisation	Attached to fetal monitor
Increase in caesarean and instrumental delivery rates	CTG not specific
Fetal trauma and infection	Use of internal electrodes

monitoring, but to date they have not been adopted as routine practice. Many clinicians hold the opinion that, for normal labour, intermittent auscultation is as effective (or ineffective) as any electronic method but the adverse effects are less common.

WHEN PROBLEMS ARISE

Complications can arise in any pregnancy and at any stage. It is important to have written guidelines for the commonest and most serious problems and trainee clinicians need to have easy access to senior obstetricians for advice and support. An example of such written guidelines, for the management of pre-eclampsia, is given at the end of this chapter.

Fetal and Maternal Medicine

Fetal medicine is a new subspeciality of obstetrics. It is simply the treating of the fetus as a patient. Just like adult medicine, it involves diagnosis, prognosis, treatment and monitoring. It differs only in that the fetus is hidden from view. The general examination of the fetus is by detailed ultrasonography. **Maternal medicine** is an older concept. Indeed, one of the reasons for the introduction of antenatal care was the detection and treatment of maternal conditions.

When caring for a woman with pre-existing or de novo medical conditions herself, it is essential to consider the effect of the complication and its potential treatments on both the mother and the fetus. It is also important to bear in mind that pregnancy complications may generate great anxiety for the mother and her partner and that careful, frank explanations are essential. For very serious problems, particularly those associated with severe fetal disease and those requiring prolonged hospital admission, it may help to include social workers and trained counsellors to give support and advice.

Liaison with Neonatal Team

Many pregnancy complications continue into neonatal life. It is essential, therefore, to have good communication between the maternity unit and the special care baby team. In addition, the parents may find it helpful to meet the neonatal doctors and nurses before delivery and to visit the special care nursery.

POSTNATAL CARE

For many women, the days and weeks after delivery are a time of emotional contentment and physical wellbeing, but there is a real chance of serious physical and psychological disease. Follow-up care is initially by the midwife and GP, and later the health visitor starts to visit regularly.

More and more women deliver in the community, and, of those who deliver in hospital, many wish to return home within a few hours of delivery. Others need a longer stay in hospital because of poor support at home, need for analgesia, etc.

In the first few days after delivery it is important to detect signs of infection, venous thrombosis, anaemia and pre-eclampsia. The healing of any scars can also be examined easily. The mother's mood and ability to care for the child should also be assessed. Transient low mood (the baby blues) is very common, but a small proportion of women develop profound depression or even delusional reactions. Education remains an important goal, especially for first-time mothers, and advice about breast feeding, washing, etc., should be continued.

Screening checks and health prevention are as important as ever. Women who are non-immune to **rubella** are offered the live-attenuated vaccine and advised to avoid conception. For women who are **rhesus (D) negative**, a series of tests are undertaken to determine the need for anti-Rh (D) gammaglobulin. The baby's blood rhesus group is typed on cord blood and, if negative, no further action is required. If the baby's group is rhesus positive, anti-Rh(D) is needed if the mother is not sensitised. The dose of anti-Rh(D) depends on an estimate of the feto-maternal haemorrhage by counting the number of fetal red blood cells in a sample of maternal blood (**Kleihauer test**). Even if the Kleihauer test is negative, anti-Rh(D) is still given.

It is also appropriate to offer advice about **contraception**. The combined oral contraceptive pill (OCP) is contraindicated in lactating mothers, but the progestogen-only pill (PoP) is satisfactory, and an IUCD can be inserted very soon after delivery. Two important pieces of information for women are that lactation is not highly effective, as a contraceptive, when the frequency of feeding declines and that many women ovulate before they menstruate.

The Postnatal Visit

It has been a tradition for many years that women visit their GP for a health check about 6 weeks after delivery. Many women do find this very helpful, and it is a good opportunity for gaining advice about cervical smears and contraception. The ritual of the routine pelvic examination has been strongly questioned, however. It is very uncomfortable for many women, and the chance of finding a problem if there are no symptoms is very low.

Some women will have concerns about their labour or delivery, and questions about future pregnancy. Our perspective of the nature of the peripartum period can be very misleading. Some women with apparently normal labours have great anxieties which merit careful consideration. The opportunity should be given to all women to make comments or to ask questions. If necessary an appointment should be requested with the hospital team.

COMMON DRUG THERAPIES

Tocolysis

Tocolytic agents are drugs which reduce uterine activity. They are primarily used in the prevention or management of preterm labour. They are also used to relax the uterus during external cephalic version and to reverse uterine hypertonus (excessive contractions) during induction of labour. The efficacy of these drugs is not well established in terms of hard endpoints such as arresting preterm labour and improving neonatal outcome, but they are thought to be valuable in preterm labour by allowing time for maternal transfer to a specialist unit and for the administration of corticosteroids to enhance fetal lung maturity. Agents used include β-adrenergic agonists (**ritodrine**), calcium channel blockers (**nifedipine**) and prostaglandin synthetase inhibitors (**indomethacin**). Complications include: maternal arrhythmias, pulmonary oedema, hypokalaemia and destabilisation of maternal diabetes (ritodrine); hypotension and vascular headache (nifedipine); premature closure of ductus arteriosus, fetal oliguria and fetal pulmonary hypertension (indomethacin). Contraindications include maternal cardiac disease, fetal distress, antepartum haemorrhage, pre-eclampsia, gestation greater than 34 weeks and cervical dilatation greater than 3 cm.

Oxytocics

Oxytocics are drugs used to stimulate uterine activity. They are used to induce termination, induce or augment labour and to prevent or treat postpartum haemorrhage. Agents used include synthetic oxytocin (Syntocinon), prostaglandins and prostaglandin analogues, and ergometrine. **Prostaglandins** are very useful for induction of labour and midtrimester termination of pregnancy, as they both soften the cervix and initiate uterine contractions. They may precipitate uterine hypertonus, which is difficult to reverse, and they should therefore be used with caution in highly parous women and those with uterine scars, because of the risk of uterine rupture. **Syntocinon** is used by infusion to augment spontaneous and induced labour. It is very safe provided that the labour and fetus are monitored carefully. Caution again is important with previous uterine surgery. Discontinuation of the infusion leads to a rapid cessation of effect. A combination of Syntocinon and ergometrine (**Syntometrine**) is routinely given in the third stage of labour to prevent postpartum haemorrhage. It may induce nausea and, more importantly, acute hypertension. It is therefore to be avoided in pre-eclampsia.

Dexamethasone

Corticosteroids are used to enhance fetal lung maturity when preterm delivery is inevitable or desirable. Dexamethasone prevents respiratory distress syndrome and, secondarily, other complications of prematurity. A course consists of two doses, 12 to 24 h apart. Effect is maximal 24 h after the second dose and lasts for about one week. Courses can be repeated. It is generally very safe but may cause worsening or precipitation of maternal diabetes. In conjunction with tocolytic, it has been associated with pulmonary oedema. It does not increase the chance of fetal/neonatal infection. It is used in preference to prednisolone, which crosses the placenta poorly.

Dopamine Agonists

Women who suffer a perinatal loss (stillbirth or neonatal death) may wish to avoid lactation. Suppression of prolactin with a dopamine agonist prevents milk production. Bromocriptine was used for many years but this had to be taken for 2 weeks, and there is a concern that it may increase the chance of cerebrovascular accident postpartum. A single dose of carbergoline is effective in 80% of women. Its safety is not established for this indication, however.

Antihypertensive Therapy

Hypertension is one of the commonest complications of late pregnancy (see Chapter 31). Control of blood pressure does not necessarily remove maternal and fetal risk but it may limit the chance of intracranial bleeding, particularly in pre-eclampsia. **Methyl dopa** has been used for many years, and it appears to be very safe. It takes up to 24 h to have effect, and so other agents may have to be used in emergency situations. It can lead to lethargy and depression but these are not usually a great problem, because of short time scale of use. The calcium-channel blocker **nifedipine** is useful for controlling acute rises in blood pressure but must be used with caution because of the risk of precipitating hypo-

tension and underperfusion of the placenta. It may cause flushes and vascular headaches in the mother. It interacts with magnesium sulphate and causes neuromuscular blockade. **β-blockers** may cause fetal growth and neonatal complications such as hypothermia and hypoglycaemia, but agents such as labetalol can be very useful for the control of severe hypertension in the peripartum period. **ACE inhibitors** are contraindicated because of adverse effects on fetal renal function. **Diuretics** appear to worsen the condition of women with pre-eclampsia, who already have a contracted circulation, and their use is advised against.

Anticonvulsant Therapy

The presence of convulsions in association with pre-eclampsia is called eclampsia and is a major cause of maternal and fetal mortality. The first step is to arrest the fit. This can be undertaken using **diazepam** or **magnesium sulphate**. Diazepam has the advantage of being simple to use and very effective. However, it is of little benefit for the prevention of further fits, and magnesium sulphate is the preferred agent for this.

Anticoagulants

Standard or low-molecular-weight **heparin** does not cross the placenta, reducing the risk of fetal haemorrhage and abnormality. Prolonged heparin therapy (over 6 months) is associated with osteoporosis, limiting its duration of use. It is also known to cause thrombocytopenia and allergic reactions. **Warfarin** is a small molecule that passes the placenta and is known to be a teratogen. There is an association with fetal haemorrhage later in pregnancy.

OBSTETRIC SURGICAL PROCEDURES

Cervical Cerclage

Cerclage is a purse-string suture which encircles the cervix to prevent passive dilatation (cervical incompetence). It is also known as a Shirodkar suture or McDonald cerclage after early pioneers. The suture can be inserted before or during pregnancy and transabdominally or transvaginally. Evidence from studies looking at emergency insertion in women whose cervices are already effaced and dilated shows that it is an effective treatment, but problems exist in deciding which cases justify suture insertion. Complications include maternal infection and cervical laceration. The suture can be removed before labour to allow vaginal delivery.

Therapeutic Amniocentesis

This is drainage of amniotic fluid using a spinal needle inserted under ultrasound guidance. It is used to relieve maternal discomfort and prevent preterm labour in women with severe polyhydramnios. Complications include chorio-amnionitis (infection), amniotic membrane rupture, placental abruption and preterm labour.

Diagnostic Amniocentesis

This is aspiration of fetal liquor for investigation of suspected fetal disease. It is most commonly performed at about 16 weeks gestation for karyotype analysis of fetuses at high risk of trisomy or other chromosomal disorder. Other indications include OD450 testing for cases of Rhesus isoimmunisation and testing for suspected congenital toxoplasmosis using PCR. The needle is passed under ultrasound control, avoiding the fetus. The main complication is about 1% chance of miscarriage. Much rarer problems are fetal trauma and chorioamnionitis. For amniocentesis and all other invasive techniques, anti-Rh(D) gammaglobulin is required if the mother is rhesus negative.

Chorionic Villus Sampling

CVS is a form of placental biopsy used for prenatal diagnosis. Like amniocentesis it is performed under ultrasound control. Placental cells are aspirated into culture medium. It is mostly used to detect aneuploidy and single gene disorders. It can be performed much earlier in pregnancy than amniocentesis (about 11 weeks). If performed in the first trimester and an abnormality is found, the woman can be offered an early termination of pregnancy (TOP) which is performed under anaesthetic. In contrast, a late TOP may involve delivery of the fetus. It can be performed later in pregnancy and is useful beyond 20 weeks gestation when fetal abnormality is suspected at scan, because a result can usually be obtained within 5 days. Disadvantages are a slightly higher miscarriage rate (1–3%) and that placental chromosomal make-up is occasionally different from that of the fetus.

Cordocentesis

Cordocentesis is a method of sampling fetal blood for prenatal diagnosis. It may be combined with fetal therapy given by umbilical vein injection or infusion. The commonest indications are karyotype analysis and viral serology for investigation of fetal abnormality, and investigation and transfusion for suspected fetal anaemia. The umbilical vein is visualised using transabdominal ultrasonography and then the needle is tracked during insertion. Complications include fetal haemorrhage, rupture of membranes and miscarriage/preterm labour.

External Cephalic Version

This is manual conversion of the fetus from breech to cephalic presentation. Usually done under tocolytic cover with continuous fetal monitoring at about 38 weeks. It should only be attempted if facilities are immediately available for emergency delivery. It is known to reduce likelihood of caesarean section but not conclusively shown to improve fetal outcome. Complications include rupture of membranes and cord prolapse, preterm labour, placental abruption, umbilical cord entanglement, uterine scar rupture. Anti-Rh (D) gammaglobulin should be given if the woman is rhesus negative.

Fetal Scalp Blood Sampling

In this technique, a capillary blood sample is taken from the fetal scalp in labour to measure pH. It is used as back-up to cardiotocography for the diagnosis of fetal acidosis. Units not using scalp pH measurement tend to have a high caesarean section rate for so-called fetal distress. Performed using aminioscope and microscalpel. Complications include fetal bleeding, scalp trauma and infection, and maternal discomfort.

Instrumental Delivery

Occasionally, vaginal delivery has to be expedited with the aid of forceps or ventouse (suction cup). The main indications are suspected fetal hypoxia and maternal exhaustion. The instruments are only applied if the cervix is fully dilated, the head is presenting and the presenting part is deeply engaged within the pelvis. Ideally, there should be adequate maternal analgesia and the bladder should be emptied. Complications include maternal and fetal trauma.

Caesarean Section

This is delivery of the fetus through the maternal abdomen. Indications can be divided into fetal (hypoxia, malpresentation and macrosomia) and maternal (failure to advance in labour, placenta praevia, large abruption and severe pre-eclampsia). Complications include infection, haemorrhage, bladder trauma, and scar rupture in next labour. A classical caesarean section is now rarely performed. It involves a midline incision in the upper segment of the uterus. It is associated with heavy blood loss, closure of the uterus is difficult, and the chance of scar rupture in future labours is high (10%). Classical caesarean delivery is now reserved for cases in which the lower segment is obscured by fibroids, etc.

Lower segment caesarean section (LSCS) is the operation of choice for over 97% of cases. It involves a transverse incision through the lower segment. This is the part of the gravid uterus which balloons up in the second half of pregnancy. It arises from the upper part of the cervix and is comparatively thinner and less vascular than the upper segment. Blood loss is therefore much less on average, and the closure is much easier.

EXAMPLE OF CLINICAL GUIDELINES – PRE-ECLAMPSIA MANAGEMENT IN PERIPARTUM PERIOD

INTRODUCTION

Pre-eclampsia is a disorder of vascular endothelial function specific to pregnancy. It arises in the placenta as a result of ischaemia, of which there are several causes. It propagates throughout the maternal vascular tree, and all organ systems can be affected. Complications of pre-eclampsia can affect both the mother and fetus; it is one of the commonest underlying causes of maternal and perinatal mortality.

There is no good method of prevention for all women, and the only means of cure is delivery. It is an unpredictable condition in both its onset and rate of progression; pre-eclampsia can never be defined as mild prospectively but only classified as complicated or uncomplicated in terms of outcome, i.e. in retrospect.

It is clear that pre-eclampsia is a systemic disease and not simply a disorder of blood pressure control. Indeed, some women may develop serious complications before the onset of hypertension.

Definition

There is no comprehensive definition because the syndrome is very variable. Not all women are hypertensive, for example, and some will present highly atypically with right upper quadrant pain alone or even with pruritus.

The disorder is suggested by two or more of the following:

- hypertension (> 125 mmHg systolic pressure or > 85 diastolic mmHg)
- rise above booking diastolic blood pressure of 20 mmHg or more

- proteinuria (1+ on proper clean MSU or > 500 mg/24 h urine collection)
- elevated serum urate
- abnormal serum alanine transaminase (ALT)
- thrombocytopaenia (< 100)
- fetal growth retardation.

Pathophysiology

The focal lesion is a microangiopathy which consists of platelet aggregation and microthrombi in small vessels. These small thrombi damage the vessel locally and release vasoactive peptides which trigger damage at other sites. The damage to the small vessels makes them more permeable, hence the oedema and proteinuria. The vasoactive peptides promote vasoconstriction, hence hypertension. Vessels also become more fragile, particularly when the blood pressure is raised, and so are more likely to rupture.

Major Complications

- intracranial bleed
- pulmonary oedema and adult respiratory distress syndrome (ARDS)
- HELLP syndrome (see below) with coagulopathy
- eclampsia
- renal failure
- placental abruption with fetal hypoxia-acidosis.

Much of the emphasis has been on the prevention of the relatively rare complication of renal failure with fluid loads but at the expense of inducing life-threatening pulmonary oedema (see *Confidential Enquiries into Maternal Death*).

PRINCIPLES OF MANAGEMENT

Optimal care of women with pre-eclampsia is based on early detection, detailed monitoring, control of hypertension, and optimal timing of delivery. The exact management of any individual woman will depend in part upon the specific manifestations in her case. Some judgement must be used by the clinicians directly involved in management.

STANDARD CARE

On Admission to Delivery Suite

In addition to any standard management of labour, carry out the following.

- **Review of symptoms**
  - headache, visual disturbance, abdominal pain.
- **Institute monitoring**
  - pulse, BP, resp. rate, fluid balance
  - continuous CTG.
- **Carry out physical examination**
  - chest for crepitations
  - heart sounds for murmurs in case vasodilator therapy needed
  - abdominal palpation for tenderness (?HELLP)
  - uterus for tenderness (?abruption) and fundal height.
- **Take full blood profile**
  - FBC, U+Es, LFTs, clotting screen and G+S
  - amylase if epigastric pain.
- **Insert venflon**.
- **Consider need for corticosteroids** to enhance fetal lung maturity.
- **Contact SCBU** if appropriate.
- **Ask woman to report serious symptoms** such as headache, visual disturbance, upper abdominal pain.
- **Start critical care observation chart**.

First Stage of Labour

1. Maintain close observation of mother (see sections on observation).
2. Avoid aortocaval compression (may cause profound fall in blood pressure).
3. Avoid fluid overload (see section on fluid management).
4. Consider value of epidural anaesthesia (pain tends to increase blood pressure).
5. There is an increased risk of fetal hypoxia/acidosis and of abruption: monitor fetal heart continuously.
6. Tocolysis is contraindicated for preterm labour in women with pre-eclampsia.

7. Start oral ranitidine therapy to reduce gastric acidity because of risk of aspiration with eclampsia.

Second Stage of Labour

It is safe for the mother to have a normal active second stage provided that she does not have a severe headache or visual disturbance, and that her BP is within acceptable limits.

If the woman complains of a severe headache or visual disturbance, or if her blood pressure is very poorly controlled (repeatedly > 160 mmHg systolic or 105 mmHg diastolic between contractions), consideration should be given to instrumental delivery.

Third Stage of Labour

1. **Avoid ergometrine (and Syntometrine)**, which may precipitate extreme rises in BP.
2. Use Syntocinon (10 u as an i.m. or slow i.v. injection).
3. If particular risk of PPH (high parity, APH, etc), also give i.v. infusion of Syntocinon: (40 u/500 ml normal saline at 120 ml/h and adjust standard Hartmann's infusion down).
4. If PPH develops, give **slow** i.v. injection of Syntocinon and start i.v. infusion of Syntocinon.
5. If PPH persists, use prostaglandin (Hemabate by i.m. or direct intrauterine injection).

REMEMBER – NEVER USE ERGOMETRINE OR SYNTOMETRINE

Puerperium

Remember that pre-eclampsia can worsen several days after delivery; if symptoms arise, investigate and monitor. This may occasionally include transfer back to delivery suite.

1. **VOLTAROL** must not be given under **ANY CIRCUMSTANCE**. It precipitates renal failure.
2. Maintain close observations on labour ward for at least 12 h, longer if there are ongoing problems.
   - Monitor symptoms, pulse, BP, temperature, resp. rate, fluid balance in all women.
   - Monitor pulse oximetry and CV pressure in complicated cases.
3. Repeat blood tests about 4 h after delivery and then at about 24 h.
4. Maintain tight control of BP.
   - Can be more aggressive about this once fetus delivered.
   - Treat if BP persistently > 150 mmHg systolic or > 105 mmHg diastolic (20 min between checks).

5. Reduce Hartmann's infusion as oral intake increases.
6. Consider need for thromboprophylaxis.
   - Apply elasticated support stockings after delivery if high risk.
   - Start clexane (40 mg s.c. daily) 24 h after delivery if high risk (provided platelet count is > 100).

Standard Fluid Management

In standard fluid management, the following should be adhered to.

1. Strictly monitor fluid balance – measure all input and output.
2. Not all women will need urinary catheterisation, but a large majority will:
   - prolonged history (> 1 week)
   - caesarean section
   - epidural anaesthesia
   - prolonged labour (> 8 hours)
   - severe hypertension
   - HELLP
   - eclampsia
   - haemorrhage.
3. Infuse Hartmann's solution @ 1 ml/kg/h if prolonged period (> 6 h) without oral fluids.
4. Adjust Hartmann's infusion rate downwards for woman's increasing oral intake/other infusions.
5. Avoid solutions of water (dextrose) at all times except in diabetes.
6. Use **10% dextrose** for women with diabetes requiring sliding regimen.
7. There is no advantage from routinely using albumin/synthetic colloid solutions.

Some workers have advocated solutions of albumin or artificial colloids in preference to crystalloid solutions. They are not known to be better and they carry the risk of anaphylactoid reaction. There may be other disadvantages in pre-eclampsia.

MANAGEMENT OF COMPLICATIONS

Maternal Monitoring

The maternal condition must be monitored frequently during labour and the early puerperium. The extent of monitoring required will vary from case to case.

Women with apparently uncomplicated PET of short duration who labour quickly will simply require monitoring of pulse, BP (hourly initially), temperature (4 hourly), and fluid balance. A full blood profile should be repeated 4 to 6 h after delivery and again at about 18 to 24 h.

Those women with complicated PET will require intensive monitoring with:

1. pulse and BP half hourly
2. temperature and respiratory rate 2 hourly
3. urine output hourly
4. pulse oximetry if infusing fluids rapidly or PET very severe
5. Central venous pressure (CVP) measurement if infusing fluids rapidly or anuria.

Blood Pressure Management

The aim of blood pressure control is to prevent intracranial bleeding. Nothing more.

1. Measure initially using standard sphygmomanometer.
2. Trend of BP may be monitored using automatic device.
3. Interval checks of automatic devices are necessary against standard sphygmomanometer (do 2 hourly).
4. Measure diastolic pressure when the sounds disappear.
5. Measure to nearest 5 mmHg.
6. Measure in right arm sitting or on side, with a cuff of appropriate size.
7. Readings above the threshold should be repeated after 20 min.
8. Consider acting to lower BP if two readings > 150 mmHg systolic or > 105 mmHg diastolic.

You must be familiar with the contraindications of drugs before using them. Do not guess; read data sheet. Ideally the BP should be well controlled before the onset of labour, preferably with oral methyl dopa.

Control of acute exacerbations

If there are **acute exacerbations**, treat with **labetalol** or **nifedipine**. There is no definite advantage for either in terms of blood pressure control, but nifedipine interacts with magnesium sulphate and so labetalol is preferred by many.

There is a risk of precipitate falls in BP during acute anti-hypertensive therapy. The maternal pulse and blood pressure must be measured frequently (every 5 min), and the fetal heart must be monitored continuously. If the maternal blood pressure falls dramatically, consider rapid infusion of Hartmann's solution in 250 ml doses.

Epidural anaesthesia should not be used to control acute exacerbations of hypertension but it may be useful in preventing further rises in blood pressure due to pain. It is particularly useful for postoperative pain control and should be considered for this alone in women having caesarean delivery.

Beware of combining actions that will lower blood pressure, e.g. giving nifedipine therapy just before epidural anaesthetic is started.

Regimen for labetalol:

1. Use i.v. bolus and/or i.v. infusion.
2. **Contraindications**:
   - asthma
   - severe cardiac lesions (bradycardia/heart block)
   - liver disease/dysfunction (including HELLP syndrome).

   In this context, diabetes is **not** a contraindication.
3. **Intravenous bolus dose of labetalol**:
   - 10 mg i.v. over 1 min
   - Check BP and pulse after 5 min
   - This can be repeated after 5 min
   - Effect lasts for up to 6 h.
4. **Intravenous infusion of labetalol**:
   - 20 mg/h of neat labetalol
   - Double infusion rate every 30 min until diastolic pressure < 95 mmHg
   - Maximum rate = 160 mg/h.

Regimen for nifedipine:

1. Use as first-line agent only if labetalol is contra-indicated.
2. **Contraindications**:
   - aortic stenosis
   - use with caution if magnesium sulphate infusion is in progress.
3. **Usage**:
   - Give orally and not sublingually in first instance.
   - Use 10 mg capsule by mouth, half hourly up to three doses.
   - Sublingual nifedipine should be reserved for resistant severe hypertension.

If both labetalol and nifedipine are contra-indicated (very rare), consider hydralazine.

Resistant hypertension

1. Resistant hypertension is a feature of rapid consumption of platelets. Consider whether the woman has developed **occult HELLP syndrome** or some variant.
2. **Treatment is difficult and should be supervised by a registrar or consultant.**
3. **Regimen:**
   - Consider sublingual nifedipine (10 mg) with con-comitant infusion of Hartmann's solution (500 ml over 30 min).
   - If sublingual nifedipine fails, consider alternative antihypertensive therapy:

- hydralazine by intravenous infusion
- sodium nitroprusside (by experienced anaesthetist/ physician only).

Management of Eclampsia

(There is a separate protocol for management of eclampsia.)

There is no reliable method of predicting eclampsia. Even true hyperreflexia (extension of reflexes or release of primitive reflexes) is poorly predictive.

There is no evidence that routine primary prophylaxis is indicated. Risks may outweigh the benefits.

The diagnosis should be considered carefully in all pregnant women who lose consciousness or have a funny turn. And remember – some women will fit with no history of pre-eclampsia.

If eclampsia occurs

1. All members of the on-site obstetric emergency team should be called including the anaesthetist.
2. Remember standard ABC for unconscious patient.
3. Active eclampsia should be controlled with diazepam given as diazemules, 2–10 mg i.v. as necessary to control convulsion over 2 min. If unconscious after diazepam, intubate airway. If fitting persists, induce general anaesthesia and intubate airway.
4. Further fits should be controlled using an infusion of magnesium sulphate (see separate protocol).
5. Consideration should be given to the possibility that the fit was precipitated by an intracranial bleed:
   - Do neurological examination in all women when stable.
   - Consider CT imaging if suspicion about intra-cranial bleed.
6. Delivery should be undertaken when the mother's condition has stabilised.
7. Mode of delivery is contentious. LSCS has the advantage that if the woman fits again, the baby is no longer a concern.
8. Consultant obstetrician and anaesthetist should be informed in all cases.

Management of Oliguria and Anuria

In the majority of women with PET, the total body water is increased but the circulating blood volume is decreased. Much of the excess fluid is contained within the interstitial tissues.

Oliguria is common, in part because of intrinsic renal (glomerular) damage resulting from small vessel disease but also because of a physiological response to the stress of labour and delivery. There may be a pre-renal component from a reduced circulating volume but this is likely to be small in women who are not bleeding.

In the absence of HELLP syndrome, isolated thrombocytopaenia, severe infection and severe haemorrhage with hypotension, renal failure is extremely rare. There is no evidence that any therapeutic measure protects the kidney, and the risk of using aggressive fluid management routinely is that pulmonary oedema will develop which may progress to death (see *Confidential Enquiries into Maternal Death*).

If moderate oliguria develops.

1. Define oliguria as < 25 ml urine flow per hour.
2. Consider possibility that PET is worsening; development of HELLP syndrome/thrombocytopaenia/DIC.
3. Consider whether there is any (occult) blood loss.
4. Check fluid balance carefully.
5. Check urinary catheter not blocked.
6. Do **NOT** use diuretic therapy unless there is direct evidence of fluid overload.
7. If the woman is well generally and the **current** LFTs and platelet count are both normal:
   - Continue with standard fluid regimen and await events for 4 h.
   - At 4 h, give 500 ml of Hartmann's solution over 30 min.
8. If the woman has **ANY** of the following, seek help from consultant obstetrician and/or anaesthetist:
   - persistent oliguria (> 6 h total)
   - hypotension
   - abnormal creatinine
   - abnormal LFTs or platelet count
   - continuing significant blood loss
   - severe pyrexia (> 38°C).

Consideration should be given to more intensive monitoring (CVP measurement) and more aggressive therapy. There is a separate protocol for this.

If anuria develops

If the woman becomes anuric, it is usually as a result of HELLP syndrome or disseminated intravascular coagulation (DIC). There is no evidence of renal protection from any therapy (fluid drive, diuretics or dopamine), all of which carry risks. There may be some benefit simply from maintaining a renal output, however.

The woman with anuria should be transferred to the Intensive Care Unit or monitored by an intensive care nurse on delivery suite if a bed is not immediately available.

Fluid Management in Haemorrhage

If aggressive fluid replacement is necessary for haemorr-

hage, monitoring of CVP and pulse oximetry are advisable. Interpretation of the CVP should be undertaken with care, however; the reading is a poor guide to pulmonary artery wedge pressures. The range of acceptable CVP measurements in PET is 2–6 cm of H_2O. Equally important is the CVP response to fluid therapy, which gives a guide to whether this compartment is full or not.

Management of HELLP Syndrome

HELLP (**H**aemolysis, **E**levated **L**iver enzymes, **L**ow **P**latelets) is an extremely severe complication of preeclampsia. It carries with it a high maternal and fetal mortality. **Senior obstetric and anaesthetic input is mandatory.**

Symptoms of right upper quadrant and epigastric pain must be taken seriously in all pregnant women over 20 weeks. Occasionally, it presents before the onset of hypertension and proteinuria, and their absence does not rule out the condition. The diagnosis is made by measurement of the platelet count and serum transaminases. Sometimes these may not change for some hours after the onset of pain (c.f. rise of cardiac enzymes in myocardial infarction), and if your suspicion is strong do repeat bloods in 4–8 h.

It may be complicated by pancreatitis. **Measure amylase**.

Theme of management of established HELLP syndrome is:

- **Intensive monitoring with**:
  - pulse oximetry and CV pressure
  - strict input/output balance
  - laboratory blood profile 2 to 4 hourly.
  Transfer to ITU may be necessary in some cases.
- **And full supportive care**:
  - Oxygen as necessary.
  - Consider blood transfusion if Hb falls below 9 g/dl.
  - Transfuse fresh frozen plasma if abnormal clotting times.
  - Platelet transfusion if < 50×10^9 (use high threshold because of dynamic situation).
  - Cryoprecipitate if uncontrolled bleeding.
  - Crystalloid fluids to maintain CVP in range 2–6 cm.

Management of Pulmonary Oedema

Prevent by cautious fluid management and maintenance of upright position. If oedema does develop, inform consultant obstetrician and anaesthetist whilst

- arranging upright position
- giving oxygen therapy
- monitoring respiratory rate and pulse oximetry

• considering possibility of acute myocardial infarction (especially diabetes patients) and doing ECG
• giving frusemide (20 mg i.v. slowly) and observing response, repeating after 30 min if no effect.

If no response, transfer to ITU for possible ventilation, etc.

GUIDELINES FOR TRANSFER TO ITU

Labour ward is a high-dependency unit, and most women should be monitored here. Some women will need to be transferred to ITU, either because of difficulty with staffing levels on delivery suite or because of a need for specialist monitoring/therapy. Before a woman is transferred, ensure her condition is as stable as reasonably possible.

Medical indications for transfer:

• anuria
• oliguria with adverse features (see above)
• resistant pulmonary oedema/need for ventilation
• resistant hypertension requiring sodium nitroprusside
• intubation/ventilation needed for eclampsia.

4 Organisation of clinical management

WOMEN WITH SYMPTOMS

Traditionally the scheme of medical practice has been for a man or woman to present to a medical practitioner with symptoms. History taking, physical examination, basic and then additional clinical tests are undertaken to make a diagnosis. After diagnosis there is a discussion of prognosis with and without therapy. This is followed by explanation of available treatments, together with details of their success rates and side effects. Treatment is then monitored and reviewed. Within this framework, there will be needs for education and support.

Some clinical approaches are based on a different model of care. An example in gynaecology is early pregnancy assessment. The conventional method of care would be for the woman to be admitted to the ward, be seen by the doctor, and have investigations arranged. Much of the management is geared to the result of a pregnancy test and an ultrasound scan, however, and so some clinicians feel that it is better to do the pregnancy test and scan first and then do the history and examination in the light of that information.

SCREENING FOR ASYMPTOMATIC DISEASE

Increasingly, healthcare programmes have sought to detect disease states before they are clinically overt, so as to prevent the development of more serious problems in the future. This is called screening, and it works on the notion that prevention is better than cure. Screening programmes have to meet certain criteria (Box 4.1) before being introduced into clinical practice. The first four are the most important criteria. The issue of harm is especially critical, particularly for very rare diseases. If the prevalence of the (asymptomatic) condition is very low and the false positive rate is high, there is a very real possibility of doing more harm to healthy women than benefit to those with the disease. Programmes for the early detection of ovarian cancer provide a good example of how screening can do much harm (see Box 4.2). Because the prevalence of the condition is so low, even when **assuming** a high sensitivity and specificity, the predictive power is very low. This indicates that for every case of cancer, about 50 women would have a false positive test result. If the confirmatory test were laparoscopy/laparotomy, 50 women would be subjected to surgery for every case of cancer detected. Harm caused also includes anxiety and guilt. This particularly applies to pregnancy screening tests for fetal abnormality. Both ultrasonography and maternal serum testing identify more false positives (normal fetus) than true positives (fetus has abnormality). Additional testing by repeat scanning or amniocentesis usually discriminates between true and false positives, but the anxiety generated by the first test may take many weeks to resolve; muddy water runs downstream. Even more serious is miscarriage of a normal fetus following amniocentesis. It has been estimated that two normal fetuses are lost as a result of invasive prenatal testing for every case of trisomy 21 detected. The guilt and sadness felt by parents may never resolve fully.

Box 4.1 Criteria for screening programmes

- Disease exists in asymptomatic state.
- Early diagnosis improves outcome.
- Test has reasonable sensitivity and specificity.
- The test is not unduly harmful.
- Systems are in place to cope with counselling and treatment.
- Screening is affordable.

Box 4.2 Mathematics of screening for ovarian cancer

Prevalence	1 in 5000
Sensitivity	90%
Specificity	99%
Predictive power of positive test	2%

There are many screening programmes in obstetrics and gynaecology. Some are simple, such as the detection of anaemia in pregnancy, but others, such as cervical cytology screening, are very complex at all levels. It is only recently, with improvements in the administration of call and recall, that the programme has started to make a big impact on the incidence of cervical cancer.

5 Using clinical tests: explaining results and probability

FUNCTION OF CLINICAL TESTS

Clinical tests are used for a variety of reasons. Some are used to make or refute a diagnosis (e.g. laparoscopy for ectopic pregnancy). Other tests give a guide to prognosis (e.g. histological grading of endometrial cancer), and some are used for monitoring clinical response to treatment (e.g. use of tumour markers with hydatidiform mole). We occasionally use tests to reassure patients even though we know the result is of no direct clinical value to ourselves (e.g. parental karyotype after birth of a child with Down's syndrome). The reassurance value of a negative test should not be underestimated, however. Many women with chronic pelvic pain notice an improvement in their symptoms after a negative ultrasound scan or laparoscopy.

PATIENT'S USE OF TESTS

A patient's use of a test can be subtly different from that of doctors. This is particularly so in pregnancy. It is said that obstetricians generally use prenatal diagnostic tests to detect abnormality, whereas women tend to use such tests to gain reassurance of normality; i.e. they do not really want to detect abnormality even if it exists. This may not seem a big difference, but the result can be that some women regret having the test when their expectation of normality is not confirmed.

Another difference in the use of prenatal diagnostic tests concerns forward planning. Doctors may assume that if a woman has a screening test for Down's and the test reveals a high risk, the woman should proceed to more invasive testing. Similarly, if an amniocentesis result is performed and trisomy 21 is diagnosed, the doctor assumes that the woman will wish to have a termination. This is a natural assumption because it is the doctor's general experience, but in fact a proportion of women do the unexpected and decline amniocentesis and termination of pregnancy, respectively. There are probably several reasons for this, but an important one is that some women cannot make the decision about continuation/termination until the result of the test is known. Before that time, all they can imagine is a normal baby, and contemplation of TOP is therefore not possible. This 'suck it and see' approach is entirely satisfactory for many women and should be for doctors as well.

In gynaecology, the use of tests is usually more straightforward. One possible exception is the use of laparoscopy for the investigation of pelvic pain. Two women may have identical histories of pelvic pain and physical findings, but one chooses to have laparoscopy while the other chooses not to have laparoscopy. This may be explained by fear, but equally it may reflect how different women get reassurance in different ways. Some women feel reassured by the doctor's clinical judgement alone; others feel the need to rely on technology.

TEST INTERPRETATION

Some tests are easy for all to understand. The result is in black and white terms. A woman is either anaemic or not, sickle positive or not. Other tests give a vague assessment of chance: very unlikely, possible, probable, etc. Others give a quantified chance: 1 in 5, 1 in 50, 1 in 5000, etc. The doctor then has to consider additional tests which may confirm or refute the diagnosis.

Some tests are complex in that a positive result may be a very powerful predictor of the presence of a condition whereas a negative result does not rule it out. Serum LH measurement for polycystic ovarian disease is such a case: a raised level is highly suggestive of PCOD, but a normal level is of little value. In other situations, one test may depend on another test for accurate interpretation. Serum FSH measurement is a good example. A raised FSH concentration in a woman who menstruates erratically may be indicative of incipient ovarian failure or simply the midcycle rise. The relative concentrations of LH and FSH reveal which: an LH concentration greater than FSH is consistent with a midcycle surge, while an LH level lower than that of FSH is indicative of a degree of ovarian failure (end-organ resistance). It should also not be forgotten that an investigation may test for a variety of very different diseases, and if the result is unusual for the condition primarily being tested for, the other possibilities should be considered. An example of this is serum alpha-feto protein (AFP). Maternal serum AFP is elevated in pregnancies complicated by fetal malformation such as neural tube defects (spina bifida, anencephaly) and gut hernias (gastrochisis), but outside of pregnancy it is used as a marker of severe liver disease and yolk sac tumours of the ovary. If a maternal serum result is reported as being **extremely** elevated for pregnancy, these other, much rarer conditions must be considered.

Understanding the limitations of tests is important. It helps doctors to ensure that they are undertaken properly and interpreted with caution. This must be explained to patients, who may not be aware of the inaccuracies of testing. To give the impression of certainty when uncertainty abounds will backfire occasionally. One test that very rarely can cause great upset is fetal sexing at amniocentesis. It is extremely accurate but occasionally maternal cells will have been cultured and couples expecting a girl will have a boy instead. Their response can range from amusement to anger and sadness for the girl they have lost.

It is also important to remember that laboratory medicine is not perfect. If the test result is incongruous with the clinical picture, consider repeating the test. It might have been that a sample was taken inappropriately (e.g. from close to the site of an intravenous infusion), or the sample was mixed up with that of another patient, or the test was incorrectly performed in the laboratory. On some occasions patients fabricate evidence, e.g. putting a drop of blood into a urine specimen to mimic renal colic resulting from renal calculi.

EXPLAINING TEST RESULTS

Tests give a fact, but that information may come in various forms and with varying degrees of certainty. Many doctors take years to grasp issues such as sensitivity, specificity and predictive values even after 5 years of rigorous training. Further, many of the women to whom we offer care do not even have a rudimentary understanding of simple mathematics. That is not to be scorned but rather taken into account when discussing results. It might be pleasurable to spend time explaining test results to a statistician with a health problem, but it is probably more important to spend more time with a woman who left school at 16 years with no qualifications. The answer is not to keep information from women but to give detail in a clear form (but without being overly simplistic). In addition, it is important to try not to assume that the woman will understand terms that we take for granted.

Screening for Down's syndrome is an interesting model for the explanation of test results. Trisomy 21 is frequently talked of and written about, but many people have no real idea what Down's syndrome involves. This also applies to the understanding of numeric information. Surveys of the general population show that many cannot understand percentages: 5% is mistaken for a chance of 1 in 5.

Table 5.1 Explaining the chance of Down's syndrome	
Chance of Down's	
At 41 years	1/80
At 42 years	1/40
Chance of not Down's	
At 41 years	79/80
At 42 years	39/40
Normalised chance of not Down's	
At 41 years	79/80
At 42 years	78/80

Statistics can easily create a false picture, particularly if terms such as high-risk are used. Is a 1 in 100 chance of Down's syndrome a high or low risk? A 1% chance seems high, but 99 out of 100 (the vast majority) will not have Down's. Perhaps it is better to give only the information and not to give one's own view of the chance but to let the couple decide themselves how they see the test result. The method of presentation of numbers can also be important. Table 5.1 shows data for the chance of Down's and not Down's for a woman of 40 wishing to have a baby who asks for the data for the next 2 years. She felt the change in chance between the 2 years was large, and this panicked her. Reversing the figures to emphasise the chance of good outcome did not placate her because she was focusing on the large difference between 40 and 80 and not on the true probability. However, when the denominator was normalised, she felt the chance differed little.

A common difficulty for us all is maintaining a proper perspective on the probability and nature of the potential problem at the same time. Many complications in pregnancy have a low chance of occurring but, if they do, the effects on the mother and fetus can be catastrophic (concept of low chance / high stake). For some individuals, they can only focus on the severity of the medical problem and not the low chance of occurrence. This applies particularly to women who have had a previous pregnancy complication, but also to the general population at large. One down-side of publicity surrounding the national screening programme for trisomy 21 is that for some women the anxiety has been raised out of proportion to the chance of a fetus being affected.

It is not only the presentation of numbers that is important; even choice of the words we use may influence thought. Risk and chance have similar meanings, but chance has a much softer edge than risk. Decline and refusal are also very similar, but for a doctor or midwife to say 'The woman has refused the test' sounds a little as

Table 5.2 Estimation of car speed according to question asked after video viewing	
Question	Average estimated speed (miles/h)
'What speed was the blue car travelling at when the two cars ...?'	
made contact	31.1
crashed	35.2
collided	36.7
smashed	44.6

though the woman has made the wrong choice or that she was obstinate. It might even be best of all to say 'The woman has chosen not to have the test'. Research psychologists have demonstrated clearly how a single word change in a sentence will alter the understanding of events (Table 5.2).

GIVING PERMISSION

In addition to giving advice about probability, it is important to give support. The instinct to conform is very powerful, and some people need permission to make the decision they feel is correct for them. With decisions about termination of pregnancy, a couple may worry that doctors, nurses or relatives are sitting in judgement on their decision. Explain to them that whatever decision they make about continuation or termination of pregnancy, they will be making a decision that many others couples have made before and that they will be given your support. Equally, some couples may feel difficulty in announcing that they wish to continue with the pregnancy. Once more, words are important. Always emphasise both parts of the choice: to say 'The only things we can offer if the amniocentesis is abnormal is termination of pregnancy' will be taken by some couples to indicate that the doctor feels it is this only choice that can be made, when in fact both continuation and termination of pregnancy are on offer. For some couples it will be important for the doctor or nurse to be explicit about the nature of the dilemma which faces many couples. They themselves may feel overwhelmed by anxiety and cannot focus on the salient questions. For many, it comes down to 'What is more important for you: to avoid having a baby with Down's syndrome or to avoid the risk of miscarriage of a normal baby'. It may also help for them to know that they do not need to make a decision immediately but can return home to think things through, perhaps with a prepared leaflet

to summarise the sort of things that have been discussed (see Figure 5.1). The final interpretation of the result is for the woman (and her partner) to decide. Their response may seem difficult for us to understand but we are primarily advisors; we cannot enforce healthcare but only give advice about the benefits and disadvantages.

ASSESSMENT OF OUTCOME

In addition to offering advice and support, we should also pay close attention to the woman's psychological responses to the information she is being offered. This issue probably applies more to maternity care than to most other branches of clinical medicine, because of the unusual relationship between mother and fetus, and because of myths and superstitions about reproduction.

Doctors often refer to good and bad pregnancy outcomes in absolute terms, but to do so may be to overlook subtle and complex reactions to pregnancy loss. Few of us could perhaps imagine that death of a baby shortly after birth is a good outcome, but it may be just that for the parents who comforted the infant in the last hour of life, having chosen to continue with the pregnancy in the knowledge of a lethal malformation, and having worried that the fetus might have died before birth, before they saw him alive. Such an experience can be sad and good simultaneously. Reactions simply cannot be predicted. Some parents will suffer a greater sense of loss of a pregnancy at 6 weeks than others do at term. Others will suffer great sadness at the birth of a healthy child because it brings back memories of a previous stillborn baby; happiness might not be felt for some time. Mothers of twins who lose one child at birth while the other survives may have great difficulty loving the healthy baby when grieving for the loss of her other child, the child whose kicks she felt during pregnancy. It is not our role to sit in judgement on the nature or extent of their grief. As health professionals we should aim to observe and respond to need. To ask a woman how she feels may seem to be a silly, even clumsy question, but it allows the woman to express herself directly, and then the doctor, nurse or midwife can respond more appropriately.

The use of words is so important for both doctors and patients. Some words or phrases can be described as softer and are, therefore, more palatable to the patient. A common example is the use of miscarriage and abortion. They have similar meanings and are used interchangeably by doctors and nurses, but women probably find 'delayed miscarriage' better than 'missed abortion'. That is not to say that doctors or nurses should avoid saying things that upset patients. It is much better to discuss important issues if the patient is willing than to hide

AMNIOCENTESIS

Most babies are born perfectly healthy but, just like a child, a fetus may develop problems with his or her health while still in the mother's womb (uterus). Although they are very rare, some of these illnesses can be very serious, and it is useful to be able to diagnose any problems during the pregnancy. Many of the problems can be detected on ultrasound scan but others can only be found by a sample being taken of the fluid surrounding the baby (amniocentesis) or the placenta (chorion villus sampling).

For most women, the reason for having an amniocentesis is so that they can consider having termination of pregnancy if the result is abnormal. Termination in this part of pregnancy would be by delivery and not an operation.

The Technique

Amniocentesis is a technique in which a small amount of fluid is taken from around the baby. The fluid can be tested in many different ways depending on the particular circumstance.

The technique of amniocentesis involves aspiration of a very small amount of the fluid which surrounds the baby, using a very fine needle. The needle is passed towards the fluid while we watch using an ultrasound scanner.

Local anaesthetic is used to make things comfortable for you. The test usually takes about three minutes to do, and the doctor will show you the baby's heartbeat after it is over.

Disadvantages

The main disadvantage of amniocentesis is that there is a small chance of miscarrying a normal baby. This is thought to be about 1 in 150 (less than 1%). It follows that 149 women out of 150 would not miscarry.

Any miscarriage would not occur immediately but usually about two weeks after the test.

The Result

The result takes about three weeks to come through. The results are very accurate but no test in medicine is 100% accurate. Amniocentesis is thought to be more than 97% accurate, which is very good. The chance of accidental termination of a normal baby is extremely remote.

It is important to realise that the amniocentesis test is only looking for a limited number of problems. If the test is normal, it does not necessarily mean that the baby is entirely normal, only that a certain number of serious problems have been excluded.

Very rarely the cells in the fluid do not grow and a result cannot be obtained. This occurs in less than 1% of cases. If it does happen the test can be repeated if you wish.

You will receive a normal result by letter. If the test is abnormal you will be contacted directly.

The test will also reveal the **probable** sex of the baby. The test is very reliable for this but not perfectly so. If you would like to know the likely sex of the baby, please ring my secretary when the result is through.

After the Test

You will rest for about twenty minutes after the test and then you will go home. It is essential that you have somebody who can accompany you home. We advise that you do not drive yourself.

We advise that you rest in the afternoon, but by the next day most women are fine to return to normal activity. Cramping (period) pains and spotting of blood are both very common. You do not need to worry about these. It is safe to take paracetamol for any moderate discomfort, but avoid aspirin and other painkillers. You should contact your GP or midwife if you have severe pain, heavy bleeding or fever.

If you have a special blood group (rhesus negative) you will be given a small injection to try to stop you producing antibodies.

Our role is not to tell you to have the test but to give you information and to support your decision.

Robert Fox
July 1998

Fig 5.1 *Patient information leaflet on amniocentesis.*

away from them. If the doctor appears not to want to talk of a previous stillbirth, the woman may become inhibited, and an opportunity may be missed to let her tell her story of the loss. As well as the words and non-verbal signals that we use, affecting women and men we care for, it is important for us to realise that words can instantly give rise to powerful images for doctors too. On hearing that a child has cerebral palsy, many of us would think of an immobile child unable to communicate. That picture can be so wrong. A famous poster by the Society for Cerebral Palsy ran: 'My son with cerebral palsy has a mental age of 8 years; he's 6 next birthday'.

PATIENT'S CHOICE

In years gone by, the medical model was that doctors decided and patients complied. With changes in society, this model is less appropriate, and choice has become a central part of good care. The Chair of the GMC has recently said:

> Patients have certain fundamental rights, including the right to be fully involved in decisions about care, and the right to refuse treatment.

Many doctors have found this hard to accept. They find it difficult to understand that a patient could understand the intricacies of medical care. Remarkably, many people grasp quite complex issues if they are explained clearly and simply. With advice, most people are able to choose a specific car from a range of fifty or more models available but without any understanding of how a car is designed or built. The same is true of medical care.

If a patient does choose not to undergo a certain treatment it is important that the doctor maintains a professional stance and follows certain guidelines (see

---

Box 5.1). It should not be forgotten that people make decisions for a variety of reasons: misunderstanding of explanation, fear of the treatment, antipathy to the doctor. It should also be borne in mind that the woman might feel great anxiety that the decision she has taken will upset the doctor and she might assume that the doctor would not wish to offer further care.

The effects of removing choice are that drugs will be prescribed that are not wanted and operations performed that are unnecessary. Compliance is likely to be less good, and if complications arise, the woman is more likely to feel resentment towards her carers. Worse still, if the doctor is stubborn and unable to negotiate care, the woman may choose to default from care altogether, and opportunity for further discussion is lost.

Allowing choice should not alter the basic message that a doctor gives. The doctor is not obliged to offer bad treatments as well as good ones. Advice should be based on the best available evidence. Allowing choice simply alters the way we deliver care.

RESPECTING PATIENTS

There is a tendency by some healthcare workers to treat the needs of a patient as secondary to the needs of the staff. This approach can lead to an enclave mentality with the patient being treated as an outsider, a nuisance. Clearly this is unacceptable. It makes patients vulnerable, anxious and angry. In some situations this tendency is manifest as a lack of understanding and even derision towards the people we care for. This includes mocking of physical traits, responding aggressively to patients' anger, even chastising people because they are late for appointments (and without finding out a reason for any delay), or because they express too much pain after surgery.

Our role is to show respect for people and their individual needs. If a woman has more pain than expected after hysterectomy, with no obvious cause, perhaps she is unusually anxious or even upset because she can have no more children. If a woman shows anger in the clinic, it might be because she is frightened that her symptoms are a sign of cancer. Alternatively, she might be under pressure from an employer to return to work quickly, or perhaps the children are about to come out of school.

People who have certain habits should not be ridiculed or derided. It is appropriate to advise people about obesity and smoking, but it is wrong to rebuke them. Humiliation is not a motivating force. Moreover, such comments will generate anger, and the woman will then fail to attend for further care. To criticise heavily a woman with a growth-retarded fetus for smoking may mean that she does not attend to have her fetus monitored.

Box 5.1 When a woman chooses not to have treatment

- Acknowledge that it is satisfactory for her to make her choice.
- Do not show anger, and emphasise that you are not displeased.
- Offer to continue with care and state she may return at any time.
- Discuss other options for treatment.
- Offer a second opinion.
- If the woman does get better without your treatment, be gracious and show pleasure.

Clinical Problems in Gynaecology

6 Bleeding in early pregnancy

CLINICAL SIGNIFICANCE

Pain and bleeding in the first trimester of pregnancy are the most common gynaecological emergencies.

50% of women with bleeding in early pregnancy have a viable intrauterine pregnancy with a low risk of pregnancy loss. However, the remaining pregnancies will be non-viable and a correct diagnosis with prompt treatment will help to minimise the physical and psychological morbidity of these conditions.

Miscarriage is a common complication of pregnancy. It is rarely life threatening, but can be extremely distressing to the woman, with potentially serious complications. Whilst the words abortion and miscarriage may be synonymous, the general public often associate abortion with termination of pregnancy; because of this, miscarriage will be used throughout this chapter.

Ectopic pregnancy is a potentially life-threatening complication of pregnancy whose incidence is increasing worldwide. It is the single largest cause of first trimester maternal mortality in the UK, with an initial incorrect diagnosis being made in up to 50% of cases.

DIFFERENTIAL DIAGNOSIS

MAIN CATEGORIES	DIAGNOSIS
1. *Normal pregnancy*	
2. *Miscarriage*	Threatened
	Missed
	Blighted ovum
	Complete
	Incomplete
	Septic
3. *Ectopic pregnancy*	Tubal
	Other pelvic sites
4. *Hydatidiform mole*	
5. *Non-pregnancy-related*	Cervical (ectropion, carcinoma)
	Vaginal (trauma)
	Urethral (haematuria)

There is an enormous range in the severity of pain and bleeding: from the shocked woman with a ruptured ectopic pregnancy to the more common slight vaginal bleeding, often less than a period, with niggling period-like pain. The majority of women who present are not acutely unwell, and emergency resuscitation is uncommon.

CLINICAL ASSESSMENT

Diagnosis relies very heavily on ultrasound scanning.

Rapid Emergency Assessment

The pallor and sweating accompanying shock can be late signs in fit young women, and the extent of the haemorrhage may not always be fully revealed. Therefore, all women with any signs of shock should be aggressively resuscitated: large bore intravenous access, cross-match 4 units of blood, start colloid fluid replacement and make arrangements for theatre.

Hypotension due to bleeding which may be vaginal or intra-abdominal will be accompanied by a tachycardia. Hypotension accompanied by a bradycardia suggests 'cervical shock', which is a reflex vagal stimulation secondary to products of conception (PoC) in the cervix. This can rapidly be reversed by removing the PoC.

Severe abdominal pain, shoulder tip pain and peritonism all suggest intra-abdominal blood and an ectopic pregnancy which requires immediate surgery.

A pregnancy test is helpful in making a diagnosis, though surgery should not be delayed in a woman with shock.

Relevant History

Presenting Complaint

MAIN COMPLAINT - **Pain and bleeding** are the most common complaints. The majority of women have very little in the way of signs and symptoms. However, there are a few pointers to the diagnosis. **Heavy bleeding** (> normal period) characterises miscarriage, and **products of conception** (PoC) may be seen within the bleeding. In contrast, the bleeding associated with an ectopic pregnancy is usually lighter and there are no PoC seen. Remember, a decidual cast is sometimes seen and mistaken for PoC and up to 50% of ectopic pregnancies are initially incorrectly diagnosed. This is not primarily due to medical incompetence, but is because the presentation of ectopic pregnancy can be extremely variable and often 'silent' with few signs and symptoms. Miscarriage is characterised by central, cramping, period-like **pain** in association with the bleeding. The pain of an ectopic pregnancy often **precedes the bleeding** and is usually more lateral. If the bleeding is intraperitoneal, there may be more generalised abdominal and shoulder tip pain.

COMMONLY ASSOCIATED SYMPTOMS - **Amenorrhoea** associated with ectopic pregnancies generally presents at an earlier gestation than intrauterine pregnancies, i.e. 6-8 weeks gestation compared with the 8-12 weeks gestation of a miscarriage. Exaggerated **symptoms of pregnancy** suggests a molar pregnancy, i.e. hyperemesis, caused by the high levels of β-hCG. Occasionally, there are also signs and symptoms of hyperthyroidism where the high β-hCG levels can mimic thyroid-stimulating hormone (TSH) stimulating the thyroid. **A reduction in the symptoms of pregnancy** may indicate a failed pregnancy, i.e. blighted ovum or complete miscarriage.

Gynaecological History

GYNAECOLOGICAL DISEASE - Pelvic inflammatory disease predisposes to ectopic pregnancy secondary to tubal damage. Previous tubal surgery increases the risk of ectopic pregnancy both because of the initial indication for surgery, i.e. tubal damage, and also the scarring caused by surgery itself. Uterine abnormalities, i.e. uterine septum, can predispose to miscarriage. Assisted reproduction techniques predispose to both ectopic pregnancy and miscarriage.

CONTRACEPTION - The risk of an ectopic pregnancy is increased where there is a slow transport of the fertilised ovum or a blockage in the tube. The progestogen-only pill predisposes to ectopic pregnancy, though the excess risk is small. This is due to a reduction in the tubal cilial motility. Use of an IUCD does not increase the rate of ectopic pregnancy per se, but if a pregnancy does occur it is more likely to be an ectopic pregnancy, as the IUCD is ineffective outside the uterus.

FERTILITY REQUIREMENTS - In women who have not completed their family the Fallopian tubes should be conserved if possible when dealing with an ectopic pregnancy.

Obstetric history

DELIVERIES - A previous history of ectopic pregnancy increases the risk in subsequent pregnancies, and similarly a previous history of molar pregnancy increases the risk of recurrence.

Medical history

MEDICAL CONDITIONS - A history of diabetes mellitus, anti-phospholipid antibodies or PCOD may all predispose to miscarriage.

SURGERY - Previous pelvic surgery may prevent the use of laparoscopy to deal with an ectopic pregnancy.

Drug history

MEDICATIONS - Chemotherapy, especially with cytotoxic drugs, can cause fetal loss because of teratogenesis.

SMOKING AND ALCOHOL - Not only has cigarette smoking been identified as a risk factor for miscarriage for the smoker herself, but also the miscarriage rate is increased in daughters of smokers even where they do not smoke themselves.

Social History

AGE - All complications of the first trimester are increased with advancing maternal age.

LIFESTYLE - When the pregnancy is viable and spotting continues, the woman is usually advised to take time off work.

Relevant Clinical Examination

General Features

GENERAL DEMEANOUR - Remember that most women who present will be haemodynamically stable. However, be aware of these more sinister findings: sweating and pallor are characteristic of shock. Check the pulse and BP for the features noted above.

Abdomen

CONTOUR - May be distended from bleeding.

OLD SCARS - Check for abdominal scars, including laparoscopy scars, as previous surgery or investigation for subfertility will predispose to an ectopic pregnancy.

PALPATION – **Tenderness** and signs of peritonism are a feature of intra-abdominal bleeding. A miscarriage does not usually present with any abdominal features except mild central tenderness and a palpable fundus after 12 weeks gestation. There are unlikely to be any abdominal findings in the first trimester of pregnancy. An abnormally enlarged uterus which is palpable abdominally suggests a molar pregnancy.

BOWEL SOUNDS – Should be present unless bowel involvement has occurred.

Pelvis

VULVA/VAGINA – PoC or vesicles may be seen in the vagina.

CERVIX – Products may be seen in the os or heavy bleeding. Opening of the cervix is a sign of incomplete or inevitable miscarriage.

BIMANUAL EXAMINATION – Cervical excitation is pain on cervical movement and is characteristic of tubal or parametrial pathology. The pain is produced by lateral displacement of the cervix, which stretches the tube and parametrium. The pain is secondary to inflammation of the tube or parametrium secondary to the tubal pregnancy. The **uterus** enlarges in early pregnancy secondary to the hormonal stimulation, not physical stretching; because of this the uterus may be an appropriate size for the gestation in an ectopic pregnancy. The uterus is larger than expected by dates for a hydatidiform mole. Ectopic pregnancies may be palpated as tender **adnexal masses**, but more commonly the adnexa are too tender to palpate.

RELEVANT INVESTIGATIONS

Haematology

HB – A full blood count should be completed as part of the initial investigation.

RHESUS STATUS – Anti-D is still necessary in rhesus negative women irrespective of gestation to avoid rhesus isoimmunisation. Therefore a blood group should be determined even where cross-match is not required

PLATELET COUNT – May be reduced after severe haemorrhage.

CLOTTING STUDIES – Required after severe haemorrhage or when monitoring large blood transfusions.

Endocrine Tests

β-hCG – A pregnancy test is essential. Urinary pregnancy tests are now very sensitive, to 25–50 IU/L β-hCG, which will be positive at the time of a missed period, i.e. 4 weeks gestation. Serum β-hCG is also used where an ectopic pregnancy is suspected. Where the serum β-hCG is >1500 then an intrauterine pregnancy should be seen with 95% confidence if it is present. Therefore, a β-hCG >1500 and an empty uterus on scan would suggest an ectopic pregnancy, and a laparoscopy should be undertaken.

Diagnostic Imaging

ULTRASOUND – Ultrasound scan (USS) is the most useful of all investigations in early pregnancy. See individual conditions for findings. Transabdominal scans require a full bladder and are most useful after 9–10 weeks gestation.

Transvaginal ultrasound scans (TVS) can very accurately demonstrate intrauterine pregnancies from 5–6/40 and allow visualisation of the adnexa. The features that should be noted at TVS to confirm an early intrauterine death, i.e. a pregnancy that will end as a miscarriage:

- If the gestation sac has a mean diameter greater than 20 mm, with no evidence of an embryo or yolk sac, this is highly suggestive of a blighted ovum.
- If the embryo has a crown-rump length greater than 6 mm, with no evidence of heart pulsations, this is highly suggestive of a missed abortion.

Retained products of conception (RPoC) consistent with an incomplete miscarriage can also be visualised (Figure 6.1).

An empty uterus at > 6/40 gestation should prompt exclusion of an ectopic pregnancy, though it can also be normal after a complete miscarriage. Other suggestive

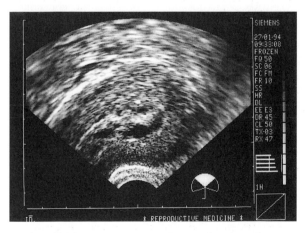

Fig 6.1 *TVS demonstrating uterus with retained products of conception.*

findings are an adnexal mass or fluid (blood) in the Pouch of Douglas. Occasionally, a live ectopic pregnancy can be visualised in the adnexa on scan.

Molar change or degeneration is diagnosed on USS. The vesicles are seen as sonolucent areas inside the uterus. The oft-described 'snowstorm' appearance is now rarely seen using modern ultrasound scanners. A fetal pole is often missing, although, with a partial mole, a fetal pole may be present. Women with bleeding in early pregnancy often present out-of-hours but, unless there is a clinical suspicion of an ectopic pregnancy or evidence of shock, there is no need for immediate admission. Early Pregnancy Assessment Clinics provide facilities for an immediate ultrasound scan and gynaecological review. They are generally available on a daily basis, and most women can then be reviewed and treated in office hours, reducing the need for unnecessary admission.

Histopathology

PoC – Any products seen in the vagina should be sent to confirm a miscarriage.

Direct Visualisation

LAPAROSCOPY – This is the gold standard investigation for suspected ectopic pregnancy. The pelvis can be directly visualised, including the Fallopian tubes.

DETAILS OF COMMON CONDITIONS

1. Miscarriage

Background

DEFINITION – Expulsion of products of conception before viability. In the UK a miscarriage is a pregnancy loss prior to 24 completed weeks gestation. In most medical textbooks miscarriage is termed as abortion, although this can be very easily misinterpreted by patients. Miscarriage is used throughout this chapter.

AETIOLOGY – The incidence of chromosome imbalance is at least 50% in first trimester miscarriage. This may account for at least part of the increased miscarriage rate in older women. Uterine abnormality such as fibroids or congenital uterine malformations may result in pregnancy loss. Antiphospholipid antibodies and anticardiolipin antibodies and 'lupus' anticoagulant are both found in autoimmune disorders. Diabetes mellitus is associated with increased fetal loss.

MAKING THE DIAGNOSIS – There are different categories of miscarriage which are defined by the clinical and ultrasound findings.

Table 6.1 Diagnosing miscarriage	
Making the diagnosis	Miscarriage
History	Vaginal bleeding prior to abdominal/pelvic cramping the onset of pain
Examination	Uterus may be enlarged with non-tender adnexa
	The state of the cervix will depend on type of miscarriage
Investigations	
– Pregnancy test	Positive
– Ultrasound	Intrauterine products or fetus confirmed
– Histology	Confirms products of conception

- **Threatened:** Bleeding and pain with closed cervical os. Now also used to mean a history of bleeding with a viable pregnancy seen on USS.
- **Inevitable:** Bleeding and pain with an open cervical os.
- **Incomplete:** Miscarriage history with an open os and PoC seen on USS.
- **Septic:** A complication of an incomplete miscarriage where the remaining PoC become infected by ascending organisms. Septic complications are more common where there has been instrumentation of the uterus, i.e. 'back street abortions', or even after evacuation of retained products of conception (ERPC).
- **Complete:** A history of pain and bleeding; often PoC are seen, followed by a diminution as the PoC are completely expelled. The USS shows an empty uterus.
- **Missed:** An ultrasound diagnosis of a non-viable pregnancy. If a sac develops to > 20 mm diameter without a fetal pole, or a fetal pole of > 5 mm is seen without a fetal heart, then these are termed a blighted ovum and a missed abortion, respectively.

MAIN COMPLICATIONS – The main complications are haemorrhage and infection.

SCREENING/PREVENTION – There are few effective clinical interventions. Aspirin has a protective effect in women with antiphospholipid antibodies. Progesterone has been used, though clear benefit has not been established.

Treatment Options

REASSURANCE – Treatment aims to reduce the potential complications of miscarriage, i.e. prolonged pain and bleeding, sepsis and rhesus isosensitisation. Miscarriage is a common complication of pregnancy all over the world; the most common treatment worldwide is expectant, i.e. spontaneous expulsion of PoC. However, the pain and bleeding can be both severe and prolonged, which is unacceptable to many women, and RPoC can also predispose to infection (endometritis), therefore surgical intervention has been advocated. Although this seems a quick and easy option, there are also complications associated with surgery and general anaesthetics – see below. Conservative treatment has been advocated for the initial management of incomplete miscarriage. After 3 days most women will have successfully passed the PoC, and the complication rate was halved compared with surgical management, in a recent study.

DRUG THERAPY – Prostaglandins have been used to make the uterus contract and expel the PoC, avoiding surgery and reducing the infection risks. The pain and bleeding can still be unacceptable to some women. This is still an experimental technique and not in general use.

SURGERY – An ERPC is still the most common form of treatment for miscarriage, including incomplete, missed abortions and blighted ova. The cervix is dilated and the PoC removed using a suction curette. Complications include perforation of the uterus either with the dilator or the curette, infection and incomplete emptying of the cavity. There are also potential anaesthetic complications.

Overview

Miscarriage is a common and distressing complication of early pregnancy. A sympathetic attitude is essential along with appropriate management.

Information for the Patient

PROGNOSIS – The prognosis after an ultrasound scan which confirms the presence of a fetal heart is good. 95% will not miscarry. For those women who have had a miscarriage, the risk of another miscarriage is low. Over 70% of subsequent pregnancies will be successful.

Follow-up

SHORT TERM – Those women who elect for medical or conservative treatment of miscarriage need follow-up, usually after 3 days, though the exact scheme can vary. Otherwise, no routine follow-up is required unless the index pregnancy was the third consecutive miscarriage, when an appointment should be made as an outpatient.

LONG TERM – Women or couples with three or more consecutive miscarriages merit further investigation: parental karyotyping, antiphospholipid antibodies and hysteroscopy.

2. Ectopic Pregnancy

Background

DEFINITION – The implantation of a fetus outside the uterine cavity. The incidence is increasing, though this may be partly due to more accurate and earlier diagnosis. The frequency ranges from 1:150 up to 1:28 in a hospital-based population from Jamaica.

AETIOLOGY – Anything that slows the transport of the fertilised ovum to the uterine cavity.

- Tubal damage:
  - PID
  - Adhesions
  - Endometriosis
  - Previous tubal surgery
  - Congenital diverticula.
- Slow transport: Progesterone slows cilial action; progestogen–only pill.
- Assisted fertilisation: gamete intrafallopian transfer (GIFT) and IVF.

MAIN COMPLICATIONS – There is considerable morbidity and mortality associated with ectopic pregnancy, both associated with surgery and from the disease itself. There is an increased risk of further ectopic pregnancies and also of subfertility secondary to tubal damage. Ectopic pregnancies most commonly implant in the Fallopian tube, in descending order of frequency: ampulla, isthmus, fimbrial end and, rarely, the cornua (Figure 6.2). There are rare reports of ovarian (< 0.5% of total) and cervical pregnancies. Tubal abortion is separation of the pregnancy from the tubal wall. It is one of the most common progressions of ampullary and fimbrial pregnancies. The natural history is variable: there can be absorption of the ectopic, which can be

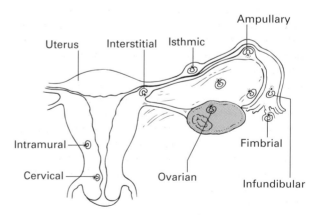

Fig 6.2 *Sites of ectopic pregnancy implantation.*

Table 6.2 Diagnosing ectopic pregnancy	
Making the diagnosis	Ectopic pregnancy
History	Lower abdominal pain may be localised
	Amenorrhoea possibly followed by vaginal bleeding
Examination	Very tender adnexae/cervical excitation
Investigations	
– Pregnancy test	Positive
– Ultrasound	No intrauterine pregnancy; ectopic pregnancy may be seen
– Laparoscopy	Necessary for definitive diagnosis
– Histology	Confirms pregnancy

managed conservatively, or retrograde bleeding into the peritoneal cavity, which may need more active intervention. A tubal rupture occurs when the pregnancy erodes through the tube and can cause heavy bleeding. This is more common where the fallopian tubes are less distensible, i.e. isthmus, and will require operative treatment.

SCREENING/PREVENTION – Women who have had a previous ectopic or undergone tubal surgery or fertility therapy should have early transvaginal ultrasound scans to confirm an intrauterine pregnancy.

MAKING THE DIAGNOSIS – See Table 6.2.

Treatment Options

REASSURANCE – Treatment is as conservative as possible, with removal of the pregnancy and reconstitution of the tube. Where there is evidence of shock, the management is resucitation, followed by immediate laparotomy. Improvements in the early diagnosis of ectopic pregnancy have allowed more conservative management regimes to be used. A minority of ectopic pregnancies will reabsorb spontaneously and can be followed by falling β-hCG levels.

DRUG THERAPY – Systemic **methotrexate** has been used with > 95% success rate. Although side effects were rare, they could be troublesome, i.e. transient alopecia. However, whilst these schemes may avoid tubal surgery, they are not 100% effective, and prolonged follow-up is sometimes necessary. Hyperosmolar glucose, prostaglandins and potassium chloride have also been used with less success overall.

SURGERY – Surgery is currently the mainstay of treatment, either **laparoscopically** or by laparotomy. Laparoscopic techniques have been recommended because of the decrease in associated morbidity and possibly increased fertility rates compared with open techniques. **Salpingostomy** is a small incision over the ectopic pregnancy and a shelling out of the pregnancy followed by repair of the tube. **Salpingectomy** is used where there is a tubal rupture or there is irreparable tubal damage. The whole tube is removed.

OVERVIEW – For smaller ectopic pregnancies, laparoscopic techniques should be employed, but with larger ectopic pregnancies or severe haemorrhage, laparotomy is the method of choice. Trials of drug treatment are currently underway.

Information for the Patient

PROGNOSIS – Women with ectopic pregnancies should be advised that there is a risk of salpingectomy and there is also a risk of impaired fertility following treatment – approximately 30% of women will have a subsequent successful pregnancy. The risk of a further ectopic pregnancy is also increased, and they will need an ultrasound scan and assessment early in any future pregnancy.

Follow-up

SHORT TERM – Those women who are treated either conservatively or medically require follow-up to ensure the levels of hCG are falling to zero. Approximately 10% of women treated by laparoscopic salpingostomy will also require follow-up because of residual trophoblastic activity.

LONG TERM – Long-term follow-up is rarely necessary. Subfertility may require follow-up and possibly assisted fertilisation.

3. Trophoblastic Disease/Hydatidiform Mole

Background

DEFINITION – Abnormality of early trophoblast development can result in the formation of a molar pregnancy. Hydatidiform mole consists of hydropically dilated trophoblastic villi, forming vesicles. A complete mole is formed from paternal genetic material. A partial mole shows evidence of a fetus as part of the same conception.

AETIOLOGY – The incidence is 0.7 per 1000 pregnancies, with a much higher incidence in SE Asia. There is an increase with maternal age and in women with blood groups AB or B.

MAIN COMPLICATIONS – The complications of molar pregnancy are twofold: haemorrhage and subsequent malignant change. There is an increased risk of uterine perforation and haemorrhage at the time of evacuation

Table 6.3	Diagnosing hydatidiform mole
Making the diagnosis	Hydatidiform mole
History	Excessive nausea and vomiting Vaginal bleeding
Examination	Uterus may be bulky for estimated gestation
Investigations	
– Serum β-hCG	Much higher than expected value for gestation
– Ultrasound	Typical grape-like vesicles seen in uterus
– Histology	Confirms diagnosis; should be examined for chromosomes

of the uterus. 5–10% of women with molar pregnancy will progress to frank choriocarcinoma.

MAKING THE DIAGNOSIS – See Table 6.3.

Treatment Options

SURGERY – Treatment is by evacuation of the uterus, with appropriate precautions in case of bleeding: i.e. Syntocinon infusion and cross-matched blood available.

Information for the Patient

PROGNOSIS – The prognosis is excellent: even in the small group of women who progress to malignant disease, there is a 90% recovery rate after chemotherapy (methotrexate, in the first instance).

Follow-up

SHORT TERM – Follow-up is essential in this group of women. After 2 weeks the woman should be reviewed and a further ERPC performed where the bleeding is still excessive. Weekly urine tests for hCG should be performed to ensure a reduction in the levels to normal. Those women with elevated levels after 10 weeks should be considered for further assessment at a specialist centre. Choriocarcinoma characteristically produces early metastases, predominantly lung, liver and brain, and follow-up of women with persistently high levels of hCG should include a chest x-ray and also a brain CT scan. These metastases can be symptomatic, i.e. haemoptysis. Chemotherapy is the mainstay of treatment, though hysterectomy can be considered in older women who do not want further children.

LONG TERM – The oral contraceptive pill should not be used for at least a year after a hydatidiform mole, and barrier methods should be employed, as pregnancy is also contraindicated over the same period. Pregnancy does not exacerbate the disease, but the high hCG levels associated with normal pregnancy obscure any underlying changes in hCG potentially produced by the molar pregnancy.

EXAMPLE OF CLINICAL GUIDELINES – EARLY PREGNANCY ASSESSMENT

Background

Early pregnancy failure is a common clinical problem, with about 15% of clinical pregnancies ending as miscarriage and almost 1% implanting at an inappropriate site, most commonly the Fallopian tube.

Expert care is essential to avoid evacuation of a normal pregnancy and oversight of an ectopic pregnancy.

The ideal facility is a daily **Early Pregnancy Assessment Clinic (EPAC)** run by trained clinicians and sonographers. An EPAC has the advantages of reduced hospital stay for many women, and of cost savings for the hospital. Nevertheless, if there is suspicion of ectopic pregnancy or pelvic infection, assessment should not be delayed until the next morning.

On arrival, the woman should be greeted and the plan of care should be outlined. A Specialist Gynaecology Nurse should do a rapid assessment (triage) including enquiry about pain and measurement of pulse, BP and temperature. A urinary pregnancy test should be undertaken if it has not already been done. Any tissue brought in should be sent to histology, as decidua (endometrium) can look just like products of conception. If the woman's condition appears stable, an ultrasound scan is then arranged. Ideally this is transvaginal for greater precision. The woman can be informed that she herself will have a better image to interpret and she can be reassured that the power setting for TVS is lower than that for TAS.

The clinical findings are then reviewed by the nurse or gynaecologist. Remember, it is also important to consider the psychological needs of the woman both immediately and in the longer term.

Clinical Scenarios

There are six common clinical scenarios.

1. Singleton Viable Pregnancy

* If normal temperature, moderate blood loss and moderate pain, consider suitable for discharge.
* Review need for anti-(Rh)D gammaglobulin.
* Consider need to examine cervix.
* Explain findings and prognosis to woman (give leaflet).
* Return to GP with instructions to report any heavy loss or severe pain.

2. Fetal Pole, No Cardiac Activity

- < 10 mm – home and rescan in 7–10 days.
- > 10 mm – missed abortion: evacuation of uterus.

3. Empty Gestation Sac

As above plus:

- < 20 mm mean sac diameter – home and rescan in 7–10 days;
- > 20 mm mean sac diameter – blighted ovum; evacuation of uterus.

Also, remember that pseudosac with ectopic pregnancy occasionally occurs.

4. Retained Products of Conception

- < Inquire about blood loss.
- Consider possibility of infection.
- Consider need for evacuation of uterus if
  - heavy or prolonged bleeding
  - infection
  - large amounts of RPoC (> 30 mm diameter).
- Send any tissue for histology.

5. Empty Uterus

- Possibilities include:
  - very early pregnancy
  - complete miscarriage
  - ectopic pregnancy.
- Consider dates very carefully.
- Have **definite** products of conception been seen?
- Consider previous history – PID, ectopic or tubal infertility.
- Examine for signs of ectopic pregnancy.
- Do serum β-hCG measurement:
  - v**<1000 iu/l** – ectopic possible but unlikely to rupture in next 48 h; if all else well, review in one week;
  - v**> 1000 iu/l** – ectopic or complete abortion; consider laparoscopy or clinical and biochemical review in 48 h.
  (NB: values relate to TVS. Critical value is 5000 iu/l for TAS.)

6. Possible Hydatidiform Mole

- Discuss with consultant.
- Measure blood pressure and test urine for proteinuria (? early pre-eclampsia).
- Examine for evidence of severe thyrotoxicosis.
- Send blood for β-hCG.
- Send blood for FBC, U+Es, LFTs, G+S.
- If ? partial mole, consider need for chorionic villus sampling.

Additional Clinical Problems

There are two additional clinical problems.

1. Threatened Miscarriage with Raised Temperature

- Causes:
  - Small rises are common, possibly because of prostaglandin release.
  - Uterine infection may coexist with normal pregnancy at scan. Should not be forgotten.
  - May be due to unrelated cause: head cold, UTI, etc.
- Management:
  - < 37.5°C – Admit for observation/investigation unless there is obvious cause.
  - < 37.5°C – Repeat temperature in 1 h. Do serum CRP. Review by SHO. If all normal, allow home but review in 48 h.

2. Threatened Miscarriage in Intrauterine Pregnancy with Abdominal Pain

- Pain is a common feature of threatened miscarriage.
- It is usually mild but can be severe. It is usually described as being like period pain.
- Management depends on severity:
  - mild – explain and advise rest at home with paracetamol if necessary.
  - moderate – SHO to review in EPAC. Consider other causes. Admit.
  - severe – admit as likely to miscarry. Consider other causes and give analgesia.

Additional Points about Ultrasonography

1. When β-hCG > 1000 iu/l, an intrauterine pregnancy should be identifiable at transvaginal scan.
2. Ectopic pregnancies are generally not visible even on transvaginal scan.
3. Other findings such as low sac, irregular sac, possible second sac, and intrauterine haematoma should not alter clinical management.
4. Small unilocular ovarian cysts (< 5 cm) are common in early pregnancy. They nearly all represent corpora lutea. They rarely need surgery.
5. Small fibroids (< 5 cm) are commonly misdiagnosed in early pregnancy. Do not inform the woman unless confirmed at a later scan.
6. A low-lying placenta in early pregnancy (< 16 weeks) is very common and is irrelevant to the management of pregnancy.

Additional Clinical Points

1. After complete miscarriage, the β-hCG level should fall to about 20% of original value by 48 h.
2. A decidual cast can be passed and appear very much like products of conception.
3. Women occasionally need to be admitted for other reasons than surgery, including the need for pain relief and observation if blood loss is heavy.
4. Infection is a serious complication of pregnancy. If you have any suspicion, do bacteriology and consider broad-spectrum antibiotic cover.

GOLDEN POINTS

1. An ectopic pregnancy should be excluded in all women with pain in early pregnancy.

2. All women with complications of early pregnancy need to be treated compassionately.

3. Resuscitation is essential where there are signs of shock.

4. Ultrasound scans are invaluable in the management of bleeding in early pregnancy.

5. An ERPC is not necessary for all women with a miscarriage.

6. Prolonged follow-up is essential after a molar pregnancy to ensure a reduction of the hCG levels.

7 Heavy periods

CLINICAL SIGNIFICANCE

Excessive menstrual bleeding may cause physical problems such as anaemia, but perhaps more importantly it is a highly distressing symptom which frequently leads to loss of self-esteem, absence from work, and sexual dysfunction. Psychological disorders may also present as menstrual disturbance, and it is interesting that many women with so-called menorrhagia have a less than average blood loss.

Menstrual disorder forms the commonest reason for referral to gynaecological outpatients in the United Kingdom, and over half of the hysterectomies performed are undertaken for heavy and/or painful periods.

Occasionally, women with genital tract cancer will complain of regular heavy periods alone.

DIFFERENTIAL DIAGNOSIS

MAIN CATEGORY	DIAGNOSIS
1. *Idiopathic*	Dysfunctional uterine bleeding
2. *Pelvic pathology*	Uterine fibroids Adenomyosis Mucosal polyps of the endometrium Pelvic inflammatory disease Cancer of the endometrium Uterine sarcomas
3. *Endocrine disorders*	Hypothyroidism Polycystic ovarian disease Ovarian endocrine tumours
4. *Systemic disorders*	Coagulopathies Thrombocytopaenia
5. *Pregnancy*	Threatened miscarriage Ectopic pregnancy Hydatidiform mole
6. *Iatrogenic*	Intrauterine contraceptive device Progestogen-only contraceptives Anticoagulant therapy

Dysfunctional uterine bleeding is the commonest cause of heavy irregular periods, accounting for 60% of cases. The diagnosis is made by the exclusion of all other causes.

Normal menstruation involves a cycle of between 21 and 35 days, with bleeding lasting from 2 to 7 days. The average blood loss is between 35 and 40 ml. Excessive blood loss (menorrhagia) is defined as greater than 80 ml and may be regular or irregular.

Sinister causes such as cancer of the endometrium generally occur in women over the age of 40 years, but they should be considered in younger women with prolonged oligomenorrhoea (indicative of polycystic ovarian disease) and in those with abnormal discharge or bleeding (intermenstrual or postcoital).

Complications of pregnancy rarely present as heavy periods per se, but these should be considered if the history is short (< 3 months).

CLINICAL ASSESSMENT

Most women will present to the GP, who will assess the need for referral to a specialist and the degree of urgency. Many women are cared for entirely in the community. The chance of malignancy increases with age, and if the woman is over 40 years old prompt referral is appropriate. The initial assessment should include a full blood count, thyroid function tests and cervical smear.

Assessment of the endometrial cavity for premalignant disease (hyperplasia), cancer and focal benign lesions (polyps etc.) has changed in recent years. D&C was previously very commonly performed, but this was a blind technique which could miss small cancers and benign polyps. Hysteroscopy then became popular enabling direct vision of the endometrial cavity. It had the additional advantage that it could be performed in outpatients, but it requires a significant capital outlay. More recently, there has been a move to performing endometrial aspiration together with a transvaginal scan of the uterus and ovaries. Hysteroscopy can then be performed if there is any difficulty or if a polyp needs removal.

Relevant History

Presenting Complaint

MAIN SYMPTOM – The **length of the cycle and duration of menstrual flow** gives some idea of the severity of the problem. The regularity of the cycle indicates whether the woman is likely to be ovulating or not. Many women find cycle irregularity causes great uncertainty because they cannot predict when their periods will commence. The degree of blood loss is very difficult to quantify, particularly because a woman's perception of her menstrual loss is highly subjective and objective methods are cumbersome. The number of tampons and/or pads used, together with the passing of **clots and flooding**, gives a crude indication. Details of the last menstrual period are important if endometrial sampling is being considered. A recent episode of amenorrhoea should alert to the possibility of pregnancy.

COMMONLY ASSOCIATED SYMPTOMS – Intermenstrual and postcoital bleeding should raise the possibility of a genital tract tumour. Abnormal vaginal discharge is also suggestive of tumours, and in young women it may be a feature of pelvic infection. Severity and timing of pain associated with the menstrual cycle may give some indication of the cause. Spasmodic pain during menstruation is often present if large clots are being passed. In contrast, premenstrual pain is more suggestive of endometriosis and adenomyosis. **Dyspareunia** is sometimes indicative of organic disease such as pelvic infection, endometriosis and pelvic tumours, but the possibility of psychosexual problems should not be overlooked.

Premenstrual symptoms do not assist in diagnosis but should be taken into consideration when considering treatment. Lethargy is rather non-specific but it may be evidence of anaemia.

EFFECT ON LIFESTYLE – Absence from work or being confined to the house when bleeding gives some indication of the severity of the condition.

Gynaecological History

GYNAECOLOGICAL DISEASE – There may be a known history of **fibroids**. Previous pelvic inflammatory disease (PID) raises the possibility of recurrent infection and may also influence the route of hysterectomy because of pelvic adhesions.

CERVICAL CYTOLOGY – The need for a cervical smear should be determined and any previous abnormalities noted, especially if hysterectomy is being considered; the possibility of premalignant disease of the cervix must be fully investigated before surgery is undertaken. In addition, the woman may consider hysterectomy a good treatment option if she has both cervical intra-epithelial neoplasia (CIN) and heavy periods.

CONTRACEPTION – The combined oral contraceptive pill helps to control menstrual loss, but the menstrual cycle is frequently abnormal in the first few months after discontinuation. The progesterone-only pill or depot progestogens can lead to heavy erratic bleeding. IUCDs are associated with increased menstrual loss.

FERTILITY REQUIREMENTS – Women who have completed their family have a wider range of treatment options.

Obstetric History

DELIVERY – The first few cycles after miscarriage or delivery may be dysfunctional. High parity has associations with heavy menstrual loss.

OBSTETRIC COMPLICATIONS – If surgery is contemplated, a history of caesarean section may influence the type of hysterectomy undertaken.

Medical History

MEDICAL CONDITIONS – A history of excessive bruising or bleeding after previous surgery or dentistry may indicate a bleeding tendency. Thyroid disease, particularly hypothyroidism, is associated with heavy periods. Previous thromboembolism should be taken into account when considering both medical and surgical treatments.

SURGERY – Previous operative complications should be recorded in case surgery is undertaken.

PSYCHOLOGICAL DISORDERS – Depression commonly coexists with menstrual disturbance, although it is not fully understood if it is caused by or influences the woman's perception of her menstrual loss.

Drug History

MEDICATIONS – Drug treatments already used should be reviewed in detail. Anticoagulation therapy may be the underlying reason for the heavy bleeding.

Social History

AGE – Young women (< 20 years) often have heavy periods which resolve spontaneously. The chance of malignancy increases with age.

OCCUPATION – Women with work or family commitments may wish to avoid hysterectomy in the short term because of the prolonged postoperative recovery period.

LIFESTYLE – There can be a serious effect on quality of life, and the treatment should be tailored to the activity of the woman.

Relevant Clinical Examination

General Examination

GENERAL CONDITION – Examine for signs of anaemia, hirsutism and thyroid dysfunction.

BODY-MASS INDEX – Weight loss alone may be beneficial in obese women with heavy periods.

BREASTS – Examine only if sex-steroid therapy is contemplated.

Abdomen

CONTOUR – There may be abdominal distension because of uterine fibroids or an ovarian mass.

PALPATION – Tenderness may suggest pelvic inflammatory disease or endometriosis.

MASSES – Large uterine fibroids and ovarian tumours may be felt abdominally.

Pelvic

VULVA/VAGINA/CERVIX – During menstruation, blood loss can be assessed, particularly in women admitted acutely. The vagina should be examined for any haemorrhagic lesions or abnormal discharge. The cervix should also be examined for malignant tumours, and for endocervical and endometrial polyps which may be seen protruding from the cervical os.

BIMANUAL EXAMINATION – Uterine size should be assessed. Fibroids may be evident, and a globular uterus is characteristic of adenomyosis. An adnexal mass may indicate an ovarian tumour, a chocolate cyst (endmetrioma) or, more rarely in this context, a pelvic abscess. Cervical excitation may indicate acute pelvic infection, and a tender uterus is a sign of adenomyosis. Poor mobility of the uterus is a feature of pelvic inflammatory disease and severe endometriosis

Relevant Initial Investigations

Haematology

Hb – Persistent menorrhagia may lead to iron deficiency anaemia.

WCC – The neutrophil count may be raised in women with pelvic infection and more rarely in those with pelvic tumours.

PLATELET COUNT – Thrombocytopaenia is a rare cause of excessive menstrual bleeding.

CLOTTING STUDIES – Not routinely performed but should be undertaken if there is a personal or family history of bleeding problems or if there is a history of liver disease or alcoholism.

SERUM FERRITIN – To confirm iron deficiency if haemoglobin concentration is low.

Endocrine Tests

TSH – Thyroid disease is often occult and should be tested for in all cases (serum TSH measurement).

LH/FSH - A raised LH/FSH ratio is diagnostic of polycystic ovarian disease. A raised FSH concentration (> LH concentration), possibly indicative of incipient ovarian failure, may influence a woman's choice of treatment.

Microbiology

BACTERIAL CULTURE – High vaginal, endocervical, urethral and rectal swabs should be taken for microscopy and culture if there is a history of vaginal discharge or of pelvic pain and tenderness. An endocervical swab should be sent for chlamydial ELISA (enzyme-linked immunosorbent assay). Tuberculosis is a rare cause of menorrhagia in the United Kingdom but, if suspected, **premenstrual** endometrium should be sent for specialist culture.

Diagnostic Imaging

TRANSVAGINAL ULTRASOUND – Some clinicians do not perform this on all women, but it should certainly be considered if the pelvic examination is technically difficult or if there are any unusual features. The pelvic organs can be examined in detail using a transvaginal scanning transducer. Uterine enlargement, fibroids, endometrial polyps or ovarian tumours may be evident.

Cytology

CERVICAL – A cervical smear should be performed if it has been over 3 years since the last test.

Histopathology

ENDOMETRIAL – This is used to detect premalignant (adenomatous hyperplasia) and malignant lesions of the uterine cavity. Endometrial malignancy should be excluded in all women over 40 years and in those under 40 years who have suspicious symptoms (erratic bleeding and abnormal discharge). Traditionally, the endometrial sample was taken under general anaesthetic by dilatation of the cervix and curettage of the uterine cavity (D&C). This is a blind technique, and focal lesions (polyps and small cancers) were easily missed. More recently, fine disposable catheters (samplers) have allowed a simple method for biopsy of the endometrium. When combined with transvaginal ultrasonography, the uterus, endometrium and ovaries can be examined at one single outpatient visit.

CERVICAL - Endocervical and prolapsing endometrial polyps can be removed in outpatients.

Direct Visualisation

HYSTEROSCOPY - Hysteroscopy was introduced to enable direct vision of the endometrial cavity. It had the additional advantage that it could be performed in outpatients, but requires a significant capital outlay.

DETAILS OF COMMON CONDITIONS

1. Dysfunctional Uterine Bleeding (DUB)

Background

DEFINITION - Heavy periods for which no organic cause can be found.

AETIOLOGY - There are probably two main subgroups. **Anovulatory DUB** makes up 20% of cases and tends to occur at the extremes of reproductive life. The cycle is chaotic and this is usually due to failure of follicular development. There is failure of the progesterone rise, resulting in unopposed oestrogen stimulation of the endometrium, which in turn results in cystic hyperplasia.

Ovulatory DUB is probably a disorder of prostaglandin metabolism within the endometrium. The concentration of prostaglandin E2, a potent vasodilator, is known to be increased, whereas that of prostaglandin F2, a vasoconstrictor, is reduced. This may be an occult form of polycystic ovarian disease.

DIAGNOSIS - The diagnosis is made by exclusion of all other pathological causes.

MAIN COMPLICATIONS - Most women simply present with menstrual disorder; a small proportion will complain instead of vague symptoms such as lethargy. Anaemia is probably the only common physical complication, but the social inconvenience can be very debilitating.

SCREENING/PREVENTION - None known, but maintenance of normal body weight may be important.

Treatment Options

ADVICE - The benign nature of DUB should be explained. The knowledge that no serious pathology exists may be all that is required for some women. If surgery is considered, the major and minor risks must be outlined.

CHANGE OF LIFESTYLE/DIET - In the obese patient weight loss may help and will also reduce the risks if surgery is required.

DRUG THERAPY - There are a wide variety of drugs available, but little evidence to support their use. The only drugs that have been shown to be efficacious are **antifibrinolytic** agents (e.g. tranexamic acid), **prostaglandin synthetase inhibitors** (e.g. mefenamic acid) and the combined oral contraceptive pill. The latter is particularly useful for young women, but many over 35 years prefer not to take it because of media scares.

Inhibitors of fibrinolysis prevent the breakdown of blood clots. This is seen in women with DUB, fibroids and some clotting disorders. There are reports that up to 50% blood reduction can be achieved using tranexamic acid (3–6 g daily).

Prostaglandin synthetase inhibitors inhibit uterine prostaglandin production. Mefenamic acid (500 mg t.d.s.) is the most effective and if taken whilst menstruating reduces the blood loss, by up to 50% of women suffering from heavy menstruation. It is also beneficial for the pain associated with menstruation.

Progestogens, such as norethisterone and medroxyprogesterone acetate, are prescribed frequently, but there is no good evidence to support their use.

Danazol is a complex synthetic steroid which causes atrophy of the endometrium, but its use is often limited by side effects.

Gonadotrophin-releasing hormone analogues act by down-regulating the pituitary, inhibiting the ovarian cycle. They induce oestrogen-deficient amenorrhoea and therefore cannot be used in the longer term because of bone mineral loss.

The new **progestogen-containing IUCD** reduces menstrual loss to very low levels in many women. About 10% of women request removal of the device in the first year. More data are awaited, but it seems as many as 80% of women previously requiring hysterectomy can avoid this with the new device.

SURGERY - **Endometrial ablation** involves destruction or resection of the endometrium using electrocoagulation, a resectoscope or laser. Prior to the procedure the endometrium is prepared using either GnRH analogues or progestogens which make it atrophic, allowing easier resection. Other methods with similar results involve ablating the endometrium using laser or diathermy. The advantages of endometrial ablation is that it can be performed as a day case procedure allowing the woman to return to normal activities quickly (1–3 weeks). Unfortunately, only 30% become amenorrhoeic, with another 50% having lighter periods. Over 20% return to have repeat surgery. Endometrial ablation is poor for the control of associated symptoms such as dysmenorrhoea. It is not contraceptive, and sterilisation should be advised at the same time.

Hysterectomy is highly effective for the control of most symptoms associated with DUB. Hysterectomy, together with bilateral oophorectomy and ocstrogen-only HRT, is also a good option for those women who are troubled by severe premenstrual syndrome. Hysterectomy involves a longer stay in hospital than for endometrial ablation, and it can take 3 months before normal activities are resumed. Satisfaction rates at 9 months are very high.

OVERVIEW – In younger women the oral contraceptive pill generally proves to be very successful. In older women with regular cycles, medical treatment with tranexamic acid is often helpful, but this will not help regulate erratic cycles. Ultimately, many women prefer a more permanent surgical solution once their family is complete. In the future, the progestogen-containing IUCD may provide a simple alternative to hysterectomy.

Follow-up

SHORT TERM – Results from clinic investigations can be sent by letter to the GP. Women initially choosing medical management should be followed up at least once to make sure their therapy is effective. If a patient later wishes to consider surgical treatment she can be referred back to outpatients.

LONG TERM – Postoperative follow-up after hysterectomy can be undertaken in the community by the general practitioner.

2. Uterine Fibroids

Background

DEFINITION – Fibroids are benign smooth muscle tumours arising from the myometrium (leiomyomas) (Figure 7.1).

AETIOLOGY – The exact aetiology is unknown, but they are noted to be more common in the Afro-Caribbean population. The blood supply to the uterus is increased in relation to the number and size of the fibroids. When they are located under the endometrium, the surface area of the mucosa is increased, as is the blood loss.

MAKING THE DIAGNOSIS – See Table 7.1.

MAIN COMPLICATIONS – In addition to heavy periods, fibroids may cause discomfort or **pain** due to pressure effects on the bladder. Severe spasmodic dysmenorrhoea is a feature of submucosal polypoid fibroids. **Red degeneration** (venous infarction) is a rare cause of acute pain. Submucosal fibroids may cause **subfertility** and **recurrent miscarriage**. A very small number (< 1%) will undergo malignant transformation to leiomyosarcoma. Very rarely, women with fibroids develop polycythaemia, which disappears after removal. If there is any serious doubt about the nature of apparent uterine enlargement, the diagnosis should be confirmed at laparoscopy or by hysterectomy.

SCREENING/PREVENTION – Hormone replacement therapy (HRT) and OCP usage may be associated with rapid increase in fibroid size.

Treatment Options

ADVICE – Provided they are not associated with massive bleeding, uterine fibroids can be managed conservatively.

CHANGE OF LIFESTYLE/DIET – Nil relevant.

DRUG THERAPY – The short-term relief of heavy periods can be gained with **tranexamic acid** or **mefenamic acid**. **GnRH analogues** have been used to reduce the size of the fibroids, but their long-term use is not advisable because of the risk of osteoporosis and the fibroids regrow quickly after discontinuation of treatment.

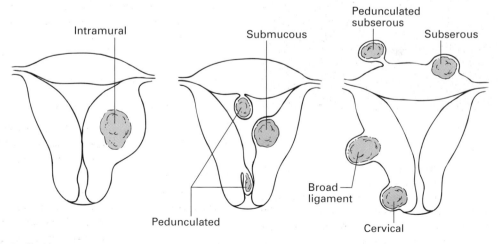

Fig 7.1   *Uterine fibroids.*

Table 7.1	Diagnosing fibroids
Making the diagnosis	**Fibroids**
History	Heavy menstrual bleeding
	There may be associated pain or urinary symptoms
Examination	Bimanual examination will reveal large uterine fibroids, but smaller or submucosal fibroids are unlikely to be found
Investigations	
– Hb	Anaemia may be present; rarely polycythaemia
– Ultrasound	Most useful diagnostic tool clarifying size and position but also allowing growth to be monitored (Figure 7.2)
– Histology	Normal endometrial sampling
– Hysteroscopy	May help to confirm submucosal fibroids
– Laparoscopy	Only required if there is doubt as to the nature of the tumour

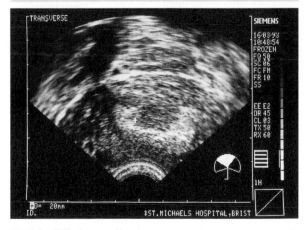

Fig 7.2 *TVS of uterine fibroid.*

These drugs may be useful prior to surgery to reduce the size and vascularity of very large fibroids.

SURGERY – Small submucosal fibroids may be removed by using an operating hysteroscope (c.f. endometrial ablation). **Myomectomy** is reserved for younger patients who wish to maintain their fertility. **Endometrial ablation** may be used if the uterine size is less than 12 weeks' equivalent. **Hysterectomy** is the only definitive treatment for women with very large fibroids.

OVERVIEW – Medical treatment will give symptomatic relief to some women, but hysterectomy remains the mainstay of treatment for symptomatic large fibroids.

Follow-up

SHORT TERM – The results of investigations should be relayed during a follow-up appointment in clinic.

LONG TERM – Annual review of large fibroids to check on their size.

3. Adenomyosis

Background

DEFINITION – This is the presence of endometrial deposits within the myometrium of the uterus. It was formerly known as endometriosis interna.

AETIOLOGY – Endometrial tissue imbeds into the myometrium, causing hyperplasia of the muscle and fibrous tissue around it. The underlying cause is poorly understood. Given that it is mostly seen in parous women, some authors have speculated that the decidua (gestational endometrium) is driven into the myometrium during labour. It is not associated with true endometriosis.

MAKING THE DIAGNOSIS – Suspect in women with heavy, regular, painful periods and a globular enlarged uterus but no obvious fibroids (see Table 7.2).

MAIN COMPLICATIONS – Dysmenorrhoea (painful menstruation) and anaemia are the main problems. There is no significant malignant potential.

Treatment Options

ADVICE – Provided the patient is not anaemic and no other pathology has been identified, the woman may decide against active treatment.

Table 7.2	Diagnosing adenomyosis
Making the diagnosis	**Adenomyosis**
History	Regular heavy painful periods
Examination	Large globular uterus which may be tender to palpation
Investigations	
– Ultrasound	Fibroids absent
– Histology	Strictly, the diagnosis can only be made after histological examination of the uterus

DRUG THERAPY – Medical treatment of suspected adeno-myosis is notoriously poor. Mefenamic acid may well control some of the pain by reducing prostaglandin production. There is no method of treating the adenomyosis per se.

SURGERY – The only definitive treatment is hysterectomy. The ovaries can be conserved. Endometrial ablation will not help the pain.

OVERVIEW – The diagnosis is difficult to make but, if it is suspected strongly and the symptoms are severe, hysterectomy is a good option.

4. Endometrial Polyps

Background

DEFINITION – Benign pedunculated tumours of the endometrium or endocervix. They may be single or multiple.

AETIOLOGY – They are lined with functional epithelium with a connective tissue core, causing them to be extremely vascular and leading to excessive bleeding as well as to intermenstrual and postcoital spotting. They can occur at any age but are more common in later reproductive life. They are benign tumours or simply infoldings of normal endometrium. They are rarely malignant, but removal for analysis is usually advised especially if the patient is over 35 years old. They have a small tendency to recur but, unless the symptoms return, further investigation is not necessary.

MAKING THE DIAGNOSIS – See Table 7.3.

MAIN COMPLICATIONS – Usually they cause little more than inconvenience with irregular menstrual spotting and occasionally postcoital bleeding. Very rarely they may be malignant.

Table 7.3 Diagnosing endometrial polyps	
Making the diagnosis	Endometrial polyps
History	Intermenstrual and heavy erratic bleeding
Examination	Polyps may be seen protruding from the cervix. Uterus normal size
Investigations	
– Ultrasound	Polyps may be identified or a very thickened endometrium seen
– Hysteroscopy	Visualisation of the polyp(s)
– Histology	Confirms the benign nature

Treatment Options

SURGERY – Removal at hysteroscopy using resectoscope, or removal by polyp forceps at D&C.

OVERVIEW – Removal by resection under direct vision using a hysteroscope is the preferred treatment. The specimen should always be sent for histological investigation.

Follow-up

SHORT TERM – The woman should report any recurrence of symptoms.

5. DUB Associated with Intrauterine Contraceptive Device

Background

DEFINITION – Heavy periods associated with IUCD-usage in which other causes have been excluded, particularly pelvic infection and ectopic pregnancy.

AETIOLOGY – The IUCD causes local effects within the endometrium, altering prostaglandin metabolism.

Treatment Options

ADVICE – If the IUCD has just been inserted, the woman may wait to see if the bleeding settles spontaneously. If the symptoms arise sometime after insertion, infection and endometrial pathology should be considered, particularly if there are other symptoms such as vaginal discharge and postcoital bleeding. If no cause is identified and the bleeding persists, consideration should be given to changing to a progestogen-containing IUCD which generally leads to reduced menstrual loss. Many women choose to have the IUCD removed.

DRUG THERAPY – Treatment with mefenamic acid or tranexamic acid may reduce flow.

6. Uterine Sarcomas

Brief Background

Very rare malignant tumours of the uterus. Seen at any age. Leiomyosarcoma is the most common. Often a surprise finding in women having hysterectomy for suspected fibroids. Generally grow rapidly and tend to spread early by blood-borne route. Prognosis is very poor, with recurrence being common and with radiotherapy and chemotherapy having little effect.

7. Congenital Coagulopathies

Brief Background

In-born deficiencies of clotting factors. von Willebrand's disease is the most common, but overall the incidence is very low. Not all women should be tested, but those with symptoms of regular heavy periods since puberty or with a history of other bleeding problems should be considered for detailed haematology investigation. Treatment of the coagulation disorder may improve the menorrhagia. Preoperative cover with clotting factors is often necessary.

8. Pelvic Inflammatory Disease

See Chapter 16.

9. Endometrial Cancer and Hyperplasia

See Chapter 9.

GOLDEN POINTS

1. If the duration of symptoms is short, pregnancy should be excluded.

2. Investigate for occult thyroid disease and anaemia.

3. Investigate for endometrial cancer if there are adverse features or age > 40 years.

4. Medical options, including the levonorgestrel IUCD, should be considered before resorting to surgery.

5. Nature and risks of major surgery should be explained carefully.

8 Non-menstrual vaginal bleeding

CLINICAL SIGNIFICANCE

Non-menstrual (postcoital and intermenstrual) bleeding is extremely common, with virtually every woman experiencing infrequent sporadic episodes.

Most women with frequent, recurrent non-menstrual bleeding have no identifiable cause or have benign lesions such as endocervical polyps. It is, however, an early symptom of genital tract cancer, particularly of the cervix.

Carcinoma of the cervix is the second commonest gynaecological malignancy, with about four thousand new cases and two thousand deaths each year in the United Kingdom.

DIFFERENTIAL DIAGNOSIS

MAIN CATEGORY	DIAGNOSIS
1. *Physiological*	Midcycle bleed
	Cervical ectropion
2. *Pregnancy*	Implantation bleed
	Early miscarriage
	Ectopic pregnancy
3. *Dysfunctional cycles*	Ovulatory/anovulatory
4. *Benigh tumours*	Endocervical polyps
	Endometrial polyps
5. *Malignancy*	Cervical cancer
	Endometrial cancer
	Vaginal cancer
	Vulval cancer
6. *Inflammatory*	Pelvic inflammatory disease
7. *Iatrogenic*	Hormonal therapy (OCP, etc.)
	Following minor gynaecological surgery
8. *Trauma*	Vaginal tear during intercourse
	Rape

Carcinoma is perhaps the most serious condition but ectopic pregnancy also may first present with non-menstrual bleeding and should be considered in all women in their reproductive years.

CLINICAL ASSESSMENT

Because of anxiety, women often arrange to see their GP after a single episode. If there are no other worrisome features and if the pelvic examination is normal, such women should be encouraged to observe the next few menstrual cycles and then report back to their GP.

If the symptom(s) persist, more detailed investigation is required in gynaecology outpatients.

Rapid Emergency Assessment

Women occasionally present with severe haemorrhage intermenstrually or after intercourse. Venous access should be obtained and resuscitation for hypovolaemia instituted. Blood should be taken for full blood count, coagulation studies, and cross-match. A urinary pregnancy test should be performed.

If there is evidence of a trauma, the bleeding may be stemmed by pressure while theatre is arranged.

Equally serious is the issue of rape. The woman may simply present with the gynaecological symptoms alone. If she is acting unusually or there are signs of trauma, sexual assault should be considered a possibility.

Relevant History

Presenting Complaint

MAIN SYMPTOM – Bleeding is often the only symptom.

The volume is usually very small. The LMP should be recorded to help exclude pregnancy. A **full menstrual history** of their periods should be acquired noting any recent alterations or past problems. If the bleeding is midcycle then it is most likely dysfunctional. Regular **postcoital** or irregular intermenstrual bleeding is more typical of pathology such as an ectropion or polyp, but carcinoma should always be suspected. The amount of blood loss and inconvenience caused may alter management.

COMMONLY ASSOCIATED SYMPTOMS – Offensive **vaginal discharges** are caused by primary infection but may be a feature of malignant disease. **Pelvic** or **leg pain** is a symptom of pelvic infection but can be an ominous sign of invasive cervical carcinoma. More sinister symptoms are **haematuria** suggestive of bladder invasion and **loin pain** from ureteric obstruction. **Rectal bleeding** may be suggestive of rectal involvement, especially if associated with tenesmus.

EFFECT ON PATIENT – It is usually seen as an inconvenience, preventing intercourse and altering daily routine. Women from certain cultural groups are not allowed to prepare food on days in which they bleed. Frequent intermenstrual bleeding may therefore be very disruptive.

Gynaecological History

GYNAECOLOGICAL DISEASE – A history of endometrial or cervical polyps, cervical ectropion or previous menstrual irregularity may reoccur.

CERVICAL CYTOLOGY – Previous cytological abnormalities, whether or not they have required treatment, increase suspicion of cervical carcinoma.

CONTRACEPTION – Starting or changing oral contraceptive pill, especially the progesterone-only pill (PoP) can, initially, lead to intermenstrual bleeding. The combined oral contraceptive pill (COC) is associated with cervical ectropion formation. Similarly, the new levonorgestrel-containing IUCD leads to irregular bleeding initially. A low-lying copper-containing IUCD is a cause of intermenstrual bleeding (IMB).

FERTILITY REQUIREMENTS – On account of the age group, the women may not have completed their family, and this should be considered when treatment is discussed.

Obstetric History

DELIVERY – Multiparity at a young age is associated with an increased chance of cervical carcinoma, but this is of no value clinically. A large cervical ectropion is very common in pregnancy. The first few cycles after a recent miscarriage are often dysfunctional, and spotting is common.

Drug History

SMOKING AND ALCOHOL – There is an association with smoking and cervical carcinoma, although it is not causal.

Social History

AGE – Under 30 years of age the risk of carcinoma is small, and the complaint is most likely to be due to pregnancy, polyps, cervical ectropion or dysfunctional bleeding. Cervical carcinoma is commonest between 50 and 60 years of age. Serious pathology needs to be considered in all ages, however.

OCCUPATION – Cervical carcinoma has an increased incidence in lower social classes.

LIFESTYLE – Multiple sexual partners is linked with cervical cytological abnormalities and carcinoma, but again this is not helpful clinically and the question should not be asked.

Relevant Clinical Examination

General Examination

GENERAL CONDITION – Anaemia may be due to blood loss or carcinoma.

BODY-MASS INDEX – Severe weight loss may be a sign of advanced malignant disease.

LYMPH NODES – Cervical carcinoma spreads to the pelvic nodes, but the groin nodes may be enlarged with concurrent disease or infection.

Abdomen

CONTOUR – Swelling due to pregnancy or ascites.

OLD SCARS – Large scars from previous surgery for malignant disease.

PALPATION – Tenderness is a common sign of pelvic infection. **Hard, irregular** or **fixed** lesions are suggestive of malignant disease. An enlarged uterus may be palpated in pregnancy or fibroids.

Pelvic

PERINEUM/VULVA – Exclude vulval lesions and signs of excoriation. A urethral caruncle is a cause of bleeding.

VAGINA – The cervix and vagina should be carefully examined for bleeding areas, especially on contact.

CERVIX – Purulent discharge coming from the cervix may be endometrial or pelvic in origin, but it is sometimes seen covering a large tumour on the cervix. Frank carcinoma on the cervix may present with minimal symptoms.

BIMANUAL EXAMINATION – The cervix and surrounding tissue should be examined bimanuall. Malignant tumours tend to be hard and craggy with parametrial spread if advanced. Fixation is suggestive of invasion. Pelvic infection leads to generalised tenderness. Malignant disease tends to be site specific.

RECTAL EXAMINATION – Rectovaginal examination allows posterior and parametrial spread to be assessed.

Relevant Initial Investigations

For most women the investigation is simple, with an assessment of the cervix and endometrium.

Microbiology

BACTERIAL CULTURE AND CHLAMYDIAL ELISA – Swabs of the vagina and endocervix should be taken if a discharge is present.

Cytology

CERVICAL – A smear should be taken if one is due, but it is not truly a diagnostic test. Visible lesions on the cervix of suspicious or uncertain nature should be biopsied. It should be remembered that cervical smears can be reported as normal even when carcinoma is present.

Histopathology

CERVICAL – Tumour should be biopsied for a histological diagnosis. This may be taken with a punch biopsy forceps with or without local anaesthetic.

ENDOMETRIAL – If there is no evidence of cervical pathology, endometrial sampling should be taken.

VAGINAL – Biopsy any suspicious areas, especially if they spread from the cervix.

Endoscopy

OUTPATIENT HYSTEROSCOPY – Endometrial polyps (Figure 8.1) are a common cause of IMB in all age groups. They can be missed by endometrial samplers and diagnostic

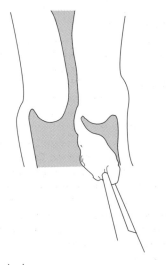

Fig 8.1 *Cervical polyp.*

hysteroscopy should be considered especially if the history is of persistent erratic IMB.

DETAILS OF COMMON CONDITIONS

I. Cervical Carcinoma

Background

DEFINITION – Carcinoma of the cervix involves malignant change of the cervical epithelium. Squamous cell carcinoma is the commonest histological type at 90%, most of the remainder being adenocarcinoma.

AETIOLOGY – The exact cause of cervical carcinoma is unknown, but there is an association with sexual behaviour. Age of first intercourse (under 20) and number of sexual partners appear to be relevant factors. Smoking has also been shown to have a strong association, with a ten times increased risk of cervical malignancy which may be due to the influence on the immune system. There has been no clear evidence implicating the combined oral contraceptive pill but the reduced risk in those using the diaphragm suggests a transmissible cause.

Human papilloma viruses (HPV) are a group of small DNA viruses that have been shown in cell culture to have the ability to cause cell transformation and tumour growth in immunocompromised animals. There have been 50 types of HPV identified, some of which are found in the female genital tract and are known to be passed by sexual contact. HPV type 16 has been found in up to 70% of women with known cervical pre-malignancy (CIN), but it also occurs in the normal population, so some other factor must be present.

MAKING THE DIAGNOSIS – Histology of biopsy.

MAIN COMPLICATIONS – Spread is usually by direct invasion or lymphatic permeation. Direct spread to the uterus or upper vagina leads to abnormal bleeding, typically after intercourse. Invasion into the parametrium and posteriorly may lead to tenesmus and rectal bleeding, whereas anterior spread into the bladder causes haematuria and urinary frequency or ureteric obstruction and eventually renal failure. Fistula formation may occur between the rectum or the bladder. Other signs of malignant disease such as weight loss and anaemia are also common.

Additional Investigations

Haematology

Hb – Anaemia is common with malignant disease.

Biochemistry

SERUM **U+Es** – If a cervical tumour is seen, invasive disease may involve the distal ureters, leading to obstruction.

SERUM LFTs – The liver may be involved with advanced disease, although it is not a common site for metastasis.

Diagnostic Imaging

PLAIN RADIOLOGY – Chest x-ray for secondaries or pleural effusions.

ULTRASOUND – Tumour bulk, renal dilatation and normal structures may be identified, but it is not possible to stage the disease or assess invasion by ultrasound.

CONTRAST RADIOLOGY – Intravenous urography (IVU) should be performed in cases of invasive cervical disease to demonstrate the level, if any, of ureteric obstruction.

AXIAL IMAGING – For visualising tumour size and node involvement, but it is not very specific and is non-contributory in most cases.

Surgical Staging

All tumours are clinically staged before treatment can be decided (Table 8.1). In cases of early invasive disease, clinical evaluation with bimanual and rectal examination is adequate, but larger tumours may be best assessed with the patient asleep. Clinical staging under general anaesthesia allows a more thorough examination of the tumour spread into the parametria. **Cystoscopy** and **sigmoidoscopy** should be performed to look for

Table 8.1		FIGO staging for cervical cancer
Stage	**0**	Cervical intraepithelial neoplasia (CIN)
Stage	**1**	Invasive carcinoma confined to the uterus
	1a	Invasive lesion less than 5 mm deep and 7 mm across (microinvasion)
	1b	Invasion greater than in 1a but still confined to the uterus
Stage	**2**	Extending to the upper third of the vagina or into the parametria
	2a	Carcinoma has extended to the upper third of the vagina
	2b	Extension to the parametria but not reaching the pelvic side wall
Stage	**3**	Carcinoma has extended further within the pelvis
	3a	To the lower third of the vagina
	3b	To the pelvic side-wall or ureteric involvement
Stage	**4a**	Carcinoma has spread to the mucosa of bladder or rectum
	4b	Tumour has spread to distant organs

bladder and rectal involvement, with further biopsies being taken if required.

SCREENING/PREVENTION – The **cervical cytology programme** was set up to detect premalignant disease and reduce the incidence of cervical carcinoma. It has taken 30 years to show any benefit from the screening programme. **Education** on sexual behaviour and the risk of cervical abnormalities in association with barrier methods of contraception may reduce the influence of transmissible factors. Avoidance of smoking may also benefit. The OCP and HRT do not increase the chance of cervical cancer.

Treatment Options

Depends on stage of disease at presentation and histological type.

ADVICE – Stage 0 disease (CIN – see Chapter 10) may be observed or undergo local excision.

DRUG THERAPY – Chemotherapy does not play a major role in the treatment of primary disease but it has been shown to induce remission in a small proportion of cases with advanced metastatic disease.

SURGERY – Similar results as radiotherapy but the treatment of choice for younger women and early invasive disease.

Microinvasion (Stage 1a) carries a low risk of lymphatic spread (less than 3%). Cone biopsy may be used for women wishing to complete their family. Simple hysterectomy is preferred for those with no fertility requirements, and some authorities advise node sampling as well.

Radical (Wertheim) hysterectomy is performed for invasive disease up to stage 1b or 2a and involves removal of the uterus, cervix, a large cuff of vagina and pelvic node dissection.

Recurrent disease not responding to radiotherapy may be treated by **pelvic exenteration** which involves radical dissection including removal of the bladder and rectum. Surgery is preferable in younger women, as there is a lower incidence of vaginal stenosis and the ovaries may be preserved, but it is a major procedure and does lead to shortening of the vagina.

RADIOTHERAPY – Used for elderly patients or invasive disease not suitable for surgery, for advanced disease (stage 2b and above) and after surgery for node positive patients. Radiotherapy is given via two routes. Para-cervical disease is treated by intrauterine and intra-vaginal caesium, and the pelvis receives external beam radiation. Radiotherapy has several drawbacks including vaginal stenosis (80%), fistula formation, bladder and bowel inflammation.

PROGNOSIS – The **size** of the initial tumour on the cervix

Table 8.2 Survival by FIGO stage for cervical cancer

Stage	5 year survival
1	90%
2a	80%
2b	65%
3	35–45%
4	15%

is the most important prognostic factor but it should be remembered that over 50% of all women diagnosed with invasive disease die within 5 years of diagnosis (Table 8.2). Histology is involved, with **adenocarcinoma** having a worse prognosis than squamous. The stage and prognosis will alter after surgery if the **pelvic lymph nodes** are involved. **Recurrent disease** usually has a poor outcome.

OVERVIEW – Surgery and/or radiotherapy form the mainstay of treatment. For Stage 1b disease, mortality rates are similar but morbidity is less with surgery. Surgery should be carried out in appropriate centres with the staff experienced in dealing with the problems that may arise.

Follow-up

SHORT TERM – Initially the patients are reviewed every 3 months in a joint clinic with a multidisciplinary team to look for recurrence and to screen for surgical or radiotherapy complications. HRT may be given if there is a radiation-induced menopause. Sexual problems are common. HRT may help to some extent. Advice should also be given that intercourse is safe and will help to prevent stenosis and it will improve shortening of the vagina.

LONG TERM – The women take great comfort from their follow-up appointments and usually will be seen in the joint clinic every 6 months for 5 years, with yearly smears being performed to exclude vault recurrence. Long-term effects of radiotherapy can be difficult to manage because of the fibrosis and tissue necrosis. Inflammation of the bowel and fistula are common complications.

2. Cervical Ectropion

Background

DEFINITION – An area of columnar epithelium extending from the endocervix on to the ectocervix.

AETIOLOGY – Caused by an outgrowing of the squamo-columnar junction. This may be congenital but it is more commonly induced by oestrogen from the oral contraceptive pill or during pregnancy.

MAKING THE DIAGNOSIS – Typical fleshy area on the cervix with a normal cervical cytology. Biopsy rarely necessary.

MAIN COMPLICATIONS – Usually asymptomatic but may cause a heavy vaginal discharge or postcoital/intermenstrual bleeding.

Treatment Options

ADVICE – This is a non-malignant condition and, if asymptomatic, requires no treatment.

SURGERY – Seldom required, but cryotherapy or diathermy to the cervix usually resolves the situation, albeit only temporarily.

GOLDEN POINTS

1. Persistent postcoital and intermenstrual bleeding should always be investigated.

2. In younger women, pregnancy should be considered before invasive tests.

3. In most women, a specific cause will not be found, but vaginal, cervical and endometrial tumours must be excluded.

4. The management of cervical carcinoma should be undertaken by specialist gynaecological oncologists together with a team of specialist counsellors, nurses and radiotherapists.

9 Postmenopausal bleeding

CLINICAL SIGNIFICANCE

Postmenopausal bleeding (PMB) is the loss of blood per vaginam 6 months or more after the cessation of menstruation. It is very common. The large majority of women do not have serious disease, but it is the commonest first symptom of endometrial cancer.

Endometrial carcinoma accounts for about 25% of gynaecological malignancies in the United Kingdom, with 3500 new cases each year. The overall 5 year survival rate is 70%, but this is because most cases are diagnosed at an early stage. The prognosis for advanced disease is similar to other gynaecological cancers.

DIFFERENTIAL DIAGNOSIS

MAIN CATEGORY	DIAGNOSIS
1. *Neoplasia*	Cervical cancer
	Endometrial cancer
	Uterine sarcomas
	Vaginal cancer
	Vulval cancer
	Fallopian tube cancer
	Oestrogen-secreting tumour of ovary
	Secondary deposits
	Endocervical polyps
	Endometrial polyps
2. *Atrophy*	Oestrogen-deficiency senile vaginitis
	Urethral caruncle
3. *Infection*	Vaginal
	Endometrial
4. *Iatrogenic*	Bleeding on HRT
	Bleeding on tamoxifen
	Ring pessary
	IUCD
5. *Miscellaneous*	Trauma during intercourse (associated with atrophy)
6. *Spurious*	Haematuria
	Rectal bleeding

CLINICAL ASSESSMENT

Organisation of Care

The history is usually a very simple one of passage of a small amount of blood. Diagnosis largely relies on investigation which can now nearly always be done as an outpatient.

Rapid Emergency Assessment

Very rarely the bleeding can be severe with life-threatening haemorrhage. Emergency admission is necessary. Intravenous access should be secured and basic resuscitation measures undertaken. Blood samples should be sent for cross-matching and full blood count.

Emergency exploration of the genital tract is occasionally necessary to arrest the bleeding. Rarely, emergency hysterectomy is required to secure haemostasis.

Relevant History

Presenting Complaint

MAIN SYMPTOM – **Bleeding** is often the only symptom. It is very variable in character from a slight brown discharge, indicating old blood, to a bright red loss. The amount can also vary widely from a smear on the toilet paper to life-threatening haemorrhage. The nature of the loss is largely irrelevant, and all cases should be investigated fully. However, it is important to ask the woman if she is sure of the source of the bleeding.

Postcoital bleeding tends to suggest a cervical lesion but may also be a feature of an atrophic vagina.

COMMONLY ASSOCIATED SYMPTOMS – Vaginal discharge is common and may indicate infection or cancer, or both. Pyometra, for example, carries a 50% risk of underlying carcinoma. Vaginal irritation or dyspareunia may be a feature of atrophic vaginitis which can bleed especially after sexual intercourse. Abdominal pain or swelling and weight loss are features of advanced carcinoma. Urinary and bowel symptoms should be asked about because some women mistake haematuria and rectal bleeding for PMB.

EFFECT ON PATIENT – Women are usually aware of the potential implications. For most the bleeding is simply an anxiety and inconvenience, but for others the loss is heavy.

Gynaecological History

GYNAECOLOGICAL DISEASE – A history of pelvic cancer and/or radiotherapy is important partly because it may hinder investigation. Hysterectomy does not exclude vaginal tumours, and if the cervix has been left in situ a small amount of endometrium may still remain.

MENSTRUAL HISTORY – Early menarche or late menopause are associated with a higher chance of endometrial carcinoma, but this does not aid management.

CERVICAL CYTOLOGY – A recent history of an abnormal cervical smear result increases suspicion of cervical or endometrial cancer.

CONTRACEPTION – These women will usually have stopped using contraception but they may have a forgotten IUCD.

Obstetric History

DELIVERY – There is an increased incidence of endometrial carcinoma in nulliparous women, but this does not aid management.

Medical History

MEDICAL CONDITIONS – Women with endometrial cancer are more likely to be morbidly obese, hypertensive and diabetic. This has implications for surgical treatment. Women with a history of breast cancer often have received treatment with tamoxifen, which has been shown to induce endometrial hyperplasia and, more rarely, carcinoma.

SURGERY – A history of bowel cancer might suggest recurrence. Diverticular disease can lead to discharge of pus through the vaginal vault.

Drug History

MEDICATIONS – Prolonged unopposed oestrogen therapy is associated with a seven-fold increased risk of developing endometrial carcinoma. This is still sometimes given mistakenly to women with an intact uterus. If HRT is being taken it should include a progestogen. Tamoxifen – see above.

Social History

AGE – Elderly women may have been widowed or be caring for sick partners, which should be taken into account when arranging investigations and treatment.

LIFESTYLE – The treatment options should consider the woman's overall quality of life.

Relevant Clinical Examination

General Examination

GENERAL CONDITION – Evidence of cachexia, lymphadenopathy and jaundice suggests metastatic disease.

BODY-MASS INDEX – Obesity is associated with endometrial malignancy due to excessive conversion of androgens into oestrone, in peripheral fat, leading to endometrial hyperstimulation.

INGUINAL LYMPH NODES – Not usually enlarged but the inguinal nodes should be palpated.

BREASTS – Not necessarily examined unless a breast tumour is suspected.

Abdomen

CONTOUR – Swelling may represent ascites or tumour.

PALPATION – Uterine fibroids or malignant tumours may be found. Free fluid is an uncommon feature of endometrial carcinoma, but ascites is often present in women with ovarian tumours. The umbilicus is a rare site for metastasis from pelvic tumours.

Pelvic

PERINEUM/VULVA/VAGINA/CERVIX – The colour, nature and site of the discharge should be noted. Evidence of blood is confirmation that the loss is from the vagina. Excessive blood loss can make visualisation of the cervix and vagina difficult, so care should be taken to clean the area. Thinning and dryness of the vaginal epithelium that bleeds on contact is usually due to vaginal atrophy. The vulva, vagina and cervix should be clearly visualised to exclude polyps, ulcers and foreign bodies. An IUCD should be removed if strings are seen.

NB – vaginal atrophic changes do not rule out the possibility of upper genital tract disease.

BIMANUAL EXAMINATION – Uterine enlargement or fixation occurs with invasive malignancy or fibroids. Pelvic tenderness may be present in both infection and invasive tumour.

RECTAL EXAMINATION – Only to assess any invasion or posterior fixation of a tumour.

Relevant Initial Investigations

The principal aim of investigation is to exclude the possibility of cancer. Traditionally this was performed by D&C but this required hospital admission and its accuracy was poor. Currently, most units undertake outpatient investigation using endometrial sampling and transvaginal scan. Some units incorporate hysteroscopy at the same visit, but this is probably unnecessary if endometrial histology is negative and the endometrium is thin at scan. If outpatient investigation is not possible because of discomfort or cervical stenosis, etc., inpatient hysteroscopy is arranged.

Haematology

Hb – Anaemia due to blood loss or malignant disease.
WCC – Raised in infection and malignant disease.
PLATELET COUNT – For thrombocytopenia.

CLOTTING STUDIES – Only if a bleeding diathesis is suspected.

Microbiology

BACTERIAL CULTURE – Vaginal and endocervical swabs should be taken for standard bacterial culture if a discharge is seen on examination.

Diagnostic Imaging

ULTRASOUND – TVS allows visualisation of the myometrium, endometrium and ovaries. The principal reason for TVS in PMB is to measure the endometrial width. If less than 5 mm, the cavity is empty (Figure 9.1). The myometrium and ovaries should also be visualised for evidence of tumours.

Cytology

CERVICAL – A cervical smear should always be taken. Occasionally, this will provide evidence of a tumour which is missed by the other tests.

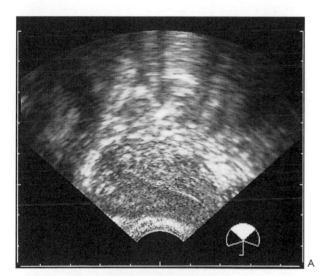

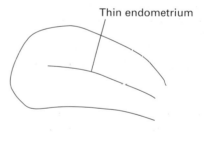

Thin endometrium

A

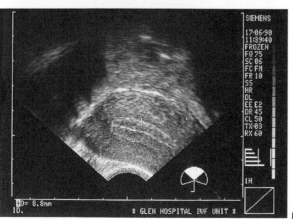

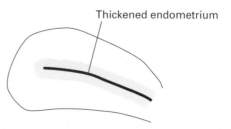

Thickened endometrium

Fig 9.1 *TVS of uteri demonstrating (A) a thin atrophic endometrium and (B) thickened endometrium.*

B

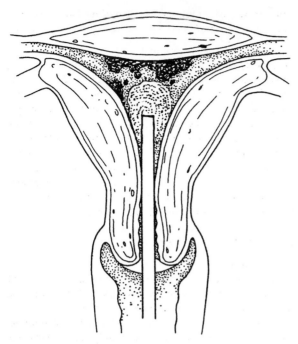

Fig 9.2 *Hysteroscopy of uterine cavity.*

Histopathology

ENDOMETRIAL – Endometrial sampling using a fine catheter.
CERVICAL, VAGINAL & VULVAL – Punch biopsies should be taken if evidence of tumour is found at examination.

Direct Visualisation

HYSTEROSCOPY – Many gynaecologists feel that hysteroscopy can be reserved for those cases in which the scan shows endometrial development but no sample is obtained at aspiration. Others undertake this routinely in outpatients (Figure 9.2).

DETAILS OF COMMON CONDITIONS

1. Endometrial Carcinoma

Background

DEFINITION – Epithelial cancer of the endometrium makes up about 25% of all gynaecological malignancies and it accounts for up to 1200 deaths a year in England and Wales. Adenocarcinoma is the commonest histological type but 10–20% have a squamous element.
AETIOLOGY – The precise cause of endometrial carcinoma is unknown, but there is an association with prolonged exposure to oestrogen, particularly when it is unopposed by progesterone. Endometrial hyperplasia with cytological atypia is a premalignant condition, but not all endometrial cancers arise from hyperplastic tissue. There is also an association between endometrial cancer and obesity, hypertension and diabetes. The link is probably polycystic ovarian syndrome, an ovulatory disorder in which endogenous ovarian androgens are converted to oestrogen in subcutaneous tissues.

MAKING THE DIAGNOSIS – See Table 9.1.

MAIN COMPLICATIONS – Abnormal perimenopausal or postmenopausal bleeding and abnormal vaginal discharge are the commonest clinical features. In extreme cases an emergency hysterectomy is made necessary by torrential haemorrhage. Rarely, the endometrial cavity may become filled with necrotic tissue (pyometra).

SCREENING/PREVENTION – There is no national screening programme for the detection of endometrial carcinoma but every woman with intermenstrual or postmenopausal bleeding/discharge should be investigated. Some clinicians argue that all women receiving tamoxifen therapy

Table 9.1 Diagnosing endometrial carcinoma	
Making the diagnosis	Endometrial carcinoma
History	Postmenopausal bleeding
Examination	Usually nothing to find
Investigations	
– Ultrasound	Endometrial thickening
– Histology	Diagnostic
	Staging is performed clinically

Table 9.2 FIGO staging for endometrial cancer		
Stage	**0**	Atypical hyperplasia (premalignant disease)
Stage	**1a**	Tumour limited to the endometrium
	1b	Invasion less than 50% into the myometrium
	1c	Invasion greater than 50% into the myometrium
Stage	**2**	Cervix involved
Stage	**3**	Tumour extends out of uterus but confined to the pelvis
	3a	Breech of serosa, involvement of adnexa, or +ve washings
	3b	Vaginal involvement
	3c	Metastases to pelvic or para-aortic nodes
Stage	**4**	Invasion to bladder, bowel or distant metastases

should have yearly endometrial sampling. Women taking hormone replacement therapy who still have a uterus must also be given progestogen to prevent the development of endometrial hyperplasia.

ADDITIONAL INVESTIGATIONS – **Blood glucose** – Type 2 diabetes is common in women with endometrial cancer and should be screened for prior to surgery or radiotherapy. **Serum LFTs** – as a test for liver metastases. **Serum oestradiol** – oestrogen-secreting tumours causing endometrial cancer are very rare. **Plain radiology** – chest x-ray for metastatic disease. **Axial imaging** – MRI scans can predict the degree of invasion into myometrium, but as yet this is not routine clinical practice.

Treatment Options

Treatment is according to clinical stage (see Table 9.2) and fitness of the woman.

DRUG THERAPY – Cytotoxic therapy is ineffective for most endometrial cancers and is reserved for recurrent disease in young women. Symptoms from metastatic disease have been said to respond to high-dose progestogen therapy but this is not proven conclusively.

SURGERY AND RADIOTHERAPY – Traditionally, a hysterectomy and bilateral salpingo-oophorectomy has been the treatment of choice for tumour limited to the uterus (Stage 1). This is followed by pelvic radiotherapy for all but a small minority with well-differentiated tumours confined to the endometrium. The management of Stage 2 is controversial; some advocate radical hysterectomy with pelvic and aortic lymphadenectomy, whereas others prefer radical radiotherapy. For Stage 3 disease, surgical debulking is followed by radiotherapy. For women with very advanced (Stage 4) disease, treatment tends to be palliative. Pelvic radiotherapy may help arrest uterine bleeding.

OVERVIEW – The mainstay of treatment for the large majority of women who present with Stage 1 disease is simple hysterectomy and bilateral oophorectomy together with postoperative radiotherapy. The management should involve a multidisciplinary team including a gynaecological oncologist, medical oncologist and oncology nurse specialist.

Information for the Patient

PROGNOSIS – The majority of cases present after the cessation of periods but up to one-third present before the menopause. Direct spread is rare. Lymph node involvement to the pelvic and para-aortic chains is the first site of spread. Distant metastases occur late. Usually the prognosis depends on various factors, including age, tissue type and differentiation, and stage. Squamous elements within the usual adenocarcinoma worsen the prognosis. Stage 1 survival is as high as 85% at 5 years in some series, which is good considering that it presents in elderly women. Survival for advanced disease is about 15% at 5 years.

Follow-up

SHORT TERM – Initial follow-up should be with the specialist team to review the wound and examine the pelvis for recurrent disease. There are no tumour markers at present, and imaging techniques have not been shown to be of value for follow-up. Oestrogen hormone replacement therapy should be avoided initially. Low-dose progestogen therapy can be used to help control flushes and give some protection against osteoporosis in younger women.

LONG TERM – After 5 years of follow-up the patients can be discharged to the general practitioner.

2. Vaginal Carcinoma

Background

DEFINITION – Malignant disease of the vagina. The majority of malignant tumours are squamous (> 90%). Some of the others may arise in embryological remnants.

AETIOLOGY – There are associations with cervical carcinoma and CIN, and the aetiology is probably similar. Previous radiation has also been associated with an increased chance of malignant change. The majority of cases arise in the menopause.

MAKING THE DIAGNOSIS – Histology of vaginal biopsy.

MAIN COMPLICATIONS – Abnormal vaginal bleeding and vaginal discharge. Rarely, bleeding may be life-threatening. Vaginal discharge may reflect infection which may lead to septicaemia. Invasion into the urethra, bladder or anal canal is relatively common (see Table 9.3).

SCREENING/PREVENTION – Premalignant disease of the vagina (VaIN) is similar to CIN in the cervix. All women undergoing colposcopy should have the upper vagina inspected also. Women with a history of CIN who have a hysterectomy should have at least two negative vault

Table 9.3		FIGO staging of vaginal cancer
Stage	0	Vaginal intraepithelial neoplasia
Stage	I	Tumour confined to the vaginal mucosa
Stage	2a	Subvaginal infiltration not to the parametrium
	2b	Parametrial infiltration but not to pelvic wall
Stage	3	Pelvic wall involved
Stage	4a	To mucosa of bladder and rectum
Stage	4b	Spread out of pelvis

smears before follow-up is discontinued. VaIN may be treated by laser.

Treatment Options

DRUG THERAPY – Not sensitive to cytotoxic chemotherapy.

SURGERY – Radical resection with hysterectomy, vaginectomy and pelvic lymphadenectomy has been used especially for young women, but the tumour is often too advanced. Some teams have used pelvic exenteration for advanced disease.

RADIOTHERAPY – For advanced disease or disease recurring after surgery. This may lead to fistula formation.

OVERVIEW – These tumours are rare, and management should be determined by regional specialists. Early detection may allow surgical removal.

Follow-up

SHORT TERM – The multidisciplinary team should follow up after surgery. There will be a special need for psychological support, particularly for young women. Hormone replacement therapy should be considered, especially for young women.

LONG TERM – After 5 years of disease-free follow-up, the general practitioner fully takes over.

GOLDEN POINTS

1. Postmenopausal bleeding should always be investigated to exclude neoplastic disease.

2. Atrophic vaginitis does not rule out the possibility of uterine cancer.

3. Investigations can now be undertaken in outpatients for most women, using endometrial samplers and transvaginal ultrasonography.

4. Women with endometrial cancer should be managed by a multidisciplinary team including gynaecologists, oncologists, specialist nurses and counsellors.

5. Oestrogen-based HRT must be opposed by progestogen in women with an intact uterus to prevent endometrial hyperplasia and neoplasia.

10 Abnormal cervical cytology

CLINICAL SIGNIFICANCE

Cervical cancer, the second commonest cause of death from gynaecological malignancy in the United Kingdom, accounts for about two thousand deaths each year. The cervical cytology screening programme was set with the aim of identifying asymptomatic premalignant disease of the cervix (cervical intraepithelial neoplasia, CIN) and reducing the mortality rate from cervical cancer. It has now been in operation for over thirty years and is thought to have reduced the incidence of cervical cancer by 25% and the mortality rate by 40%.

Most women with abnormal cervical cytology would never have developed cancer, but such a finding causes untold anxiety for many women.

DIFFERENTIAL DIAGNOSIS

MAIN CATEGORY	DIAGNOSIS
1. *Inadequate*	Insufficient squamous cells No glandular cells
2. *Inflammatory*	Non-specific inflammatory cells Bacterial vaginosis Human papilloma virus Herpes simplex virus Trichomonas vaginalis Candida albicans
3. *Premalignant disease*	Mild dyskaryosis Moderate dyskaryosis Severe dyskaryosis Atypical glandular cells
4. *Suggestive of malignant disease*	Squamous cells Glandular cells

The main focus of this chapter is the care of women with smears that show dyskaryosis.

THE SCREENING PROGRAMME

Cervical cytology is usually carried out by the general practitioner or the practice nurse according to recommendations of the national screening programme:

- First cervical smear when the woman becomes sexually active. Smears are not usually performed before 20 years of age.
- 5-yearly smears thereafter if both normal, although regional variation means they may be repeated every 3 years.
- Carry on until the age of 65 years.

There is a computerised system for routine call and recall for all women registered with a general practitioner.

All women should be advised of the nature and significance of the test. Information leaflets are often helpful.

At the clinic, a brief history is taken to ensure the woman has no current symptoms. The cervix should be inspected to look for overt pathology.

Smears must be performed by a trained practitioner. The optimal time for taking a smear in young women is midcycle. There are a variety of small devices for taking the sample of cells from the cervix. Most CIN arises within the transformation zone (TZ), the area on the cervix where columnar epithelium is being covered by squamous cells. The ideal sample is taken from this area which includes the current squamocolumnar junction (SCJ). The transformation zone runs from the old SCJ to the new SCJ (Figure 10.1). The smear should contain plentiful squamous and glandular cells, the glandular cells indicating that the smear has been taken from the correct part of the cervix. A wooden **Ayre's spatula** is the most commonly used sampler. With one part fixed within at the external os, the spatula is swept around the cervix, removing cells as it passes. If the SCJ is high in the endocervix, a special brush device is also used which can take cells from within the endocervical canal. The sample is immediately smeared onto a labelled glass slide and fixed with alcohol. The slide is later prepared for viewing with the Papanicolaou solution which stains the nuclei blue and the cytoplasm pink. At microscopy the technician looks for signs of **dyskaryosis**; an increase in the size of the nucleus

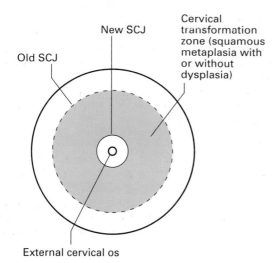

Fig 10.1 *The transformation zone (TZ) lies between the old and new squamocolumnar junctions (SCJ).*

compared with the cytoplasm. There may also be evidence of mitosis in the nuclei or lobulation; these changes are described as dyskaryosis.

If the result is abnormal (dyskaryosis) the women should be referred to a colposcopy clinic for diagnostic testing to determine the presence and extent of any premalignant disease. Rarely, intraepithelial neoplasia involves vagina (VaIN) as well as the cervix (CIN). The degree of cytological abnormality (mild, moderate or severe dyskaryosis) correlates poorly with the changes that are found at histology (CIN I, CIN II and CIN III).

Although cervical cytology is primarily used to screen for premalignant disease of the cervix, non-neoplastic abnormalities are frequently detected, including common vaginal infections. These may obscure any abnormal squamous cells and prevent the detection of cervical intraepithelial neoplasia.

It is important to remember that cervical cytology is a method of screening for premalignant disease and not a diagnostic test for cervical cancer. Indeed, cervical smears from a cervix with an invasive lesion often contain inflammatory cells only. If at the time of pelvic examination a woman is thought to have an established cancer of the cervix the appropriate test is a biopsy and histology.

CLINICAL ASSESSMENT – THE COLPOSCOPY CLINIC

Colposcopy is a simple method of examining the cervix (and vagina) for evidence of pre-malignant disease using light magnification and special stains (acetic acid and iodine). The cervix is inspected and washed with saline before being stained. Acetic acid stains CIN white, and iodine stains normal epithelium brown. The pattern of staining can be used to direct cervical biopsy. A satisfactory colposcopic examination involves:

- full view of the vagina and cervix, including the whole of the transformation zone;
- identification of the new squamocolumnar junction in the endocervix;
- adequate biopsies to confirm the diagnosis.

Colposcopy is also used to direct ablative therapy such as laser and cryotherapy. In many units, diagnosis and treatment are now combined at a single visit using diathermy to excise the whole of the transformation zone (large loop excision of the transformation zone, LLETZ).

For several reasons colposcopy is a very upsetting experience for many women. To help reduce any anxiety, the woman should receive a leaflet explaining the nature of the test with the letter advising her of her appointment. It may also help if she is able to bring a companion.

Relevant History

Presenting Complaint

MAIN SYMPTOM – Premalignant disease of the cervix is a subclinical condition, and so women with cervical dyskaryosis are nearly always asymptomatic. A very small proportion will already have an invasive lesion, however, and it is important to inquire about symptoms suggestive of cervical cancer. If these women have been in a cervical smear programme elsewhere in the country the results should be requested.

COMMONLY ASSOCIATED SYMPTOMS – **Vaginal discharge** is a common symptom of cervical cancer and **intermenstrual, postcoital and postmenopausal bleeding** are also suspicious symptoms. **Last menstrual period** – The date of the last period should be added to the request form if a repeat smear is taken. In addition, special consideration must be given to cervical examination and biopsy in pregnancy. There is a risk of excessive bleeding and infection.

EFFECT ON PATIENT – The publicity surrounding the smear programme mean anxiety levels are high until a diagnosis is found.

Gynaecological History

GYNAECOLOGICAL SURGERY – **Previous** cervical surgery may make colposcopic interpretation more difficult.

SEXUAL HISTORY – A history of **multiple sexual partners** and **teenage pregnancy** are risk factors for cervical pathology, but these features do not help with the management of women with abnormal cervical cytology, and there is a risk of inflicting guilt upon the woman.

MENSTRUAL CYCLE – Women with menstrual problems may feel that hysterectomy cures both the menstrual problems and the cervical problem.

CONTRACEPTION – An **IUCD** may lead to cervical discharge and inflammatory cells on the smear. The strings of the device may interfere with any future treatment.

FERTILITY REQUIREMENTS – If the woman has not completed her family, more conservative treatment should be considered in order to avoid cervical damage and an increased chance of cervical incompetence in future pregnancies.

Obstetric History

PREVIOUS DELIVERY – A history of recent delivery may make colposcopy more uncomfortable, and it can often be delayed for a few weeks.

Relevant Clinical Examination

Abdomen

PALPATION – To be sure there is no obvious tumour of the upper genital tract.

Pelvis

VULVA/VAGINA – The vagina should be examined for any **haemorrhagic lesions** and for **abnormal discharge**. If there is a strong suspicion of active pelvic infection, swabs should sent for bacteriology, and treatment should be initiated before a biopsy is taken.

CERVIX – The cervix should also be examined for **ulcers, raised lesions or benign polyps**.

BIMANUAL EXAMINATION – **Tenderness** may be a feature of pelvic infection. **An enlarged uterus** should raise the possibility of an unsuspected pregnancy. The cervix should be felt for any indurated areas. The opportunity should be taken to feel for any ovarian tumours.

Relevant Initial Investigations

Microbiology

BACTERIAL CULTURE – **High vaginal, endocervical, urethral** and **rectal swabs** should be taken for microscopy and culture if there is a vaginal discharge or any other signs of genital tract infection. An endocervical swab should be sent for **chlamydial ELISA**. Some units do this routinely for all women attending a colposcopy clinic because there is a higher rate of sexually transmitted disease in women with CIN.

Cytology

CERVICAL – It is usual to take a repeat **cervical smear** at the time of colposcopy. If the smear is repeatedly abnormal but no disease is found on the vagina or cervix, consideration must be given to exploration of the endocervical canal and endometrial cavity. Sometimes abnormal cells from an upper tract tumour have been detected on a cervical smear.

Histology

CERVICAL – Binocular microscopy or **colposcopy** allows direct vision of the cervix. Suspicious areas can be clearly identified and biopsied.

ENDOMETRIAL – If the woman is over 35 years of age with abnormal vaginal bleeding or has had abnormal endometrial cells seen on the smear, then endometrial biopsy should be undertaken.

DETAILS OF COMMON CONDITIONS

I. Cervical Intraepithelial Neoplasia (CIN)

Background

DEFINITION – Cervical intraepithelial neoplasia (CIN) is a histological diagnosis used for the older terms dysplasia and carcinoma-in-situ of the cervical epithelium.

MAKING THE DIAGNOSIS – The features are of large abnormal nuclei, reduced cell cytoplasm together with loss of cell stratification and maturation throughout the thickness of the cervical epithelium.

CIN 1 – the nuclear abnormalities are confined to the inner third of the epithelium with a few mitotic figures.

CIN 2 – mitotic figures are seen in the lower two thirds, but the upper 50% of the epithelium is well differentiated.

CIN 3 – only the upper third of the epithelium is well differentiated, and abnormal nuclei and mitotic figures are seen through the full thickness.

AETIOLOGY – An association exists with multiple sexual partners and an early age at first sexual intercourse. This is thought to reflect the action of human papilloma virus (HPV) on rapidly dividing squamous cells. Cigarette smoking may also play an important role.

MAIN COMPLICATIONS – Up to 30% of women with CIN 3 will progress to invasive carcinoma of the cervix.

PREVENTION – Education from an early age about sexual behaviour and sexually transmitted diseases. This should include information about condoms, which may limit the spread of HPV and reduce the incidence of CIN. For those women who do develop CIN, the cervical cytology screening programme is vital in order to prevent progression to cervical carcinoma.

Treatment Options

ADVICE – The prognosis of CIN is good, as it is a premalignant condition, so its removal should result in a cure. The difficulty arises in deciding which lesions should be treated. CIN 1 is thought to be a mild form that is probably safe to watch rather than remove. Provided that repeat smear and colposcopy examination is normal the woman may then be reassured. CIN 2 and 3 require treatment, but the results of therapy are good.

DRUG THERAPY - None yet identified.

SURGERY - These are divided into excisional and ablative techniques.

Ablation - these techniques have gone out of fashion and tend only to be used with the mild abnormalities or where the excisional techniques are not possible. They can be used as long as there is no suspicion of micro-invasion, the cytology and histology match and the whole of the lesion is within the TZ. They have an advantage in that they are performed on an outpatient basis with low morbidity and risk of cervical trauma.

Laser vaporisation - this is well tolerated with the cervix healing within a month of treatment. The laser can reach a depth of 7 mm.

Cold coagulation - a hot probe is used to burn the abnormal area. It can ablate to a depth of 7 mm and is more accessible than laser. There is a higher incidence of discharge and secondary haemorrhage.

Electrocoagulation diathermy - this technique requires a general anaesthetic.

Cryotherapy - this involves freezing the cervix using liquid nitrogen and is seldom used these days except in the treatment of an ectropion.

Excision - excisional biopsies are required if there are suspicious areas or unsatisfactory colposcopy, but they have a higher incidence of haemorrhage and cervical stenosis. The degree of excision will also depend on the age of the patient because of the fertility problems associated, so lesions may be watched for longer if the woman has not had children.

Knife cone biopsy - this is largely being succeeded by newer techniques but is still used for difficult lesions. A general anaesthetic is required and sutures are inserted into the cervix for haemostasis. Unfortunately, heavy blood loss can occur, and there is also a 10% risk of cervical stenosis.

Laser cone biopsy - this is essentially similar to the knife cone biopsy but can be performed using local anaesthetic and allows excellent control, with a shallower cone being taken. There is a much lower blood loss and risk of cervical stenosis. Unfortunately the equipment is expensive and requires more training to use.

Large loop excision of the transformation zone (LLETZ) is one of the most popular methods (Figure

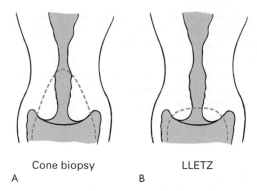

Cone biopsy   LLETZ
A   B

Fig 10.2 *The difference between (A) cervical cone biopsy and (B) large loop excision of the transformation zone (LLETZ).*

10.2). A wire loop connected with diathermy is used to excise the whole of the transformation zone. Its advantages are that it is easily learnt, acceptable to the patients and less traumatic, causing cervical stenosis in only 2% of cases.

Hysterectomy - this used to be the treatment of choice for CIN until the rate and speed of progression to carcinoma was known. It still has a place if the woman has recurrent lesions or if she has finished her family and has other gynaecological problems such as menorrhagia.

OVERVIEW - As the understanding of CIN lesions improves, the trend for treatment is becoming more conservative.

Follow-up

SHORT TERM - If the colposcopic examination has been normal the patient may be followed up with cervical smears. After excisional biopsy, colposcopy is usually repeated after 6 months with a repeat smear. As mentioned above, the trend is to treat CIN 1 conservatively with colposcopic follow-up.

LONG TERM - Providing the follow-up smear is normal the woman should have yearly smears for 5 years before entering the screening programme again.

2. Inadequate Smear

Background

DEFINITION - The slide does not contain sufficient numbers of cervical cells for interpretation.

AETIOLOGY - Any condition which results in reduced oestrogen levels leads to atrophy of the vaginal and cervical epithelium, and the SCJ lies very high in the endo-cervical canal. As a result, only a few cells are sampled. In contrast, conditions associated with a raised oestrogen level, such as pregnancy or the oral contraceptive pill, may lead to the formation of a large ectropion which consists mostly of columnar epithelium. If the smear is not taken carefully a large number of glandular cells are obtained but very few squamous cells.

MAKING THE DIAGNOSIS – A smear should contain a representative sample of the two main types of cervical cells: **squamous** and **columnar** (glandular).

MAIN COMPLICATIONS – Anxiety and inconvenience for the woman, who will be asked to attend for repeat testing.

PREVENTION – Careful technique while performing the smear.

Treatment Options

ADVICE – The woman should be reassured that this is not an abnormal finding but simply a technical problem. The smear should be repeated after 3 months, preferably at about midcycle when the cervix is more open.

DRUG THERAPY – Atrophic changes can be reversed using either oral oestrogen in the form of HRT or topical vaginal oestrogen cream/pessaries.

OVERVIEW – Inadequate smears will usually be sorted out by the GP, but, if the problem persists, colposcopy is advised (for reassurance alone, one hopes).

Follow-up

SHORT TERM – Providing the repeat smear is negative the woman may rejoin the routine screening programme.

3. Inflammatory Smear

Background

DEFINITION – The presence of bacterial, viral, fungal, protozoal or inflammatory cells which make cytological interpretation difficult.

AETIOLOGY – All common vaginal and cervical infections. Bacterial vaginosis and candida are the commonest.

MAIN COMPLICATIONS – Surgical treatment of CIN in the presence of certain pelvic infections may lead to an acute exacerbation.

PREVENTION – Condoms will prevent transmission of human papilloma virus.

Treatment Options

ADVICE – It should be explained that a follow-up smear is very important, but that repeat cytology is usually normal.

DRUG THERAPY – The infection should be treated with antibiotics if appropriate. Viral infections cannot be treated, but the interval of 3 months often allows viral shedding to reduce.

Follow-up

SHORT TERM – Repeat 3 months later, after treatment if appropriate. If the repeat smear is negative, the woman can return to the routine screening programme.

LONG TERM – If two smears are reported as inflammatory, the woman should be referred to the colposcopy clinic.

4. Atypical Glandular Cells

Background

DEFINITION – The presence of glandular epithelial cells with abnormal nuclei and/or atypical cytoplasmic features.

AETIOLOGY – These may reflect premalignant or malignant disease in the upper genital tract (endocervix, endometrium, Fallopian tube or ovary).

ACTION – If no obvious cause is evident, the upper genital tract should be explored using hysteroscopy, endometrial and endocervical curettage, and laparoscopy as appropriate.

GOLDEN POINTS

1. Cervical cytology is a screening test; do not use if you suspect invasive disease.

2. The vast majority of women with abnormal cytology do not have invasive cervical cancer.

3. Avoid irrelevant questions which create anxiety and guilt for women with CIN, e.g. how many sexual partners have you had?

4. The diagnosis of CIN is made by colposcopically directed biopsy.

5. Remember, abnormal cells on a cervical smear sometimes reflect disease in the upper genital tract.

6. Sexually transmitted disease is common in women with CIN; consider routine screening.

11 Urinary incontinence

CLINICAL SIGNIFICANCE

Urinary incontinence is extremely common, with about 50% of women having urinary leakage from time to time. About 15% of women between 18 and 65 years, upwards of 2.5 million women in the United Kingdom, find their symptoms intolerable. The prevalence increases with age. This places huge financial demands on health resources, with 2% of the total budget being spent on incontinence services alone. Many women will not seek advice because of embarrassment.

Aside from the great distress and social inconvenience this condition causes, in a small proportion of cases incontinence is the presenting feature of serious pelvic pathology or degenerative neurological diseases.

DIFFERENTIAL DIAGNOSIS

MAIN CATEGORY	DIAGNOSIS
1. *Genuine stress incontinence (GSI)*	Bladder neck hypermobility Urethral sphincter failure
2. *Detrusor instability*	Idiopathic Secondary to neurological disease (hyperreflexia)
3. *Retention with overflow*	Motor neurone lesions Drugs Pelvic mass Severe prolapse
4. *Fistulae*	Ureteric/vesical/urethral
5. *Congenital*	Bladder extrophy Ectopic ureter
6. *Miscellaneous*	Functional (no identifiable cause) Urinary infections

---

Genuine stress incontinence and detrusor instability are by far the two most common diagnoses in women under the age of 70. In many women the two conditions exist together.

Mechanism of continence – Continence depends on relaxation of the bladder (detrusor muscle) during filling, and urethral closure pressure which is assisted by the pelvic floor muscles. If the bladder neck and proximal urethra remain within the abdominal cavity, any increase in the intra-abdominal pressure will be transmitted to the urethra, raising the closure pressure.

CLINICAL ASSESSMENT

Urinary incontinence, the involuntary leakage of urine that becomes a social or hygienic problem, is not of itself a life-threatening condition. The general practitioner (GP) should be alert to the possibility of serious underlying pathology, including pelvic tumours and neurological disorders. It is also important to exclude urinary infection and gross urinary retention. For mild symptoms, the GP can give preliminary advice about pelvic floor exercises and biofeedback therapy.

Relevant History

Presenting Complaint

MAIN SYMPTOM – The pattern of incontinence may give some indication of the cause of the problem, but in the vast majority of women this can only be accurately defined during urodynamic studies. The real importance of the history is to gain some idea of the nature and severity of the woman's symptoms and to try to detect any serious underlying pathology. Incontinence is often accompanied by other equally distressing urinary symptoms such as urgency and nocturia. Any therapeutic regimen needs to take all symptoms into account. **S**tress incontinence is urine leakage with exertion, most commonly coughing. Its severity is indicated by the activity required to cause it; leakage during very strenuous exercise would not be as significant as from walking, coughing or laughing. It usually reflects bladder neck weakness (genuine stress incontinence) but it is also a common feature of detrusor incontinence. **Urge incontinence**, the leakage of urine associated with urinary urgency, is more typical of detrusor instability but may be present in women with genuine stress incontinence. **Dribbling incontinence** is suggestive of a fistula or retention with overflow. The number of protective pads used by the woman has a poor correlation with the severity of the incontinence. COMMONLY ASSOCIATED SYMPTOMS – **Urgency** is a sudden desire to void (with fear of leakage). **Increased frequency**, the voluntary passage of urine more than seven times in a day, may reflect a reduced bladder capacity (interstitial cystitis or pelvic tumours), bladder hypersensitivity (bladder calculi, tumours or infection), increased urine production (diabetes, diuretics, or excess intake), or detrusor instability. In some women, frequency indicates nothing more than the desire to keep the bladder empty to avoid incontinence. Increased frequency may or may not be associated with **nocturia**, which is defined as waking more than twice in the night to pass urine. In isolation in elderly women, nocturia is often a feature of congestive cardiac failure with dependent oedema returning to the circulation during recumbency. Nocturia is a particularly serious symptom in elderly women because of the risk of falls and bone fracture. **Dysuria** or painful micturition may be caused by bladder infection, calculi or tumour. **Haematuria** may be a feature of bladder infection, tumours and calculi. **Hesitancy and poor stream** may indicate some form of bladder outlet obstruction. Some women will report that this can be overcome by temporarily returning their prolapse into the vagina. **Sensation of prolapse** may be a significant symptom which requires separate consideration. It does not necessarily indicate genuine stress incontinence. **Neurological symptoms** such as leg weakness or paraesthesia may reflect an upper or lower motor neurone problem such as multiple sclerosis. BACKGROUND INFORMATION – **Fluid intake** – the volume, nature and timing of fluid intake will effect bladder function. A high intake of caffeine-containing drinks causes increased frequency. The risk of nocturia is increased if a drink is taken near to bedtime. EFFECT ON PATIENT – Women with severe symptoms may feel unable to leave their homes. Psychosexual upset is common.

Gynaecological History

GYNAECOLOGICAL DISEASE – A history of bladder neck surgery may make repeat surgery difficult and less likely to succeed. Previous pelvic surgery, especially if complicated, should also raise the possibility of a fistula. FERTILITY REQUIREMENTS – Completion of their family is relevant, especially if surgery is to be performed, as further pregnancy is likely to reverse any therapeutic benefit.

Obstetric History

DELIVERIES – There is an increasing association of incontinence and number of vaginal deliveries, especially with prolonged labours, large babies (> 3.5 kg) or assisted vaginal deliveries. In practice, however, this makes little difference to any management. A history of recent complicated vaginal delivery should raise the rare possibility of fistula.

Medical History

OPERATIONS – Any previous bladder or pelvic surgery. MEDICAL CONDITIONS – **Chronic constipation or chest disease** will lead to a rise in the intra-abdominal pressure and put extra strain on the already weak urinary sphincter. **Diabetes** may lead to a peripheral neuropathy, and incontinence may rarely be its presenting feature. **Other neurological conditions** such as multiple sclerosis may lead to damage to the nerve supply to the bladder. PSYCHOLOGICAL DISORDERS – Low intelligence and severe depressive disorders are associated with a higher incidence of functional incontinence.

Drug History

MEDICATIONS – Diuretics, which increase urinary output, can lead to frequency and worsen incontinence already present. Anticholinergic agents and tricyclic antidepressants may cause urinary retention. SMOKING AND ALCOHOL – Both may promote or worsen detrusor instability.

Social History

AGE – Urinary incontinence is more commonly seen in middle to old age, with an increased incidence after menopause. OCCUPATION – Women with jobs that involve great exertion may find that this makes the incontinence worse. DEPENDANTS – Dependants at home may require assistance, exacerbating the woman's symptoms. LIFESTYLE – Lack of regular exercise may be associated with increased weight gain, which may worsen any symptoms due to genuine stress incontinence.

Relevant Clinical Examination

General Examination

GENERAL CONDITION – The overall physical condition will influence the treatment options. BODY-MASS INDEX – Obesity is associated with stress incontinence. It also increases the risks of surgery with a reduction in the chance of success in the longer term. NERVOUS SYSTEM – Leg reflexes and sensation should be examined to test for evidence of neurological disease.

Abdomen

CONTOUR – Large pelvic tumours or a full bladder may be obvious.

OLD SCARS – The site of previous pelvic surgery may influence the type of procedure undertaken.

PALPATION – An enlarged tender bladder may indicate retention, although chronic retention is usually painless. A large pelvic mass is a common cause of the urinary symptoms. Renal tenderness may be a sign of urinary infection.

Pelvis

VULVA – Chronic wetness leads to vulval irritation and excoriation. Atrophy of the vaginal epithelium may also be found. Leakage on coughing is suggestive of bladder neck weakness but it does not rule out detrusor instability. Reduced sensation over the vulval skin may accompany neurological disease.

VAGINA – Prolapse of the uterus, anterior and posterior vaginal wall can exacerbate bladder symptoms. Vaginal tone and the state of the pelvic floor muscles can be assessed digitally.

BIMANUAL EXAMINATION – Uterine enlargement or ovarian tumours may be felt. Bladder tenderness may be a feature of infection and, more rarely, malignant tumours.

RECTAL EXAMINATION – Poor anal tone may be a sign of neurological disease.

Relevant Initial Investigations

Biochemistry

RANDOM BLOOD SUGAR OR GLUCOSE TOLERANCE TEST – If the woman has been troubled by increased frequency or recurrent urinary tract infections, diabetes mellitus should be tested for. U+Es should be undertaken if there is anything to indicate ureteric obstruction, including severe prolapse (procidentia).

Microbiology

URINE – A midstream specimen of urine (**MSU**) should always be sent for microscopy and culture to test for infection and to screen for tumours (indicated by sterile pyuria or haematuria). Urodynamic studies should never be undertaken before infection has been ruled out, as catheterisation may lead to a rapid deterioration.

Urinary Function Tests

FREQUENCY VOLUME CHART – This is a simple way of assessing a woman's bladder function. The timing and volume of each micturition are measured and recorded on a chart for a week, together with the pattern of fluid intake. These can be sent out with the clinic appointment card. It is particularly useful for identifying women who drink excessively. It also serves as a useful baseline against which therapy can be assessed.

PAD TEST – This estimates the volume of urine lost by incontinence using perineal towels that are weighed before and after use, the increase in weight being an index of the urine lost. The result may be an overestimate if there is a heavy vaginal discharge or if the woman is menstruating. It is a useful test if there is any doubt about the validity of the woman's story.

URODYNAMIC STUDIES – These are a group of tests that look in detail at bladder and urethral function. **Uroflowmetry** is a cheap and non-invasive test of urinary function. The patient is asked to pass urine into a vessel with a measuring device. It calculates the rate of flow and the total volume voided. In a female the minimum flow rate should be 15 ml/s and voided volume over 150 ml. Straining can lead to abnormal flow patterns with interrupted flow. **Residual volume** is a guide to the adequacy of bladder emptying. Women who cannot empty their bladder completely are at increased risk of urinary tract infections. Moreover, such women are more likely to be unable to micturate after surgery for GSI. It can be measured by ultrasonography or more directly by catheterisation. **Filling cystometry** (Figure 11.1) tests bladder function by examining the relationship between the bladder pressure and volume during filling and voiding. It is a particularly useful test of detrusor function. Urinary and rectal catheters measure the intravesical (p_{ves}) and intra-abdominal pressures (p_{abd}), respectively, and subtraction of these calculates the detrusor pressure ($p_{det}=p_{ves} - p_{abd}$). Warm saline is slowly infused into the bladder at 50 ml/min, and the patient is asked to signal when she feels the first desire to void. The detrusor pressure is monitored as the bladder fills, and any increase in detrusor pressure is noted. At the end of filling, the patient is asked to stand to look for an increase in detrusor pressure while erect and is asked to cough. Any leakage of urine is recorded on the pressure profile to determine whether or not it coincides with detrusor activity. Finally, during voiding, the woman is asked to interrupt the flow by contracting (squeezing) her pelvic floor.

- **Normal cystometry**:
  - Residual volume less than 50 ml
  - First desire to void between 150 and 200 ml
  - Capacity of greater than 400 ml
  - Minimal increase in detrusor pressure
  - Absence of abnormal detrusor contractions
  - No leaking on coughing
  - Maximum detrusor pressure of 70 cm H_2O while voiding
  - The patient should be able to stop voiding.
- **Abnormal cystometry**:
  - If leakage of urine occurs without a rise in detrusor pressure, genuine stress incontinence can be diagnosed

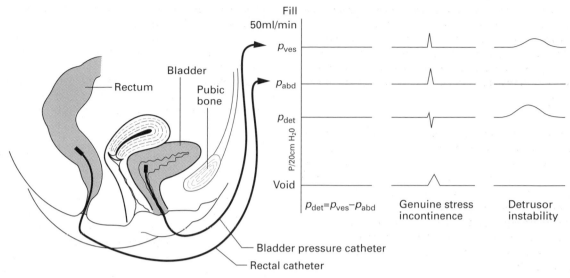

Fig 11.1 *Filling cystometry: detrusor pressure (p_{det}) = bladder pressure (p_{ves}) − abdominal pressure (p_{abd}).*

- Involuntary detrusor activity during filling confirms detrusor instability
- Small bladder capacity suggests interstitial cystitis
- High residual volume indicates incomplete bladder emptying
- High detrusor pressure during voiding is suspicious of outflow obstruction.

Micturating cystourethrography, videocystourcth-rography and ambulatory monitoring are yet more specialised tests allowing the functional anatomical relationship of the urethra, urethrovesical junction and bladder base to be visualised, thereby facilitating the diagnosis of stress incontinence in complex cases.

DETAILS OF COMMON CONDITIONS

I. Genuine Stress Incontinence (GSI)

Background

DEFINITION – GSI is the involuntary loss of urine from the urethra when the intravesical pressure exceeds the maximum urethral closure pressure in the absence of detrusor activity.

AETIOLOGY – There are two mechanisms for the development of GSI: first, prolapse of the proximal urethra and bladder neck out of the abdominal cavity means that a rise of abdominal pressure does not compress the bladder neck and therefore increases the vesical pressure but not the urethral pressure. Second, a reduction in resting urethral closure pressure, below that of the bladder, will lead to incontinence. There are several factors that lead to an alteration in these conditions. Childbirth is one of the commonest factors - vaginal delivery leading to stretching of supporting tissues around the bladder neck and, more importantly, denervation of the levator muscles which form part of the sphincter mechanism. Menopause sees a large increase in the incidence of GSI, and this is thought to be due to loss of collagen from the supporting tissues secondary to oestrogen deficiency Congenital weakness of connective tissues plays a part in a small proportion of cases. Fibrosis secondary to surgery resulting in a rigid (drainpipe) urethra occasionally plays a part.

MAKING THE DIAGNOSIS – See Table 11.1.

MAIN COMPLICATIONS – The main effect of GSI is changes in lifestyle, including loss of time from work and psychosexual disturbances. Leakage of urine sometimes causes vulval irritation which may lead to excoriation and secondary infection.

PREVENTION – As childbirth is one of the major causes of GSI one might suppose that improvements in obstetric care should lead to a lower incidence of problems. Elective caesarean section is requested by some women, but this is unproven for the prevention of GSI, as nulliparous women may still develop bladder neck incompetence. After the menopause, HRT may prevent loss of collagen, but this is also unproven.

Treatment Options

ADVICE – GSI is not life-threatening but there is a ten-

Table 11.1	Diagnosing GSI
Diagnosis	Genuine stress incontinence
History	Leakage of urine on coughing/ straining/exertion
	No urgency at the time of leakage
Examination	Urethral/bladder neck mobility
Investigations	
– Microbiology	No urinary infection
– Urethral pressure	Under 20 cm H$_2$O at rest is suggestive of urethral sphincter failure
– Cystometry	Low urinary residual volume
	Urinary leakage on straining with no detrusor pressure rise
	Urinary leakage from the urethra without straining and no detrusor pressure rise indicates possible urethral sphincter failure

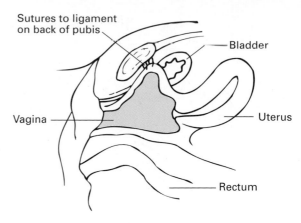

Fig 11.2 *Burch colposuspension.*

dency for the symptoms to become worse with time. Women may be referred with very mild symptoms, and reassurance that no underlying pathological process exists is all that some require.

CHANGE OF LIFESTYLE/DIET – Weight loss and decreased smoking may reduce abdominal pressure. Fluid restriction (< 1.5 L/day) and timed voiding may make the incontinence less of a problem.

PHYSIOTHERAPY – Pelvic floor exercises (PFE) are intended to build up the muscles of the levator floor. They are best taught by a specialist physiotherapist. Patients should be warned that it may take 4 months before any improvement is noticed. Weighted cones which the woman has to retain in the vagina by clenching her levator muscles are said to lead to better results. Many women like the idea of active therapy but PFE demands a continuing programme of exercises, and so compliance is often poor and relapse rates are moderately high. Electrical stimulation (inferential therapy) is a passive method of strengthening the pelvic floor.

DRUG THERAPY – Drugs do not play a major part in the treatment of GSI. HRT may have a small effect by improving the urethral mucosa in women with prolonged oestrogen deficiency.

CONTINENCE DEVICES – A variety of inventions, which act by occluding the urethra, have been developed to prevent urine leakage in women with GSI. They are particularly useful for very elderly women in whom surgery is contraindicated and for younger women who only get incontinence during extreme exercise.

SURGERY – For many, surgery provides the only means of control in GSI. There are a wide range of operations which have their individual advantages and disadvantages. Anterior vaginal repair with bladder neck buttress has been used for many years but the long-term success is poor.

Burch colposuspension (Figure 11.2) involves elevation of the vagina (and bladder neck) through a suprapubic incision. Sutures run through the vagina to the iliopectineal ligament at the pelvic brim. The Marshall–Marchetti–Krantz colposuspension is similar, but the sutures are attached to the periosteum just lateral to and behind the symphysis pubis, and up to 5% of women get bone inflammation. These procedures are suitable for treating urethral and bladder neck hypermobility.

Suburethral sling may be used to treat urinary incontinence caused by bladder neck hypermobility and urethral sphincter failure but has an increased incidence of postoperative voiding problems because of difficulties in gauging sling tension. Homologous tissue such as rectus sheath strips have shown improved success rates.

Stamey bladder neck suspension involves the passage of non-absorbable suture from the paraurethral tissue to the rectus sheath. It is done under cystoscopic control to ensure that the bladder is not perforated and to determine the degree of elevation. It is felt to be a useful procedure for older women who might not tolerate a standard colposuspension.

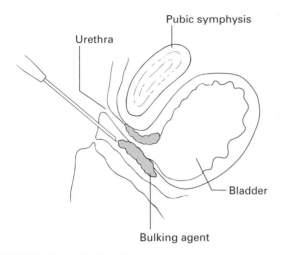

Fig 11.3 *Urethral bulking injections.*

Urethral bulking injections (Figure 11.3) used to treat urethral sphincter failure and, more recently, urethral hypermobility are proving reasonably successful. Collagen or silicon is injected into the side walls of the urethra, closing the lumen. Results are poorer than for other procedures, but it is a simple low-risk technique usually performed under local anaesthetic. The relapse rate is high, but the procedure can be repeated and the newer synthetic products may last longer.

Artificial urinary sphincters are reserved for women after multiple attempts at surgery but have a good success rate considering the major surgery involved. OVERVIEW – Optimal treatment of GSI depends upon the exact nature of the problem, associated prolapse, general physical condition of the woman, previous treatment failures and the wishes of the woman. For most gynaecologists, the Burch colposuspension is the operation of first choice for correction of GSI. Providing the diagnosis has been made correctly, and detrusor instability has been excluded, the success rates for surgery are as high as 90%, whereas pelvic floor exercises have only a short-term success of 50–60%. In general it is true to say that the greater success the procedure has at creating continence, the greater the chance of inducing chronic urinary retention. In addition to the common complications of major surgery, colposuspension may lead to chronic retention of urine in about 1% of women, with the need for long-term intermittent self-catheterisation. This can be predicted in women who have poor detrusor function on voiding demonstrated by cystometry. There is also a chance of chronic pelvic discomfort and enterocoele formation. Urethral bulking injections have a lower success rate (60%), but they carry less risk of complication and are easily repeated. When GSI coexists with detrusor instability, it is important to treat the instability before attempting surgery.

Follow-up

SHORT TERM – Immediate postoperative care after colposuspension includes monitoring bladder emptying. This is best achieved by the insertion of a suprapubic catheter at the time of surgery. The catheter is usually removed when the residual volume is less that 150 ml. It is also very important to test for urinary tract infections, which are common after this type of surgery.

LONG TERM – The results of colposuspension are good, but recurrence of the symptoms may occur as late as 5 years after surgery.

2. Detrusor Instability

Background

DEFINITION – The objective demonstration of involuntary

Table 11.2	Diagnosing detrusor instability
Making the diagnosis	Detrusor instability
History	Urgency, frequency of micturition, leading to leakage if they don't get to the toilet in time
	They may have had previous bladder surgery or neurological disease
Examination	If idiopathic the examination may be normal
	Neurological deficit may be present, e.g. spina bifida, multiple sclerosis
Investigations	
– Frequency volume chart	Daytime frequency > 8, night time > 2 and small voided volumes (< 250 ml)
– Ultrasound	No calculi but there may be a residual volume in neurological cases
– Cystoscopy	Normal epithelium, no calculi, tumours or interstitial cystitis
– Microbiology	No urinary tract infection
– Cystometry	Detrusor waves on filling with or without leakage

detrusor contraction either spontaneously or provoked during bladder filling. This diagnosis can only be made during cystometric testing at urodynamics.

AETIOLOGY – Psychological state may influence the severity of the symptoms, but the underlying cause is unknown in the majority of cases. Interestingly, abnormal detrusor contractions are found over 10% of apparently normal women. It occasionally arises as a result of bladder outlet obstruction, usually after bladder neck surgery. In a very small proportion of women, it is a sign of neurological disease such as multiple sclerosis, when it is called detrusor hyperreflexia.

MAIN COMPLICATIONS – The symptoms of urgency and frequency and nocturia are probably the biggest problem, with the woman constantly feeling the need to pass urine and with micturition not giving relief. Genuine stress incontinence is commonly associated with detrusor instability, making continence and treatment more difficult. Neurological disease may have complications that outweigh that of incontinence.

SCREENING TESTS – All women undergoing surgery for stress urinary leakage should undergo urodynamic testing to exclude associated detrusor instability.

Treatment Options

ADVICE – **Detrusor instability** is the second commonest cause of incontinence in premenopausal women and the commonest after the menopause. It is a self-limiting disorder of remissions and relapses. It is not life-threatening unless associated with neurological disease, when outlet obstruction can lead to renal failure. It is often impossible to control the manifestations completely, but judicious use of the various treatments usually leads to a great improvement in symptoms. Persistent symptoms should be investigated by cystoscopy, screening for tumours or calculi. Redness of the mucosa is suggestive of interstitial cystitis, but this can only be diagnosed on histological examination of a mucosal biopsy. For some women, **reassurance** that it can just be a variant of normal bladder function may be all that is required.

CHANGE OF LIFESTYLE/DIET – The frequency described by these women is the result of their voiding before they get severe urgency and leak. The frequency volume chart can show if large volumes are being passed (i.e. > 300 ml), and the women should be encouraged to drink less, especially drinks containing caffeine such as coffee and tea. Incontinence aids such as pads and nappies may be appropriate.

BEHAVIOURAL THERAPY – **Bladder drill** is a form of self-training. It can be done in the community, but some claim the results are superior if it is undertaken during inpatient stay. The woman is advised to hold on to urine for 1 h even if leaking occurs. When this is reached with continence maintained the period is increased gradually up to 2 h. This is not dissimilar to bladder training that parents do with their offspring in childhood. Some groups have tried **biofeedback techniques**. This involves the woman's being taught to become aware of the early part of the detrusor contraction and learning to inhibit it. Contractions usually pass off after 15–30 s and it is often safer to attempt inhibition than to dash to the toilet. Pelvic floor exercises can help but there is a high relapse rate.

PHARMACOLOGICAL THERAPY – Drugs are the mainstay of treatment for severe symptoms. They act by inhibiting detrusor contractions. The two main classes of drugs are **musculotropic relaxants** (e.g. oxybutinin) and **anticholinergic** agents (e.g. probantheline). Both groups of drugs have proved useful, with up to a 70% improvement in symptoms. **Tricyclic antidepressants** and **calcium channel blockers** have also been used but with less success. **Analogues of antidiuretic hormone** (ADH) have been used to reduce the nocturnal urine production for women greatly troubled by nocturia, but there is a real risk of pulmonary oedema in elderly women.

SURGERY – There is little place for surgery apart from exceptional cases. Small bowel may be used to increase the bladder capacity (**clam cystoplasty**) or the ureters may be implanted into an isolated loop of small bowel connected with the abdominal surface (**ileal conduit**).

OVERVIEW – Behavioural therapy is safe and reasonably successful but many women fail to gain long-term control. Drug therapy is the mainstay of treatment of severe symptoms but is often limited by the anticholinergic side effects such as dry mouth, blurred vision and dizziness. The dose has to be titrated against side effects and improvement in symptoms. Surgery is very much a last resort.

Follow-up

SHORT TERM – After urodynamic testing, initial follow-up should be at the referring unit, especially if drug treatment is being prescribed, but the GP will be more directly involved in the longer term.

LONG TERM – If symptoms recur, the initial treatments should be tried again, as secondary remission is common. The continence advisory nurse in the community should be involved in the care of women with recurrent severe symptoms. Neuropathic patients and those who undergo surgery should be followed up for life as there is a risk of voiding difficulties leading to ureteric dilatation and renal damage.

3. Fistulae

Background

DEFINITION – A fistula is an abnormal communication between two viscera lined by epithelium. In the urinary tract, a fistula may form between the ureter, bladder or urethra and the vagina, uterus or bowel.

AETIOLOGY – In the developed world, fistulae involving the ureter or bladder are commonest and these are usually secondary to obstetric or gynaecological surgery, including caesarean section and hysterectomy. Malignant tumours of the cervix account for most other cases. Some of these arise after radiotherapy. In developing countries, the commonest fistulae involve the bladder neck and/or urethra and typically they are caused by traumatic vaginal delivery or pressure necrosis after prolonged obstructed delivery.

MAKING THE DIAGNOSIS – See Table 11.3.

MAIN COMPLICATIONS – The main presentation will be with constant wetness leading to excoriation and infection. The underlying cause, especially malignant disease or irradiation, may be the overriding problem. Urinary fistulae resulting from prolonged labour are often associated with faecal incontinence secondary to fistulae involving the vagina and rectum.

PREVENTION – Good surgical technique with careful handling of tissues and attention to sterile technique and haemostasis is important. Improved understanding of radiotherapy has lead to a reduction in damage to surrounding tissues and a lower incidence of urinary fistulae. In the third world, improvements in maternity care with a reduced length of labour and avoidance of difficult vaginal delivery will prevent many fistulae, but adequately trained personnel and suitable facilities will need to be provided for caesarean delivery to be a safe option.

Treatment Options

REASSURANCE – Support forms a major part of therapy for women with large fistulae and especially for those with fistulae associated with malignant disease. A significant proportion of small fistulae will heal spontaneously, but the woman should be warned that it may take several months.

CATHETERISATION is sometimes necessary in order to allow the fistula to heal.

PHARMACOLOGICAL THERAPY – Urinary tract infections must be treated aggressively with an appropriate antibiotic.

SURGERY – **Transvaginal fistula repair** is appropriate for low vesicovaginal fistula. The fistula is dissected out and non-viable tissues are removed. The deficit is then closed in layers, care being taken not to create tension in the wound. **Higher urinary fistulae** are repaired through the abdomen. The omentum may be used to separate the bladder and vaginal walls. All repairs should be followed by catheterisation for a minimum of 10 days, and particular attention should be paid to haemostasis and maintenance of a good blood supply. It is also important to prevent infection. Occasionally **urinary diversion (ileal conduit)** is necessary if repair is not possible for women with a reasonable life-expectancy.

OVERVIEW – All but the smallest fistulae should be repaired by an experienced surgeon in a specialist referral centre.

Information for Patients

PROGNOSIS – Depending on the cause of the fistula the outlook can be very good or very bleak. Very large fistulae and those associated with malignant disease/irradiation do particularly badly. The first attempt at closure offers the best chance of success, with a 70% cure rate for non-malignant cases.

Follow-up

SHORT TERM – Close observation is necessary after surgery to detect evidence of infection.

LONG TERM – A case can be made for sterilisation if the woman has living children. If she does become pregnant again, vaginal delivery should be avoided.

4. Overflow Incontinence

Background

DEFINITION – This is the involuntary loss of urine when the

Table 11.3	Diagnosing urinary fistulae
Making the diagnosis	Fistula
History	Constant wetness and leakage of urine
	Recent traumatic delivery, surgery or radiotherapy
Examination	Excoriation of the skin. The fistula is often difficult to visualise
Investigations	
– Cystoscopy/EUA	Examination under anaesthetic may allow visualisation, but dye injected into the bladder often helps
– Cystogram/IVP	Radiological dye demonstrating site of connection

intravesical pressure exceeds that of the urethra because of an inability to void urine.

AETIOLOGY – This may be acute or chronic. Acute retention can occur postoperatively after surgery close to the bladder neck, during pregnancy, with an acutely retroverted uterus following childbirth, especially if epidural anaesthesia is used, and in association with urinary infection. Chronic retention may extend from acute retention (see below) or be associated with outflow obstruction most commonly due to procidentia in elderly women. It may also arise after colposuspension and as a complication of neurological diseases and spinal injury.

MAIN COMPLICATIONS – Acute retention may cause permanent damage to the detrusor muscle, leading to bladder atony and chronic retention. Retention is associated with an increased risk of urinary infection.

PREVENTION – Early recognition of acute retention postoperatively or following childbirth may prevent permanent damage to the detrusor muscle.

Treatment Options

CATHETERISATION – Suprapubic or urethral drainage should be used in the short term for reversible problems. Some women with spinal injuries can be taught to empty their bladder successfully by external pressure. If the woman develops permanent voiding problems, she may be required to perform taught intermittent self-catheterisation (ISC) 2–3 times each day. An indwelling catheter should be considered for women who are unable to catheterise themselves.

PHARMACOLOGICAL THERAPY – Cholinergic agonists may be used to increase detrusor activity. Alpha adrenergic blockers may help by relaxing the proximal urethra. The success rate for these is poor.

5. Temporary Disorders

Background

DEFINITION – This is incontinence caused by a reversible condition.

AETIOLOGY – Urinary tract infections cause a significant number of urological symptoms, especially symptoms of urgency leading to incontinence. Prescribed medication such as diuretics can lead to increased urine output putting further strain on an already compromised bladder neck. Faecal loading and pelvic masses pressing on the bladder cause irritation.

DIAGNOSIS – The history and physical examination play an important role along with assessment of the urine for infection.

Treatment Options

ADVICE – These conditions are usually responsive to the appropriate therapy and should not have long-term effects if they are appropriately monitored.

CHANGE OF LIFESTYLE/DIET – Constipation can be prevented by increasing the fibre in the diet and fluid intake if it is low. Medication may need altering if it is felt to be a cause.

DRUG THERAPY – Urinary tract infections should be treated with the appropriate antibiotic after culture of a midstream specimen of urine.

OVERVIEW – Treatment should result in an improvement, but, if not, the woman should be referred to the appropriate unit for investigation.

GOLDEN POINTS

1. Using posters in health centres encourages women to present symptoms.

2. Use history and urine microscopy to screen for features of urinary tract cancer. Perform renal ultrasound and cystoscopy if suspicious.

3. Examine nervous system for evidence of rare neurological diseases.

4. Examine pelvis for evidence of uterine and ovarian tumours.

5. Send MSU for culture to screen for infection in all cases.

6. Undertake urodynamic studies to diagnose functional causes: genuine stress incontinence, detrusor instability, and outflow obstruction.

7. Consider conservative treatments such as pelvic floor exercises and biofeedback before resorting to drugs and surgery.

8. Carefully explain complication of urinary retention before surgery for GSI.

12 Sensation of prolapse

CLINICAL SIGNIFICANCE

Uterovaginal prolapse is a herniation of the female genital tract. It is extremely common, with the prevalence increasing rapidly beyond the age of 50 years. Prolapse is the commonest indication for major gynaecological surgery after the menopause.

Uterovaginal prolapse is commonly associated with urinary incontinence and to a lesser extent faecal incontinence. Rarely, prolapse is precipitated by pressure from a pelvic mass.

DIFFERENTIAL DIAGNOSIS

MAIN CATEGORY	DIAGNOSIS
Other causes of vaginal lump	
1. *Bartholin's cyst*	
2. *Genital tract tumour*	Cervical fibroid
	Cervical polyp
	Cervical cancer
	Vulval cancer
3. *Neglected foreign body*	
Precipitating causes	
1. *Congenital weakness*	Abnormal collagen
2. *Acquired weakness*	(Traumatic) vaginal delivery
	Oestrogen deficiency (the menopause)
3. *Pelvic/abdominal pressure*	Uterine or ovarian tumour
	Ascites
4. *Abdominal strain*	Chronic cough
	Chronic constipation
	Heavy manual work

Prolapse is generally classified according to the herniating viscera, e.g. anterior vaginal wall prolapse with bladder attached is termed a cystocoele, posterior vaginal wall prolapse is known as a rectocoele, and prolapse of the posterior vaginal fornix containing intestine is called an enterocoele. Vault prolapse is usually restricted to descent of the upper vagina in women who have previously had a hysterectomy. Uterine prolapse is classified into three grades (I, II, III) depending on the degree of descent; I in the vagina, II to the introitus, and III outside the introitus. There is now a new classification, approved by the International Continence Society (ICS), which has standardised the terminology describing the prolapse after the most distal part and graded by degree of descent in centimetres using the introitus as point zero, with prolapse below this recorded as positive readings and above as negative. Figure 12.1 shows the supporting structures of the vagina and uterus.

Box 12.1   Type of prolapse

Vaginal prolapse	Anterior (cystocoele)
	Posterior (rectocoele)
	Vault (enterocoele)
Uterine	Above the introitus (grade I)
	To the introitus (grade II)
	Below the introitus (grade III/ procidentia)

CLINICAL ASSESSMENT

These women will present to the GP describing a swelling or discomfort in the vagina. They frequently also complain of urinary incontinence, difficulty with micturition, and difficulty with defaecation. More rarely, a woman

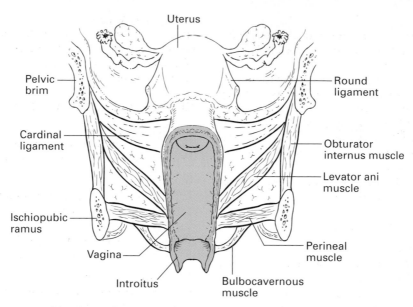

Fig 12.1 *Supporting structures of the vagina and uterus.*

may present urgently with complete uterovaginal prolapse (procidentia) requiring urgent assessment.

Relevant History

Presenting Complaint

MAIN SYMPTOM – '*I have a swelling below*' is the classical presentation, together with a dragging sensation especially towards the end of the day. If they can feel a lump, ask if they can replace it, and does it get worse after walking or coughing. This will help gauge the severity. Many women associate the prolapse with backache, but it is often difficult to be certain whether this is coincidental or not.

COMMONLY ASSOCIATED SYMPTOMS – Prolapse is associated with **genuine stress urinary incontinence** on straining due to descent and weakness of the bladder neck. **Frequency** and **hesitancy** of micturition, sometimes together with a sensation of incomplete emptying, suggests kinking of the bladder neck. Some women report that they overcome these by pushing the prolapse back in during micturition. Women may also complain of constipation and using a finger to replace the prolapse in order to defaecate. Severe pain is unusual and usually indicates acute urinary retention.

EFFECT ON PATIENT – The discomfort is usually an inconvenience, and the associated symptoms are the reason why treatment is sought, but some women are extremely fearful that the prolapse will suddenly worsen while they are in public.

Gynaecological History

MENSTRUAL HISTORY – Women are more likely to present with prolapse after the menopause, and this may in part result from oestrogen deficiency leading to loss of collagen in supporting tissues of the pelvic floor and vagina.

FERTILITY REQUIREMENTS – If surgery is to be considered, there is a line of argument that states it should be delayed until after the woman's family is completed.

Obstetric History

DELIVERY – The number and difficulty of vaginal deliveries is a factor in the pathogenesis of prolapse, but this does not aid clinical management, and indeed nulliparous women may develop prolapse. However, prolapse is sometimes severe after delivery but improves greatly with natural involution and physiotherapy.

Medical History

MEDICAL CONDITIONS – Chronic constipation or chest infections, which lead to a rise in abdominal pressure, should be controlled before any surgery. Connective tissue disorders of collagen metabolism have been implicated in weakening of the vaginal skin and pelvic floor support.

SURGERY – Previous pelvic surgery may make any future surgery more difficult.

Drug History

SMOKING AND ALCOHOL – Cigarette smoking causes chronic coughs and is associated with a reduction in tissue collagen.

Social History

AGE – Severe prolapse is very rare in women under the age of 30 years, and it should raise the possibility of a connective tissue disorder.

OCCUPATION – Manual occupations that cause abdominal strain not only put women at risk of prolapse but may also affect the results of surgery.

DEPENDANTS – Elderly or handicapped relatives often require a lot of care, including heavy lifting. Additional support for the woman will be needed to allow full recovery from any surgery.

LIFESTYLE – Women who are very active tend to maintain a stronger pelvic musculature and pelvic support.

Relevant Clinical Examination

General Examination

GENERAL CONDITION – To assess if surgery is safe, especially in very elderly women.

BODY-MASS INDEX – Prolapse is said to be more common in the morbidly obese, and the results of surgery are said not to be as good.

Cardiorespiratory System

Chronic chest infections need treating prior to anaesthesia and to improve the chances of success of any corrective surgery.

Abdomen

PALPATION – Pelvic masses and ascites are a rare cause of raised intra-abdominal pressure. The bladder may be over-distended because of urinary retention.

Pelvic

PERINEUM – The cervix or vaginal vault may be seen protruding from the introitus (procidentia).

VAGINA – Ideally the woman is examined in the left lateral position, using a Simm's speculum. It will help to ask the woman to strain. Care should be taken to examine for atrophy and to assess the site and degree of any vaginal prolapse. If a procidentia is discovered, attempts should be made to replace it gently. The introitus (see Figure 12.1) should be taken as zero, with measurement taken from the vault, anterior/posterior vaginal wall and cervix. This method allows a reproducible record, with prolapse above the introitus having negative values and below positive values. Anterior wall prolapse may have bladder closely adherent, and posterior wall descent may have rectum involved which can be assessed by digital rectal examination. Forceps can be used to put gentle traction on the cervix to assess descent and mobility of the uterus.

CERVIX – With procidentia the cervix may become ulcerated and infected. Infection should be treated before surgery is undertaken.

BIMANUAL EXAMINATION – Uterine fibroids or ovarian tumours may be pushing the uterus/vault down.

RECTAL EXAMINATION – A rectum full of hard faeces may make symptoms of a prolapse worse.

Relevant Initial Investigations

Biochemistry

SERUM U+Es – If ureteric obstruction with renal impairment is suspected in women with procidentia.

Microbiology

URINE – A midstream specimen of urine should be taken if there are urinary symptoms or if retention of urine is suspected.

BACTERIAL CULTURE – A vaginal swab should be taken if a procidentia appears ulcerated or infected.

Diagnostic Imaging

RENAL ULTRASOUND – To exclude ureteric obstruction in women with procidentia.

PELVIC ULTRASOUND – If a pelvic mass is found or suspected.

Urodynamic Studies

Women with urinary symptoms should have cystometry and uroflowmetry prior to corrective surgery (see Chapter 11).

Histopathology

VAGINAL – A procidentia may become ulcerated. A punch biopsy should be sent for microscopy if there is any suspicion of malignant change.

DETAILS OF COMMON CONDITIONS

I. Uterovaginal Prolapse

Background

DEFINITION – Downward herniation of the vagina and/or uterus toward or past the introitus with or without secondary involvement of bladder, urethra, rectum or intestine.

AETIOLOGY – The pelvic floor consists of the superficial and deep perineal muscles which are made up of numerous fibres from origins round the bony pelvis. The pelvic ligaments are thickenings of the endopelvic fascia and include the pubocervical, cervical and utero-sacral, which in combination with the pelvic floor muscles provide support for the vagina and surrounding structures. The ligaments may be congenitally weak, but this accounts for only a small percentage of cases of prolapse. **Childbirth** is a major cause of pelvic floor weakness, particularly if delivery is complicated. **Post-**

menopausal atrophy leads to a reduction in collagen with weakening of the supporting. **Chronic elevation of abdominal pressure**, either with constipation, chest infections or heavy lifting, may worsen any prolapse.

MAIN COMPLICATIONS – Vaginal **discomfort** and **dragging** are common. Anterior vaginal wall prolapse may lead to urinary urgency, frequency, hesitancy and stress incontinence. Posterior wall prolapse can make defaecation difficult because of faeces being pushed into the sac of the rectocoele. Procidentia may cause ureteric obstruction with renal failure.

SCREENING/PREVENTION – It is hoped that improvements in the management of labour with greater resort to caesarean section will reduce the incidence of prolapse. Similarly, postpartum pelvic floor physiotherapy is thought likely to prevent problems. Hormone replacement therapy in postmenopausal women may prevent prolapse by reducing the rate of loss of collagen from pelvic ligaments.

MAKING THE DIAGNOSIS – This is by examination in the clinic. Sometimes the findings vary from time to time; this particularly applies to examinations done under anaesthesia at the time of surgery. The prolapse is termed after the presenting part and may be called anterior, posterior, vault or uterine.

Treatment Options

ADVICE – A degree of prolapse is present in the large majority of parous women over 50 years. Many are asymptomatic and are simply found during routine examination. Treatment is not necessary unless there are significant symptoms.

CHANGE OF LIFESTYLE/DIET – Weight loss plays an important role in preventing prolapse and improving the success rate after surgery. Cessation of smoking and treatment of chest disease is important for similar reasons.

VAGINAL PESSARIES – In older women, especially those unfit for surgery, or those who have not completed their family, pessaries may be used to support the prolapsing tissue. The **ring pessary** is a plastic device which sits within the vagina behind the pubic symphysis tenting up the vagina. Careful assessment is required to ensure the correct size of pessary is inserted. The **Jessop** or **shelf pessary** resembles a coat hook with plate. It is retained better in women with a deficient perineum. Pessaries are well tolerated by many women, allowing them to avoid surgery. They tend to cause an inflammatory discharge and contact bleeding. Very rarely they cause pressure necrosis and fistula formation.

PHYSIOTHERAPY – **Pelvic floor exercises** have been involved in the prevention and improvement of incontinence for many years but they require good patient motivation. Physiotherapy may improve symptoms from a small prolapse but it is unlikely to help with more severe degrees of herniation.

DRUG THERAPY – **Hormone replacement therapy** may improve tissue quality by increasing collagen content. It is unlikely to rectify any existing prolapse. It is hoped that HRT will prevent further deterioration and improve the outcome of surgery, but these are not yet proven. Treatment of constipation may lead to a complete resolution of symptoms in women with a small rectocoele.

SURGERY – Numerous surgical procedures have been described for the correction of genitourinary prolapse. Both abdominal and vaginal are used depending on the site and severity of any prolapse, and on the presence or absence of incontinence. **Anterior and posterior colporrhaphy** (anterior and posterior vaginal repair) with or without vaginal hysterectomy is the most commonly performed primary procedure for prolapse alone. It is used for anterior and/or posterior vaginal wall prolapse where excess skin is removed and buttressing sutures are placed to support the vaginal walls. A **hysterectomy** is usually performed if there is marked uterine descent. Colporrhaphy has good early results but it may lead to excessive vaginal tightening and shortening which may lead to coital problems. There is also a chance of voiding problems and of urinary incontinence developing. The recurrence rate is moderately high, particularly in elderly women with severe atrophy. **Vault (enterocele) repair** is a more difficult procedure, as the herniated sac, containing bowel, has to be closed and there is a lack of tissue to provide support for the vault. More surgeons now attempt to attach the top of the vault to the sacrospinous ligament (sacrospinous colpopexy). Abdominal procedures for vault prolapse include **Yate's colposacropexy** – a synthetic non-absorbable mesh is attached to the vaginal vault and slung across the pelvis to the sacrum (Figure 12.2). **The**

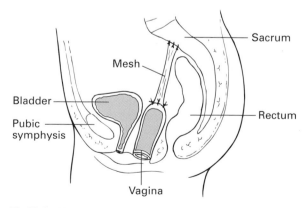

Fig 12.2 *Vaginal support surgery (colposacropexy).*

Burch colposuspension is an abdominal procedure primarily intended for women with genuine stress incontinence (see Chapter 11). It elevates the bladder neck but in doing so it corrects anterior wall prolapse at the same time.

OVERVIEW – Many elderly women are satisfactorily treated with pessaries, but for young women with a completed family, surgery offers the best solution. Prolapse is not life-threatening, however, and surgery is not without risk of vaginal stenosis and the development of urinary symptoms. The future lies in primary prevention of vaginal prolapse.

Information for the Patient
It is important to discuss the possibility of urinary dysfunction and sexual problems after surgery.

Follow-up
SHORT TERM – Review in outpatients at 3 months to assess any immediate recurrence and look for vaginal adhesions which may need dividing. Vaginal narrowing may be improved by vaginal dilators and oestrogen creams.

2. Rectal Prolapse

Brief Background
This requires management by a general surgeon.

GOLDEN POINTS

1. Procidentia requires urgent referral to avoid urinary retention and ureteric obstruction.

2. Pelvic tumours may precipitate prolapse.

3. If the woman is sexually active, discuss the possible effects of surgery on intercourse.

4. Ring and shelf pessaries will provide good control for many very elderly women.

5. Topical oestrogen therapy may alleviate associated problems such as traumatic ulceration. Systemic oestrogen therapy may also help prevent the loss of pelvic floor collagen, but this requires further study.

6. Surgery is the mainstay of treatment in younger women.

13 Vulval irritation

CLINICAL SIGNIFICANCE

Vulval irritation occurs in women of all ages, but the prevalence rises rapidly beyond 50 years. It rarely reflects serious disease, but it is an important condition because of the effect on sleep and sexual function.

In a small proportion of cases, vulval irritation is a feature of premalignant disease. Even more rarely, it may be the only outward sign of a systemic disorder such as diabetes, hepatic disease or renal failure.

DIFFERENTIAL DIAGNOSIS

MAIN CATEGORY	DIAGNOSIS
1. *Infection*	Fungal (Candida, Tinea cruris)
	Parasitic infestation (scabies, threadworm)
	Viral (herpes, wart virus)
	STDs (gonorrhoea, trichomoniasis)
2. *Intrinsic skin disease*	Lichen sclerosis
	Squamous cell hyperplasia
	Allergic or irritant dermatitis
	Atrophic changes (menopausal)
	Glandular/cystic swelling (Bartholin's)
3. *Premalignant disease*	Vulval intraepithelial neoplasia (VIN)
4. *Malignant disease*	Vulval carcinoma
	Melanoma
5. *Miscellaneous*	Trauma (scratching)
	Foreign body

The commonest conditions are lichen sclerosis and candidal infection. Malignancy is rare, but a careful examination for this should be undertaken in all women.

CLINICAL ASSESSMENT

Due to the embarrassing nature of this condition women often delay seeing their GP. The initial approach should be sympathetic. The vulva must always be examined since suspicious lesions require urgent referral. If there are no suspicious lesions seen, and simple dermatitis is suspected, the GP can start appropriate treatment and refer if unsuccessful.

Relevant History

Presenting Complaint
MAIN SYMPTOM – **Pruritus** (itchiness) is commonly described. Infection or other dermatitis usually present after a relatively short period of time. The women have often changed soap, detergent or perfume, with the irritation starting afterwards when allergic dermatitis is likely.

COMMONLY ASSOCIATED SYMPTOMS – **Vaginal discharge** may also be present; infection or malignancy tend to produce offensive loss, with dermatological conditions being inoffensive. Blood-stained discharge should be treated suspiciously, especially in older women. Swelling may be due to tumour, ulceration, gland enlargement or even genital prolapse. **Vulval pain/burning** (vulvodynia) is a related symptom but thought to be a psychological disorder. It does not often resolve with treatment.

EFFECT ON THE WOMAN – Protracted symptoms may lead to sleep deprivation and sometimes depression.

Gynaecological History
GYNAECOLOGICAL DISEASE – Previous infections or

vulvovaginal disease, especially premalignant or malignant lesions, and especially if treatment was required. Sexually transmitted diseases, especially warts, have a close association with premalignant and malignant diseases of the vulva.

MENSTRUAL HISTORY – Atrophic changes are common in postmenopausal women, when the risk of malignancy is also greater.

CERVICAL CYTOLOGY – CIN and premalignant disease of the vulva have common aetiological factors.

CONTRACEPTION – Allergies to spermicides/condoms may cause intense vulval irritation.

Medical History

MEDICAL CONDITIONS – Diabetes, hepatic and renal disease all may manifest themselves as vulval disease, especially irritation. The woman may have a generalised skin disease.

PSYCHOLOGICAL DISORDERS – Women with depressive disorders are more likely to present with vulval pain (vulvodynia).

ALLERGIES – Allergic reactions are common causes of vulval irritation, especially to soaps, detergents, washing powder and rubber.

Drug History

MEDICATIONS – A recent course of antibiotics may have led to a fungal infestation.

Social History

AGE – About 80% of cases of vulval carcinoma are in women over the age of 65. Under the age of 40, malignancy is rare, with benign dermatological and depressive conditions more common.

LIFESTYLE – Poor hygiene, particularly with faecal soiling, may lead to skin irritation or infection. Conversely, excessive hygiene may remove natural oils, causing rubbing and irritation.

Relevant Clinical Examination

General Examination

GENERAL CONDITION – The woman may appear to be in severe discomfort and have trouble sitting in the chair. The appearance and standard of hygiene should be assessed. Examine for evidence of generalised skin disorders.

BODY-MASS INDEX – Malignant disease of the vulva tends to be localised, and weight loss would be a late and very ominous sign.

LYMPH NODES – The inguinal and femoral lymph nodes drain the vulval region, with midline structures draining to both sides.

Pelvic

PERINEUM/VULVA – **Discharge** – the nature of the discharge is important with offensive loss being suggestive of malignancy or infection, and non-offensive suggesting allergy or atrophy. **Bleeding** – special attention should be paid to areas of contact bleeding. **Rashes** – the vulva, perineum and anal margin should be inspected for redness, warts or ulceration although lesions may be masked by scratch marks or other trauma. **Atrophic changes** make the skin look dry and thin. Thickened white skin (leukoplakia) is typical of lichen sclerosis, and several other conditions, but requires biopsy to exclude underlying malignancy. **Vulval swelling** is commonly due to the Bartholin's gland, which may become inflamed and infected. Ulceration may be due to malignancy or viral infection (herpes). Typically, malignant lesions will be hard and irregular with everted edges. There may be bleeding or secondary infection. Suspicious areas should be biopsied.

VAGINA/CERVIX – Should also be assessed for similar signs.

BIMANUAL EXAMINATION – The vulva may be extremely red and painful, making examination difficult.

Relevant Initial Investigations

Haematology

SERUM VITAMIN B12– There is an association between lichen sclerosis and pernicious anaemia.

Biochemistry

U+ES AND LFIS – May reveal a systemic cause for pruritus.

Endocrine Tests

THYROID FUNCTION – There is an association between lichen sclerosis and autoimmune thyroid disease.

Microbiology

BACTERIOLOGY – Vaginal swabs should be taken for bacterial and fungal microscopy and culture.

PARASITOLOGY – Evidence should be sought for threadworm infestation in young girls with pruritus.

Cytology

CERVICAL – Smear should be taken if one is due.

Histopathology

VULVAL – Areas of ulceration or other suspicious features should be biopsied, as they may conceal a malignant or premalignant condition. These can be performed using local anaesthetic.

DETAILS OF COMMON CONDITIONS

1. Lichen Sclerosis et Atrophicus

Background
DEFINITION – Thinning of the epidermis with atrophy and scarring.

AETIOLOGY – The cause is unknown but it is associated with autoimmune disorders, especially with thyroid disease, diabetes, pernicious anaemia and primary biliary cirrhosis. The skin of the vulva and perianal area becomes thinned with white plaques developing. The hypertrophic patches may coalesce, and the skin has a tendency to develop superficial ulcers.

MAKING THE DIAGNOSIS – Histology of vulval biopsy.

MAIN COMPLICATIONS – **Pruritus** is the commonest symptom, but some women complain of **dysuria** and others are troubled more by pain with intercourse. Symptoms tend to relapse and remit.

SCREENING/PREVENTION – None known.

Treatment Options
ADVICE – It is important to explain that the condition is seldom cured but that cancer is an unusual occurrence. Explain that symptoms tend to come and go from time to time. They should be advised to report any hard areas or deep ulcers.

CHANGE OF LIFESTYLE/DIET – Careful hygiene and avoidance of irritant soaps may help ease some symptoms. Women should be advised about the problems of overwashing, and also about not letting the vulval skin become too warm. Ice packs may help during the night when symptoms are sometimes at their worst.

DRUG THERAPY – If symptoms are mild, an aqueous cream should be used. Severe lesions should be treated with high-potency steroid creams with a reducing-dose regimen. There is some evidence that 2% testosterone cream may be helpful in women with a very atrophic skin. Mild sedatives at night may help improve sleep and prevent scratching during sleep.

SURGERY – Laser ablation has been used for very severe symptoms but it can be disfiguring, and symptoms often recur with time.

OVERVIEW – Self-care of the vulval skin is very important. Intermittent courses of corticosteroid creams are the mainstay of pharmacological treatment.

Follow-up
LONG TERM – Some clinicians advise yearly review to inspect the vulva for early malignancy.

2. Squamous Cell Hyperplasia

Background
DEFINITION – **Hyperplasia** and **irregular thickening** of the epidermis with associated **hyperkeratosis** and chronic inflammatory cell infiltration in the absence of atypia.

AETIOLOGY – Unknown.

MAKING THE DIAGNOSIS – The diagnosis is suspected when no other cause is evident for the irritation and histology shows squamous cell hyperplasia.

MAIN COMPLICATIONS – The labia, clitoris and interlabial sulcus are common sites for the typical white plaques. May get secondary infection because of excoriation.

PROGNOSIS – In the absence of atypia, the risk of malignancy is very small. The pruritus may pursue a chronic course.

Treatment Options
As with lichen sclerosis.

3. Vulval Intraepithelial Neoplasia (VIN)

Background
DEFINITION – Atypical hyperplasia of **squamous cells** in the vulval epithelium which may involve the full thickness of the epidermis but without evidence of stromal invasion. Atypical **glandular** cell growth is known as **Paget's disease**, with a 30% chance of underlying adenocarcinoma.

AETIOLOGY – The aetiology is poorly defined but the human papilloma virus is probably involved.

MAKING THE DIAGNOSIS – Histology of vulval biopsy. Extent of disease can be defined using colposcopy. These lesions are usually raised and either white, due to hyperkeratosis, or red due to thinning.

MAIN COMPLICATIONS – Often presents with **pruritus** although up to 40% are asymptomatic.

SCREENING/PREVENTION – Up to 25% of cases are associated with CIN, but there is no routine assessment of the vulva at present.

Treatment Options
ADVICE – The rate of progression of VIN to carcinoma is low. Attempts should be made to reassure the woman that therapy is not always necessary and follow-up with colposcopy may be preferable.

SURGERY – Surgical excision has been the mainstay of treatment, but more recently laser ablation has proved very successful.

OVERVIEW – In younger women the treatment should be as conservative as possible, as both excision and laser ablation may lead to scarring and permanent vulval pain.

Follow-up

SHORT TERM – Initially 6-monthly follow-up with colposcopy to assess the vulva for any change or recurrence.

LONG TERM – Annual colposcopy should be performed while the abnormal areas still exist.

4. Vulval Cancer

Background

DEFINITION – Epithelial cancer of the vulva. The majority (85%) are squamous. About 10% are adenocarcinomas and 5% are melanomas.

AETIOLOGY – There is an association with cigarette smoking and HPV types 16 and 18 (compare with cervical cancer).

MAKING THE DIAGNOSIS – Histology of vulval biopsy.

MAIN COMPLICATIONS – The tumour may become secondarily infected. The primary tumour is usually confined to the vulva but direct spread may occur to the urethra and anus. Lymphatic spread is common through the pelvic lymphatic chain. Rarely, inguinal lymph node deposits erode into the femoral artery.

PROGNOSIS – Without groin node involvement the 5 year survival is over 70%. With positive groin inguinal nodes the 5 year survival drops below 50% (See Table 13.1). Melanoma carries a worse prognosis of 10% if positive nodes are found.

STAGING – See Table 13.2.

ADDITIONAL TESTS – **Plain radiology** – a chest x-ray to exclude metastases prior to surgery. **Colposcopy** – the cervix and vagina should be examined for evidence of CIN and VaIN. **Standard preoperative blood tests**.

Treatment Options

SURGERY – Surgery is the first line of treatment, with radical excision and inguinal groin node dissection on the affected side. Due to the interconnecting lymphatic drainage, bilateral node dissection is necessary for midline lesions.

RADIOTHERAPY – For follow-up treatment for women with positive lymph nodes. It also has a place for palliation of advanced disease.

OVERVIEW – Surgery is the mainstay of treatment, but it is disfiguring, leading to severe psychological problems particularly in younger women.

Follow-up

SHORT TERM – Examination for local recurrence. Psychological support is essential because the surgery is disfiguring. Wound breakdown is common, and a build up of lymph (lymphoedema) may lead to leg swelling.

Table 13.1   5 year survival rates for vulval carcinoma

Stage	5 year survival (%)
1	100
2	83
3	43
4	30

Table 13.2   FIGO staging of vulval cancer

Stage	
Stage 1	Confined to the vulva/perineum. Lesion ≤ 2 cm. No groin nodes palpable
Stage 2	Confined to vulva/perineum. Lesion > 2 cm. No nodes palpable
Stage 3	Extends beyond vulva/vagina. Unilateral node metastases
Stage 4a	Involvement of mucosa of rectum or bladder, upper urethra or bone Bilateral node enlargement
4b	Distant metastases including pelvic nodes

Physiotherapy is important to maintain mobility after radical surgery.

LONG TERM – For 5 years to detect recurrent disease. Early local recurrences may be treated by wide local resection or radiotherapy.

5. Bartholin's Cyst

Background

DEFINITION – A cyst arising from the duct of Bartholin's gland (Figure 13.1) which lies subcutaneously in the lower third of the labia majorum.

AETIOLOGY – Usually caused by blockage of the Bartholin's duct.

MAIN COMPLICATIONS – The cyst can become tense and infected, leading to an extremely **painful swelling** preventing sitting and usually requiring acute admission. Infection leads to abscess formation and pointing. They should be differentiated from cysts of the duct of Skene's and the vestibular gland which are higher up. Sometimes associated with gonococcal infection and may be bilateral.

Treatment Options

REASSURANCE – Providing the cysts are not infected or tender, the woman can be reassured that they usually settle. If an abscess has burst and drained it is best treated with antibiotics.

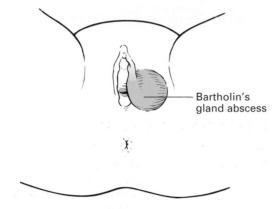

Bartholin's gland abscess

Fig 13.1 *Bartholin's abscess.*

DRUG THERAPY – **Staphylococcus** and **gram-negative bacilli** are commonly to blame, and inflamed cysts should be treated with the appropriate antibiotics.

SURGERY – Large painful pointing abscesses that are not responding to antibiotics should be incised and have the edges sown out (marsupialisation).

OVERVIEW – It is best to treat conservatively if possible, but occasionally the gland has to be excised; this is best performed as a routine operation. If the problem recurs frequently the cyst can be excised.

6. Allergic Dermatitis

Brief Background
Skin inflammation secondary to immune reaction to foreign material. Most cases are caused by detergents, soaps, perfumes or condoms.

Main Complications
Chronic irritation may lead to protracted scratching with thickening of the skin (lichenification) and ulceration. Secondary infection is not uncommon, which itself may lead to yet more inflammation and irritation.

Prevention
Avoidance of allergens (soaps and perfumes).

Treatment
Identification and avoidance of allergen. A short course of a mild corticosteroid or antibiotic cream may be needed to allow the inflammatory process to subside and break the vicious cycle. Removal of the allergen/irritant or treatment of secondary infection is usually all that is required. A mild hydrocortisone cream may be necessary initially.

7. Vulvovaginal Infections

See Chapter 14.

GOLDEN POINTS

1. Always inspect the vulva carefully for evidence of small tumours and ulcers.

2. Hyperkeratosis (leukoplakia) may obscure malignant lesions.

3. Consider possibility of systemic diseases.

4. Allergy and infection are common and easily treated.

5. Simple measures such as avoiding thick underwear, overwashing and use of cosmetics may be very effective for some women.

6. High-potency steroid creams are the mainstay of treatment for exacerbations in women with intractable vulval dystrophies.

7. Vulval cancer is a rare tumour and medical care should be undertaken in regional centres.

14 Vaginal discharge

CLINICAL SIGNIFICANCE

Vaginal discharge is one of the commonest gynaecological complaints seen in general practice. In gynaecology outpatients it is involved in up to one third of referrals.

Physiological discharge and vaginal infection account for the majority of cases, but discharge will occasionally be the first symptom of genital tract malignancy.

Vaginal fluid consists of contributions from cervical mucus, secretions from Skene's and Bartholin's gland and transudate from the vaginal vault. The vaginal fluid becomes acidic after puberty as the rising oestrogen levels increase the glycogen content of the squamous cells. Lactobacillus, a normal vaginal commensal, converts the glycogen to lactic acid. The resulting acidic vaginal fluid is said to prevent the growth of other organisms and so provide a defence against ascending infection. The squamous epithelium, apposition of the vaginal walls, and bactericidal effects of the cervical mucus are also thought to act as barriers to infection.

DIFFERENTIAL DIAGNOSIS

MAIN CATEGORY	DIAGNOSIS
1. *Physiological*	Idiopathic Pregnancy (Combined contraceptive pill)
2. *Infection*	Bacterial vaginosis Candida spp. Trichomonas vaginalis Chlamydia trachomatis Other sexually transmitted infections
3. *Atrophy*	Postmenopausal vaginitis
4. *Tumours*	Cervical polyp Intrauterine polyp Pedunculated fibroid Cervical cancer Endometrial cancer
5. *Fistulae*	Vesicovaginal fistula Rectovaginal fistula
6. *Sexual problems*	Psychosexual upset Sexual abuse (in girls)
7. *Miscellaneous*	Vaginal foreign body Intrauterine device Allergy (rare)
8. *Spurious*	Urinary incontinence Faecal incontinence

CLINICAL ASSESSMENT

Initial assessment of women with vaginal discharge should be by the GP. Women with proven sexually transmitted diseases (STDs) should be advised to attend a special STD clinic. Chronic or non-infectious discharge should be referred to a gynaecologist.

Relevant History

Presenting Complaint

MAIN SYMPTOM – **Discharge**. A non offensive clear discharge which is related to the menstrual cycle is most likely physiological. Offensive coloured discharges associated with vulval irritation or urinary symptoms are usually associated with infective causes. If the woman's normal discharge has increased recently, the possibility of pregnancy must be considered. There is an increase in alkalinity of the vaginal secretions, around menses and during pregnancy, which increases the risk of infection.

COMMONLY ASSOCIATED SYMPTOMS – **Pelvic pain** and **deep dyspareunia** are suggestive of upper genital tract infection. **Superficial dyspareunia** is suggestive of vaginitis. **Menstrual disturbance** may accompany both upper genital tract infection and tumours.

EFFECT ON PATIENT – Physiological discharge when heavy can make the woman feel unclean and be associated with loss of confidence. STDs can lead to psychosexual problems and marital discord, particularly in monogamous women.

Gynaecological History

GYNAECOLOGICAL DISEASE – A history of previous infection increases the likelihood of an infective cause. There is no benefit to be gained by asking about the number of previous partners. Such questioning will not alter management and it may lead to the woman being upset.

CERVICAL CYTOLOGY – Women with a history of STD have an increased chance of cervical neoplasia. Presentation with vaginal discharge is an opportunity to take a cervical smear for cytology.

CONTRACEPTION – Oestrogen-containing contraceptive pills raise the alkalinity of the vaginal secretions, thus reducing the protective effect of the acidic vagina. Barrier methods can set up an allergic reaction and an inflammatory discharge. Condoms give some protection against STDs but this is not absolute. Low-lying IUCDs may induce an inflammatory response in the cervix.

FERTILITY REQUIREMENTS – If the family is not completed and chronic infection is suspected, there is a high risk of tubal damage leading to subfertility. This will be relevant if STDs are found. Careful advice should then be given about the risk of ectopic pregnancy and also about contraception (avoid IUCDs).

Obstetric History

DELIVERY – A recent delivery, miscarriage or termination may be complicated by upper genital tract infection. In addition, some women appear to experience an increase in the physiological discharge after term delivery. This may reflect a change in the cervical ectropion.

Medical History

MEDICAL CONDITIONS – Diabetes mellitus is a predisposing factor for recurrent vaginal infection, especially Candida spp.

SURGERY – Recent vaginal surgery may have caused infection or fistula formation. Normal healing produces a white discharge.

ALLERGIES – Reaction to soaps or perfumes is a rare cause of vaginal discharge.

Drug History

MEDICATIONS – Recent antibiotics, by altering the vaginal flora, and corticosteroids, by causing immunosuppression, may lead to an overgrowth of Candida spp.

Social History

AGE – Before the menarche and after the menopause low levels of oestrogen reduce the acidity in the vagina, making the women more susceptible to infection. If the discharge has been present since puberty, infection is unlikely.

LIFESTYLE – Excessive vaginal douching and washing with perfumed soaps may alter the vaginal flora and lead to an overgrowth of unusual organisms such as Gardnerella vaginalis or Candida spp.

Relevant Clinical Examination

General Examination

GENERAL CONDITION – Look for signs of anaemia and systemic infection.

BODY-MASS INDEX – Obesity may make hygiene difficult and it may be associated with occult diabetes.

Abdomen

TENDERNESS – Lower quadrant tenderness which may indicate upper tract infection.

MASSES – A pelvic mass may indicate an abscess or ovarian tumour.

Pelvic

PERINEUM/VULVA/VAGINA – Inspected for the discharge noting its nature, colour, consistency and smell. Any warts or inflammation should also be identified. The urethra can be milked to release discharge if sexually transmitted disease is suspected. Vaginal atrophy may be seen in menopausal women.

CERVIX – Warts, ulcers or foreign bodies (including retained tampon). The cervix may shows signs of inflammation or of an ectropion (Figure 14.1) and endocervical or endometrial polyps may be seen protruding from the os.

BIMANUAL EXAMINATION – Bimanual examination will elicit any cervical excitation or adnexal tenderness suggestive of pelvic infection.

Initial Clinical Investigations

Microbiology

LITMUS TESTING – This determines the acidity of the

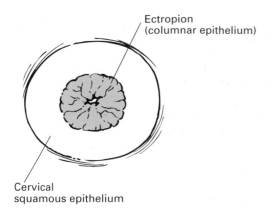

Ectropion
(columnar epithelium)

Cervical
squamous epithelium

Fig 14.1   *Cervical ectropion.*

vagina. A pH of 5 or more is relatively alkaline for the vagina and is very suggestive of bacterial vaginosis or trichomonas infection.

AMINE TEST – Two drops of 10% potassium hydroxide are placed on a slide made from the vaginal discharge. A fishy odour is suggestive of bacterial vaginosis. The potassium also destroys epithelial and white cells, allowing the pseudospores and hyphae of Candida to be seen.

MICROSCOPY OF WET SMEAR – Normal saline is run onto the slide which is then viewed under low-power microscopy revealing the flagellated mobile trichomonates. The presence of 'Clue cells' indicates bacterial vaginosis (see Figure 14.2). The spirochaetes of syphilis can be seen on dark ground illumination. **Gram staining** will help demonstrate the gram-negative diplococci of gonorrhoea.

BACTERIAL CULTURE – **High vaginal swab (HVS)**, transported in Stuart's medium, will allow microscopy and culture. It can be used to detect Candida, Trichomonas, bacterial vaginosis (BV). The standard HVS is poor for detecting gonnococcus and **endocervical, urethral** and **anal swabs** should be sent for gonnococcal culture. A special endocervical swab should be sent for **Chlamydia ELISA**. Swabs can also be sent for **viral culture** if herpes simplex is suspected.

Cytology

CERVICAL – The opportunity should be taken to do a cervical smear if one is due.

DETAILS OF COMMON CONDITIONS

1. Physiological Discharge and Cervical Ectropion

Background

DEFINITION – Vaginal discharge for which no causative agent has been identified.

AETIOLOGY – An increase in volume of the normal vaginal fluid is called leucorrhoea. It is usually odourless and clear without vaginal irritation. It may cause slight staining of underwear. Vaginal fluid is made up of contributions from cervical mucus, secretions from Skene's and Bartholin's gland and transudate from the vaginal vault. There is an increase in vaginal secretions around ovulation, associated with thinning of the cervical mucus, causing a clear and watery discharge. Some women may not realise that sexual excitement also leads to a large increase in vaginal secretions from the glands of the vestibule. An increase in oestrogen, such as in pregnancy or with the oral contraceptive pill, causes the columnar epithelium, which is normally confined to the endocervix, to grow out onto the cervix (ectropion).

DIAGNOSIS – It is a diagnosis of exclusion.

MAIN COMPLICATIONS – Chronic heavy vaginal discharge is an inconvenience for some women and may also cause psychological distress for others.

SCREENING/PREVENTION – Not relevant.

Treatment Options

ADVICE – With physiological discharges reassurance and an explanation are usually all that is required.

CHANGE OF LIFESTYLE/DIET – Advise against vaginal douching and encourage daily washing with mild soap and water.

SURGERY – Some clinicians attempt to ameliorate the discharge by applying cryocautery to any cervical ectropion but there is no evidence that this is a beneficial therapy. Moreover, it is initially associated with an increase in the volume of discharge as the cervix heals. This treatment also tends to reinforce any belief the woman has that her discharge is abnormal. Finally, the ectropion often returns within 1 year.

OVERVIEW – Medication and surgery do not play any part in treatment and are likely to make the problem worse.

Follow-up

SHORT TERM – Once pathology has been excluded care can pass back to the GP.

2. Bacterial Vaginosis

Background

DEFINITION – Bacterial vaginosis (BV) is a complex alteration in the vaginal flora with an overgrowth of anaerobic bacteria such as Gardnerella vaginalis. It is accompanied by a reduction in concentration of lactobacilli. It is not an infection but simply abnormal colonisation.

AETIOLOGY – The exact cause is not understood because the offending organism is a natural commensal of the female genital tract. There is an alteration in the normal flora, bringing about this proliferation of Gardnerella. It is associated with low social class, smoking and multiple sexual partners. Recent studies have shown that it has a prevalence of around 15% in antenatal clinics in this country; the majority of such women are asymptomatic. There is an increased prevalence in women attending termination clinics (nearly 30%). It may be discovered to play an important role in other processes such as preterm rupture of membranes and preterm labour. Emphasis should be placed on the fact that they are normal commensals but just present in a higher concentration than normal and not necessarily sexually transmitted.

MAKING THE DIAGNOSIS – See Table 14.1.

MAIN COMPLICATIONS – The **copious discharge** can lead to psychological distress and even interference with intercourse. It has been shown to play an important role in causing preterm labour and preterm rupture of membranes.

SCREENING/PREVENTION – As yet screening does not take place routinely for BV. Routine screening programmes in pregnancy are being evaluated.

Treatment Options

ADVICE – As the majority of women are asymptomatic, medical treatment is unnecessary unless it is associated with problems.

CHANGE OF LIFESTYLE/DIET – Avoidance of vaginal douches that may alter the vaginal acidity and allow a change in the natural vaginal flora.

DRUG THERAPY – Treat symptomatic women only, with either **oral metronidazole** or **topical clindamycin** cream. Metronidazole can be given as a single oral dose

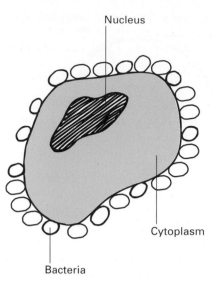

Fig 14.2 *Clue cell associated with bacterial vaginosis.*

of 2 g, or in recurrent cases 400 mg twice a day. Clindamycin cream once a day for 7 days is also effective and has fewer side effects. The colonisation tends to recur, particularly around the time of menstruation, and repeated courses of antibiotics are often needed. There is no evidence that treating the partner is of any value.

OVERVIEW – This is not infection but simply abnormal colonisation. Outside of pregnancy, treatment is only necessary if the woman is symptomatic.

Follow-up

SHORT TERM – Single-dose therapy is very effective. Recurrence is quite common but should only be treated if symptoms return.

LONG TERM – None necessary.

3. Candidal Infection

Background

DEFINITION – This is an overgrowth of Candida, a commensal of the gastrointestinal tract. Candida is a fungus; the commonest strain is Candida albicans (95%).

AETIOLOGY – Recent theories indicate that it is associated with raised concentration of oestrogen, which explains its increase premenstrually, during pregnancy and in women using oestrogen implants. The combined oral contraceptive pill has been associated with candidal infection but the new low-dose pills may be less of a problem. Any alteration in the immune system, such as that resulting from corticosteroid and immuno-supressive therapies or diabetes, increases the risk of a

Table 14.1	Diagnosing bacterial vaginosis
Making the diagnosis	Bacterial vaginosis
History	Heavy vaginal discharge
Examination	Greyish odourless discharge
Investigations	
– Litmus test	Alkaline pH (5 or more)
– Fish amine test	Positive
– Microscopy	Clue cells (squamous cells surrounded by bacteria) (see Figure 14.2)
– Microbiology	Excess of anaerobic bacilli (lactobacillus)

Candida infection. Antibiotics may also allow an over-growth of Candida.

MAKING THE DIAGNOSIS – Suspicion raised by symptoms of itching associated with white creamy discharge. Confirmed by microscopy and culture from high vaginal swab.

MAKING THE DIAGNOSIS – Vulval irritation associated with a thick, white, non-offensive discharge. The main complications are associated with the newer strains of Candida that are becoming resistant to therapy, increasing the incidence of **recurrent vulvovaginal candidiasis**.

SCREENING/PREVENTION – Women who are prone to vaginal candidiasis should be given prophylactic clotrimazole pessaries during antibiotic therapy.

Treatment Options

REASSURANCE – The woman should be reassured that candida is a common infection. Candida infections are not sexually transmitted and do not cause cancer or tubal infertility.

CHANGE OF LIFESTYLE/DIET – Improved hygiene with avoidance of tights and nylon underwear may help to prevent recurrent or chronic infection.

DRUG THERAPY – Topical antifungal therapy with a single dose of clotrimazole (500 mg vaginal pessary) is the treatment of choice. Recurrent infections may be treated monthly by inserting clotrimazole pessaries once a month after menstruation. Chronic vaginal candidiasis can be treated with oral antifungal agents such as fluconazole (150 mg monthly). There is no evidence that treatment of an asymptomatic partner is beneficial.

Follow-up

SHORT TERM – Single dose therapy is very effective, and the GP should only repeat swabs if symptoms return.

LONG TERM – None necessary if symptoms do not return.

4. Trichomonas vaginalis

Background

DEFINITION – A flagellated protozoan.

AETIOLOGY – Trichomonas vaginalis is spread by sexual transmission and is often cultured along with Neisseria gonorrhoea.

MAKING THE DIAGNOSIS – History of vulval irritation associated with watery discharged. Suspicion confirmed with microscopy and culture from high vaginal swab.

MAIN COMPLICATIONS – **Vulvovaginal irritation** and occasionally **dyspareunia** are the main problems. It is associated with other pathogens which may cause upper genital tract infection but Trichomonas causes no long-term sequelae itself.

SCREENING/PREVENTION – Screened for in STD clinics. Spread prevented by safe sex techniques. It is important to see and treat the partner(s).

Treatment Options

ADVICE – Trichomonas responds well to treatment and providing it is not associated with other infections there are no long-term sequelae.

DRUG THERAPY – This is best treated with oral metronidazole. A single 2 g oral dose is effective.

Follow-up

SHORT TERM – If other sexually transmitted diseases are suspected the patients should be seen at the special clinic. Recurrent infection is common, and a repeat assessment should be made 3 months later.

LONG TERM – Not relevant.

5. Neisseria Gonorrhoea

Background

DEFINITION – Neisseria gonorrhoea is a gram-negative diplococcus that thrives on the columnar epithelium of the urethra, cervix and Bartholin's gland.

AETIOLOGY – Transmitted by sexual intercourse. It is often masked by the presence of Trichomonas.

MAKING THE DIAGNOSIS – See Table 14.2.

MAIN COMPLICATIONS – **Vaginal discharge, vulval pain** with associated **urinary symptoms** (dysuria and urinary frequency). Passed by sexual contact, it may

Table 14.2	Diagnosing gonorrhoea
Making the diagnosis	Neisseria gonorrhoea
History	Vaginal discharge
	Vulval pain
	Associated urinary symptoms (frequency and burning)
Examination	Purulent greenish discharge from urethra and cervix
Investigations	
– Microscopy	Gram stain reveals the intracellular gram-negative diplococci
– Microbiology	Swabs taken from the endocervix, urethra and rectum are transported on Stuart's medium and cultured on Thayer–Martin plates

pursue a chronic course with salpingitis and tubal infertility and infection and blockage of Bartholin's glands. Occasionally, there may be septicaemia and pyoarthritis. If present at the time of delivery, the neonate may develop a severe ophthalmitis.

SCREENING/PREVENTION – Spread prevented by safe sex techniques. It is important to see and treat the partner(s).

Treatment Options

ADVICE – Treatment is effective. Patient is to report return of symptoms. There is a risk of tubal infertility and ectopic pregnancy.

DRUG THERAPY – A variety of treatment options are needed because of penicillin resistance and penicillin allergy. Probenecid 2 g orally with either 2.4 mega units of procaine penicillin intramuscularly or 3 g of ampicillin orally is the preferred treatment. Women with penicillin allergy or an organism resistant to penicillin should be given erythromycin.

Follow-up

SHORT TERM – Should be reviewed at the special clinic along with partner.

LONG TERM – Not relevant.

6. Atrophic Vaginitis

See Chapter 9.

GOLDEN POINTS

1. Many women complaining of discharge simply have physiological leucorrhoea.

2. Consider carefully possibility of neoplastic causes.

3. Screen thoroughly for sexually transmitted diseases and arrange contact tracing if positive.

4. Bacterial vaginosis can be missed with conventional bacteriology swabs.

5. Certain vaginal infections may increase chance of preterm labour.

6. If prescribing antibiotics to women on the contraceptive pill, advise extra precautions for that cycle.

15 Acute pelvic pain

CLINICAL SIGNIFICANCE

After early pregnancy problems, acute pelvic pain is probably the commonest reason for emergency gynaecological admission. Often there is a non-gynaecological problem or no cause is identified, but serious gynaecological causes include pelvic inflammatory disease, torsion of ovarian cyst, and ectopic pregnancy. All of these may lead to serious long-term complications if treatment is not instituted promptly.

DIFFERENTIAL DIAGNOSIS

MAIN CATEGORY	DIAGNOSIS
Gynaecological	
1. *Pregnancy related*	Ectopic
	Miscarriage
	Fibroid degencration
	Incarcerated uterus
2. *Ovarian*	Cyst accident (torsion, rupture, etc.)
	Ovarian hyperstimulation syndrome
3. *Infection*	Pelvic inflammatory disease
4. *Tumour*	Benign
	Malignant
5. *Physiological*	Mittelschmerz (ovulation pain)
	Heavy menstruation
Non-gynaecological	
1. *Urinary tract*	Calculus
	Acute retention
	Infection
2. *Gastrointestinal*	Appendicitis
	Inflammatory bowel disease
	Irritable bowel syndrome
	Constipation
	Diverticulitis
	Strangulated hernia

CLINICAL ASSESSMENT

These women may present straight to the hospital emergency department or after an urgent referral by their GP.

Rapid Emergency Assessment

Emergency assessment should be performed on arrival. It will be clear that most women are not severely ill, but a small proportion will be in cardiovascular shock because of hypovolaemia (ectopic pregnancy and ovarian cyst rupture) or septicaemia (PID). Intravenous access should be gained at two sites and crystalloid fluids infused rapidly. Blood should be sent for emergency cross-match, full blood count, urea and electrolytes, liver function tests and coagulation studies. Blood cultures are taken and broad-spectrum antibiotics are commenced if septicaemia is suspected. Oxygen is given by face mask. Full monitoring of pulse, blood pressure, temperature and urine output is commenced. Central venous pressure can be monitored later if necessary.

In women with pain and hypovolaemic shock, a urine pregnancy test should be undertaken immediately. If positive, ectopic pregnancy should be tested for quickly.

Relevant History

Presenting Complaint

MAIN SYMPTOM – **The speed of onset, nature and site of pain** should be elicited. Pain of rapid onset tends to indicate a mechanical problem such as cyst torsion or rupture, whereas pain of gradual onset is more likely to be due to infection, especially pelvic inflammatory disease (PID) or appendicitis. The site of the pain on the surface does not always indicate the origin of the underlying disease. Radiation of the pain to other sites occurs with peritoneal irritation. Shoulder tip pain is typical of subdiaphragmatic irritation associated with ectopic pregnancy. Radiation to the thigh is seen in women with ovarian problems. Loin pain may indicate either ureteric colic or ovarian torsion. A central pelvic pain with no radiation is typical of acute pelvic infection, but sometimes right upper quadrant pain is seen in association with chlamydial PID because of a perihepatitis (**FitzHugh–Curtis syndrome**). The nature of the pain is also sometimes helpful though often not conclusive. A sharp pain tends to suggest a cyst accident or tubal rupture, whereas a central colicky pain is more indicative of an intestinal problem or miscarriage. A constant dull ache is typical of pelvic infection.

COMMONLY ASSOCIATED SYMPTOMS – **Vaginal bleeding** or **brown discharge** following a period of amenorrhoea is suggestive of pregnancy-related problems. Traditionally, pain starting before the onset of bleeding is said to be due to an ectopic pregnancy, whereas pain which follows bleeding is more likely to be related to miscarriage.

Dyspareunia tends to be thought of as suggesting a gynaecological problem but may be a feature of bowel disease and urinary tract infection as well. **A purulent vaginal discharge** is a common feature of pelvic infection but may also rarely be seen in cases of diverticulitis with perforation through the vaginal vault.

Vomiting associated with acute pelvic pain often reflects nothing more than pain, but severe vomiting may be due to intestinal obstruction and mild vomiting is often seen in appendicitis and pelvic infection. **Diarrhoea** is common and may contain blood and mucus in cases of inflammatory bowel disease/diverticulitis. It is important to ask about recent foreign travel. **Haematuria** occurs in the presence of urinary tract infection or calculi and there may be a recent history of frequency and urgency.

Gynaecological History

MENSTRUAL HISTORY – The date of the last proper menstrual bleed should be checked in order to consider pregnancy-related causes. Ectopic pregnancy typically presents 6 to 8 weeks after the last period, but equally the period may not have been missed or may have been abnormal in some way. Discomfort midcycle may be due to ovulation (Mittelschmerz) and can occasionally be severe.

GYNAECOLOGICAL DISEASES – This may be an acute exacerbation of previous pain that the woman may have because of known endometriosis, adenomyosis or chronic pelvic infection. Recent pelvic surgery may have caused infection, haematoma or urinary tract trauma.

FERTILITY REQUIREMENTS – Women undergoing assisted conception treatment may develop multiple ovarian cysts (ovarian hyperstimulation syndrome). If surgery is performed, especially for ovarian disease, care should be taken to avoid removal of the ovaries in women who have not completed their family.

CONTRACEPTION – The IUCD increases the likelihood of acute pelvic infection and abscess formation. If the OCP is being used, extra protection will be required if antibiotics are prescribed.

Obstetric History

OBSTETRIC COMPLICATIONS – A recent traumatic or surgical delivery may have led to a pelvic collection (haematoma or abscess).

Medical History

OPERATIONS – Previous pelvic or abdominal surgery may lead to adhesions and intestinal obstruction. It is also important to take previous surgery into account when considering diagnostic laparoscopy.

MEDICAL CONDITIONS – A long history of constipation is a risk factor for diverticulitis and for volvulus. Inflammatory bowel diseases (ulcerative colitis and Crohn's disease) have a chronic course of remission and acute exacerbations. Poorly controlled sickle cell disease and diabetes may rarely present with acute pain.

PSYCHOLOGICAL DISORDERS – Munchausen's syndrome (presentation of fictitious symptoms to gain access to medical care) is not common but should be considered if the story is odd or if the woman has had multiple previous operations.

Drug History

RECREATIONAL DRUGS – Drug abusers may fake illness to gain access to opiates.

Social History

AGE – PID is very uncommon over 40 years, and diverticulitis is rare before 50 years.

LIFESTYLE – Recent foreign travel, especially to third-world countries, increases the likelihood of gastroenteritis or intestinal infestation. Pain coming on during vigorous exercise may be due to rupture of a rectus muscle.

Relevant Clinical Examination

General Examination

GENERAL CONDITION – Acute severe pain will prevent the woman from lying comfortably. She may be pale and sweating or even collapsed. A mildly raised temperature is compatible with appendicitis and PID but also ovarian cyst torsion.

BODY-MASS INDEX – Obesity can make examination difficult and surgery carries a higher risk.

LYMPH NODES – The groin lymph nodes may be enlarged with pelvic sepsis.

Abdomen

CONTOUR – Swelling may be due to an ovarian cyst, pregnancy, intestinal obstruction or an over distended bladder.

OLD SCARS – Signs of multiple abdominal or pelvic operations may indicate previous true pathology but may rarely be a sign of attention-seeking behaviour; old hospital records should be studied.

TENDERNESS – After the woman has indicated the area of maximum tenderness, the abdomen should be lightly palpated. A rigid, extremely tender abdomen (peritonism) is indicative of pelvic/abdominal infection, perforation or ischaemia. Deeper palpation is used to elicit the site of maximum pain. Rebound tenderness in the right iliac fossa is suggestive of appendicitis. Suprapubic tenderness with swelling my be due to acute urinary retention.

MASSES – Palpate for any mass which may be a pelvic tumour (ovary, fibroid, pregnancy).

HERNIAE – The hernial orifices should be examined.

BOWEL SOUNDS – Increased bowel activity, especially when associated with tinkling sounds, occurs with intestinal obstruction. Absent bowel sound occurs with paralytic ileus, which may be caused by infection and perforation.

Pelvic

VULVA/VAGINA/CERVIX – Excoriation with offensive or purulent discharge may be seen with vaginitis; it may come from the cervix in pelvic infection. Bleeding occurs with infection but it is suggestive of pregnancy-related problems such as miscarriage or ectopic pregnancy. The strings of a forgotten IUCD may be seen.

BIMANUAL EXAMINATION – This is often impossible, because of the severity of the pain, but exacerbation with moving the cervix is typical of pelvic inflammatory disease and ectopic pregnancy. Tenderness in one adnexus is suggestive of an ovarian problem.

RECTAL EXAMINATION – Severe finger tip pain in the right iliac fossa occurs with an inflamed appendix. Blood and mucus is suggestive of inflammatory bowel disease. Faecal loading may also be found with severe constipation.

Relevant Initial Investigations

Haematology

Hb – To assess acute blood loss.

WCC – Sometimes greatly elevated with severe pelvic/abdominal infection, but not always, and a differential count may be performed looking for a neutrophilic leucocytosis.

PLATELETS – May be lowered by severe infection.

SERUM – In acute cases blood should be cross-matched and saved.

Endocrine Tests

URINE β-hCG – Pregnancy must always be excluded in women of childbearing potential.

Biochemistry

SERUM U+ES/LFTS – Mainly as a baseline in severely ill women but also to look for hypokalaemia if there has been severe diarrhoea.

C-REACTIVE PROTEIN (CRP) – Raised, although not specifically, in cases of infection.

Microbiology

BACTERIAL CULTURE – **Urine** should be sent for microscopy and culture to exclude infection. **Vaginal** swabs taken from the fornix may be positive if vaginitis is present, but **endocervical, urethral and rectal swabs** are required if upper genital tract infection is suspected, e.g. Chlamydia and gonorrhoea. Pus can be sent directly to the laboratory in a sterile pot.

IUCD – May be removed and sent for culture if PID suspected.

SEROLOGY – Chlamydial antibodies should be checked and repeated; an increasing titre is seen in an acute infection.

Diagnostic Imaging

PLAIN RADIOLOGY – Haematuria, microscopic or macroscopic, requires a plain film of the renal tract to identify calculi. Intestinal obstruction may be seen with dilated loops of bowel or an intestine loaded with faeces. Gas may be seen under the diaphragm with perforation.

CONTRAST RADIOLOGY – Intravenous urogram (IVU) is also advised for undiagnosed haematuria when other investigations are normal.

ULTRASOUND – A simple safe investigation that may give a clear picture of the pelvis and abdomen. Tumours, cysts, pregnancy, fluid (blood or ascites), upper renal tract dilatation and renal calculi may all be observed.

AXIAL IMAGING – Provides very clear images but has little role to play in the management of acute pelvic pain.

Endoscopy

LAPAROSCOPY – In severe cases where the diagnosis is in doubt, laparoscopy allows a definitive diagnosis to be made, including that of some bowel conditions.

DETAILS OF COMMON CONDITIONS

1. Ectopic Pregnancy and Other Pregnancy-related Problems – See Chapter 6.

2. Acute Pelvic Inflammatory Disease (PID)

Background

DEFINITION – PID is a clinical syndrome most commonly secondary to ascending infection affecting the upper genital tract (cervix, endometrium, fallopian tubes and surrounding structures). Less commonly it may also be due to secondary spread of infection from the appendix or other parts of bowel.

AETIOLOGY – Numerous micro-organisms have been implicated in pelvic infection (see Table 15.1), with bacteria the commonest. Many infections are by multiple organisms. Other factors have been implicated in the spread of infection. The cervix acts as a barrier to ascending infection, aided by a thick cervical mucus plug. The mucus becomes thinned during ovulation and disappears with menstruation or after surgical procedures, thus allowing access to an ascending organism. The cervical mucus is thickened by progesterone, and women using the contraceptive pill have a lower

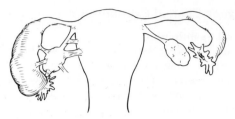

Fig 15.1 *Acute salpingitis leading to pyosalpinx.*

incidence of pelvic infection. Sexual activity, especially multiple partners, or sexually transmitted diseases are commonly associated with pelvic infection. The IUCD (a foreign body) is thought to act as a protective site for organisms, making infection more common. Strings of older IUCDs acted as a wick and allowed bacteria to pass more freely into the uterus.

MAIN COMPLICATIONS – **Acute pelvic pain** is the most common problem and may be associated with septic shock and dehydration. In severe cases the Fallopian tubes become swollen and inflamed with pus. The peritoneum becomes inflamed and adherent to pelvic organs.

Abscess formation occurs in severe disease: in the fallopian tube it is known as a pyosalpinx (Figure 15.1), and sometimes the ovary becomes involved, when it is known as a tubo-ovarian abscess. Scarring and blocking of the Fallopian tubes is common, leading to **subfertility** in nearly 15%. If the women does conceive, there is an increased chance of **ectopic pregnancy**.

Chronic pelvic pain occurs as a consequence in up to 20% of women, and some develop recurrent episodes of acute infection (chronic PID). **Septicaemia** is uncommon but may be life-threatening.

PREVENTION – The partners should be traced for screening and treatment in order to prevent reinfection and further spread. Prophylaxis at the time of surgery, particularly termination of pregnancy, reduces the incidence of postoperative pelvic infections. Barrier contraception such as the condom prevents the spread of sexually transmitted disease. The contraceptive pill has some protective effect by increasing the thickness of cervical mucus.

MAKING THE DIAGNOSIS – This is often evident from the history (see Table 15.2) but, if there is doubt, particularly if appendicitis or other bowel problems remain a strong possibility, then laparoscopy should be undertaken. Swabs for bacteriology can be taken from the Fallopian tubes at the time of the procedure.

Treatment Options

DRUG THERAPY – The first priority after initial assessment

Table 15.1	Infective agents in pelvic inflammatory disease
Organism	Problems
Neisseria gonorrhoea	Cultured in up to 40% of cases
Chlamydia trachomatis	Found in 70% of women under 25 diagnosed with PID. Potent cause of tubal damage
Bacteroides/ Peptostreptococcus	Gain access from lower genital tract and are common after previous infection
Coliforms H. influenzae	Thought to be secondary to gonococcal infection
Mycoplasma hominis Ureaplasma urealyticum	Tend to be found in younger women and lead to peritoneal inflammation rather than salpingitis

Table 15.2 Diagnosing pelvic inflammatory disease	
Making the diagnosis	Pelvic inflammatory disease
History	Acute pelvic pain
	Constant dull ache, worse with movement and intercourse
	Purulent vaginal discharge
	Hepatic tenderness (FitzHugh–Curtis syndrome)
Examination	Pyrexia is common; may be mild or severe
	Severe lower abdominal tenderness with or without rebound
	Adnexal tenderness, cervical excitation and vaginal discharge
Investigations	
– WCC	Neutrophil leucocytosis but only in minority
– Biochemistry	Raised CRP is more common
– Microbiology	Positive bacterial culture
	Positive ELISA for Chlamydia
– Ultrasound	May show abcess (ill-defined mass of mixed echogenicity) or pyosalpinx
– Laparoscopy	Reddening or swelling of the Fallopian tubes with pus and abscess formation.
	Appendix will look normal.

is to provide analgesia, bedrest, intravenous fluids and broad-spectrum antibiotic therapy. **Opiates** such as morphine together with an **NSAID** will be required initially in severe cases. **Antibiotics** should be started before the results of microbial culture are available. Long-term therapy is necessary to eradicate Chlamydia. The route of administration depends on the severity of the infection. If the woman is hospitalised with severe infection, particularly with a pelvic abscess, **intravenous therapy** is recommended until the temperature drops below 38°C. **Ciprofloxacin** and **metronidazole** is a good combination. If the infection is mild, outpatient treatment with oral ciprofloxacin and metronidazole may be satisfactory. 10 days of treatment is recommended.

SURGERY – The diagnosis can be difficult to make, and if a diagnostic laparoscopy is performed, abcesses can be drained and the peritoneum can be lavaged. Most cases will then settle with antibiotic therapy. Some women do require laparotomy if the pain and fever do not improve within a few days. The advantage of avoiding laparotomy initially is that any surgery can be extremely difficult, with anatomy being distorted and haemostasis being difficult to achieve. And most women will respond well to conservative management. At laparotomy, the whole of the abdominal cavity should be inspected, including the subdiaphragmatic spaces which can be the site of abscess formation. Large tubo-ovarian abscesses often require excision or marsupialisation with the insertion of abdominal drains. In extreme cases a hysterectomy may be required in order to clear the severely inflamed tissue, but this should be avoided in women who may want children.

OVERVIEW – Initially most women should be managed conservatively with analgesia, bedrest, intravenous fluids and broad-spectrum antibiotic therapy.

Follow-up

SHORT TERM – Women treated on an outpatient basis should be reviewed after 1 week to make sure the symptoms have improved. Contact tracing of sexual partners should be done.

LONG TERM – The women should be warned of the risk of subfertility and referred early to an appropriate unit for investigation if they have difficulty with conception. They should also be advised of the increased chance of ectopic pregnancy if they do become pregnant and to report early to their GP.

3. Ovarian Cyst Accidents

(See also Chapter 16.)

Background

DEFINITION – Epithelial-lined cysts in the ovary. They may be physiological, benign or malignant. Cysts presenting acutely are usually physiological or benign. The commonest cysts presenting acutely are small haemorrhagic corpus luteal cysts.

MAIN COMPLICATIONS – If there is rupture, blood loss may be heavy. Prolonged torsion will lead to loss of the ovary because of necrosis, and the surrounding peritonism may cause pelvic adhesions. Coagulopathy is a rare complication of cyst torsion.

MAKING THE DIAGNOSIS – These cysts can cause pain in several ways. Rupture of the cyst can lead to a sharp pain, with the cyst contents causing irritation of the surrounding peritoneum. Haemorrhage into a cyst causes a constant dull ache. The cysts may also undergo torsion which causes a pain similar to ureteric colic. Later necrosis of the ovary can lead to generalised abdominal pain and peritonism. See Table 15.3.

Table 15.3   Diagnosing ovarian cyst accident

Making the diagnosis	Ovarian cyst accident
History	Acute pelvic pain, usually unilateral often radiating to the leg or loin but with no other symptoms
Examination	Mild pyrexia is common
	Localised lower abdominal tenderness, usually unilateral
	Mass may be palpable abdominally or bimanually
	Fluid distension suggests haemoperitoneum or ascites
Investigations	
– Pregnancy test	Negative, although cyst may co-exist with pregnancy
– Ultrasound	Main diagnostic tool. Cyst will be evident
– Laparoscopy	Necessary to exclude ovarian torsion if pain persists
– Microbiology	Negative culture but pyuria may occur
– FBC/coagulation	Mild leucocytosis. May get DIC with chronic torsion

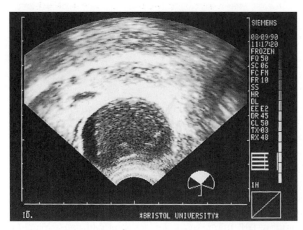

Fig 15.2   *Haemorrhage into an ovarian cyst.*

Ultrasound is the mainstay of diagnosis but even this will only give a guide (Figure 15.2). The size and nature of the cysts should be noted, and any evidence of free fluid should be recorded. This will give some idea of the likely pathology. Small (< 6 cm) cysts that are unilocular with no solid areas tend to be physiological in nature. Large multiloculated cysts with solid areas are more likely to be pathological, and if accompanied by free fluid (ascites) are more likely to be malignant. Cysts with a diameter of < 7 cm rarely undergo torsion.

Laparoscopy is not necessary for all women, particularly for those with cysts of less than 5 cm, but it should be undertaken if the diagnosis is in doubt. It should also be remembered that small ovarian cysts are common in asymptomatic women and that the presence of a cyst in a woman with pain may be a misleading finding.

Treatment Options

ADVICE – Ovulation pain and haemorrhagic/functional cysts are physiological variants with no sinister consequences. Although analgesia is occasionally required, they usually resolve spontaneously. Larger cysts (> 6 cm) or cysts with multiple loculations are more likely to be pathological and require definitive surgery.

DRUG THERAPY – Opiate and NSAID analgesia may be required for initial pain relief, but, as this settles, oral paracetamol will suffice.

SURGERY – Laparoscopy is used as a diagnostic tool but may also allow drainage and even cystectomy for medium sized (6–10 cm), simple cysts. Often laparotomy is needed. In younger women malignant disease is unlikely and minimal surgery should be performed, conserving both ovaries if possible. In older women (> 40 years), the ovary should be removed in total. If malignancy is strongly suspected, hysterectomy and bilateral oophorectomy should be performed (providing consent has been given).

OVERVIEW – The vast majority of cysts resolve spontaneously. Emergency surgery should only be undertaken for women with large cysts, torted cysts or for pain that does not settle.

Follow-up

SHORT TERM – A repeat ultrasound scan should be undertaken at 6 weeks to ensure that small cysts are resolving.

4. Acute Bowel Disease

Bowel disorders are beyond the scope of this book, but this section explains types of presentation and methods of diagnosis.

Background

COMMON PROBLEMS – **Appendicitis** is an acute non-specific inflammation of the appendix which often arises because of a faecolith blocking the opening. **Ulcerative colitis** is a chronic inflammatory disease of the rectum and colon. **Crohn's disease** is regional chronic inflammatory granulomatous condition of the ileum but can involve the jejunum, stomach and colon. Specific gastrointestinal infections and infestations also occur, especially after foreign travel. These diseases are beyond the scope of this book, but a short description of the features of acute presentation is given.

MAKING THE DIAGNOSIS – The big difference between acute bowel disease and gynaecological disorders is the frequency of gastrointestinal symptoms, particularly diarrhoea and rectal bleeding, but these can be features of PID. In addition, menstrual disorder is an uncommon, but not unknown, feature of bowel disease. Pain is, of course, common to both but is more usually colicky in nature with gastrointestinal problems.

Acute pain may be a feature of a group of **non-specific dysfunctional bowel problems** – irritable bowel syndrome (IBS) and constipation – which are probably the commonest conditions presenting acutely to the gynaecologist. The pain is generally colicky in nature, with diarrhoea or constipation but no other adverse features. **Appendicitis** has a typical history of central colicky abdominal discomfort which then changes to a sharp pain in the right iliac fossa. **Intestinal perforation** leads to sudden onset of sharp pain which is initially localised and then more diffuse. Peritonism is quickly evident. **Inflammatory bowel disease** is typically characterised by a subacute history with variable bowel habit and the passage of blood and mucus in the stools. See Table 15.4.

COMPLICATIONS – **Anaemia** and **electrolyte disturbance** are common. **Septicaemia** is rare but potentially life-threatening.

OVERVIEW – Bowel problems in women may present in a very similar way to gynaecological problems. A careful history and high index of suspicion are essential to prevent them being overlooked. If there is any doubt, an urgent surgical opinion should be requested.

5. Urinary Infection and Renal Tract Calculi

Urinary tract diseases are beyond the scope of this book but this section explains types of presentation and methods of diagnosis.

Background

COMMON PROBLEMS – **Renal calculi** are small stones that form in the renal tract. **Urinary tract infection** (UTI) is an abnormal growth of bacteria in the normally sterile urine.

AETIOLOGY – UTIs are caused by a variety of organisms, but the commonest infecting agents are bowel and vaginal flora, because of the proximity of the urethra to these structures. Women with urinary tract malformations, calculi, ureteric reflux and tumours are more prone to infection.

MAIN COMPLICATIONS – **Septicaemia. Urinary retention** may occur with infection. Recurrent infections may lead to renal damage with the **nephrotic syndrome** and **chronic renal failure (chronic pyelonephritis, CPN)**. In pregnancy, infection may initiate **preterm labour**. Calculi may obstruct a ureter leading to **hydronephrosis and/or pyonephrosis**.

SCREENING/PREVENTION – In pregnancy the risk of urinary tract infection is increased, and the urine is checked with reagent sticks at antenatal appointments.

Table 15.4	Diagnosing acute bowel disease		
Making the diagnosis	Appendicitis	Ulcerative colitis	Crohn's disease
History	Central to RIF pain	Generalised abdo pain	Generalised abdo pain
	Nausea/vomiting	Bloody diarrhoea	Bloody diarrhoea
Examination	Mild pyrexia	Fever	Fever
	Tender RIF and	Peritonism	? RIF mass
	per rectum		
Investigations			
– WCC	Mildly elevated	May be normal	May be normal
– Ultrasound	? Appendix abscess		? RIF mass
– Laparoscopy	Inflamed/infected		
– Barium enema		Ulcers	Strictures
		Loss of haustrations	
– Histology/	Inflammatory reaction	Mucosal ulcers and	Submucosal ulcers,
sigmoidoscopy Bx		crypt abscesses	fistulae, granulomas

MAKING THE DIAGNOSIS – Urinary tract pain secondary to infection and/or calculi can be severe. **Infection** can cause anything from suprapubic discomfort to severe abdominal pain and this is associated with **urinary urgency, frequency** and **dysuria**. **Microscopic haematuria** is also common as is severe **loin ache**. **Renal colic** caused by calculi passing down the ureter is said to be one of the most severe pains. It is generally unilateral and runs from loin to groin. It comes in waves which last about 2 minutes. Haematuria is common, and a stone may be found in the urine with sieving. See Table 15.5.

OVERVIEW – Urinary tract problems are very common in women and they may present in a very similar way to gynaecological problems. A careful history and high index of suspicion are essential to prevent them being overlooked. Urinary microscopy often reveals the diagnosis, but renal ultrasound and/or x-rays should be considered, even if this is negative, if the history is very suggestive. If there is any doubt, an urgent urological opinion should be requested.

Table 15.5   Diagnosing UTI and renal calculi

Making the diagnosis	UTI	Renal calculi
History	Suprapubic and loin pain	Severe loin-to-groin colic
	Dysuria/frequency/ urgency	Haematuria
Examination	Severe pyrexia	Mild pyrexia or normal
	Suprapubic/loin tenderness	Tender on affected side
Investigations		
– WCC	Neutrophil leucocytosis	Normal
– Urine	Positive culture and microscopy	Red and white cells
– Ultrasound	Normal or signs of CPN	May show hydronephrosis
– X-ray	Normal	Calculi may be visualised

GOLDEN POINTS

1. Resuscitation should be prompt, with correction of hypovolaemia.

2. Ectopic pregnancy must always be considered in women of childbearing age.

3. Non-gynaecological causes must be considered and a surgical opinion sought when necessary.

4. Always beware of women who have undergone multiple procedures; ?Munchausen's syndrome.

5. Laparoscopy is an excellent diagnostic tool, but a detailed non-invasive assessment should be performed first.

6. Cultures from vaginal swabs do not accurately predict higher genital tract infections. Endocervical swabs are essential.

7. Contact tracing of partners of women with PID helps prevent recurrent infection.

16 Chronic pelvic pain

CLINICAL SIGNIFICANCE

Chronic pelvic pain is a common presentation to gynaecology outpatients, accounting for about 10% of all referrals. Only a minority have true gynaecological disease, with many of the women having non-gynaecological pathology and a large proportion having no identifiable disease at all.

Regardless of cause, pain is a debilitating symptom even when relatively mild, and reactive depression is a common consequence. For many, this is made worse when no cause is found, particularly if the clinician creates the impression that the woman is neurotic.

It is important to stress the need for the clinician to take the woman seriously from the start, as confidence in the investigating doctor is vital if there is to be an improvement in symptoms. Long-term chronic pain causes misery to the woman and her partner.

DIFFERENTIAL DIAGNOSIS

MAIN CATEGORY	DIAGNOSIS
Gynaecological	
1. *Infection*	Chronic pelvic inflammatory disease Pelvic adhesions
2. *Endometriosis*	Minimal disease Chocolate cysts
3. *Tumour*	Any benign or malignant pelvic mass
4. *Physiological*	Mittelschmerz Premenstrual syndrome
5. *Functional*	Pelvic congestion syndrome Polycystic ovarian disease
Non-gynaecological	
1. *Psychological*	Psychosomatic Postnatal depression Somatomisation Previous child sexual abuse Munchausen's syndrome
2. *Urinary tract*	Urinary infection Urinary retention Bladder tumour (very rare)
3. *Gastrointestinal*	Irritable bowel disease Constipation Inflammatory bowel disease Diverticulitis Rectal cancer (very rare)
4. *Neurological*	Trapped nerve
5. *Orthopaedic*	Hip disease

Although gynaecological disease is actually quite rare, there is no doubt that certain pathologies of the genital tract do cause pelvic pain. These include chronic pelvic infection, pelvic tumours and severe endometriosis. Other gynaecological conditions are known to be associated with pelvic pain, such as polycystic ovarian disease and pelvic congestion syndrome, but the nature of the association is unclear.

Functional bowel disease (IBS or constipation) appears to be the commonest group of disorder, accounting for about 40% of cases. Given that many women with IBS and constipation never complain of pelvic pain, it seems likely that some other psychological condition plays a part in the presentation. This may be general anxiety, somatomisation (unusual awareness of physiological sensation) or depression. Just as many men become worried by chest sensations, some women appear to become preoccupied about the health of their internal genitalia, perhaps because of concerns over fertility or cervical cancer, or because of previous sexual abuse. Every gynaecologist should bear this in mind when dealing with any symptoms in women. A wrong explanation may induce chronic anxiety and propagation of symptoms.

One example is the use of the diagnosis of pelvic inflammatory disease (PID) without proper investigation such as bacteriology or laparoscopy. The woman then worries about the source of the supposed infection, her future fertility, etc. As anxiety increases, any pain worsens, and this in turn is treated with further antibiotics and analgesics. When the woman finally comes to laparoscopy, sometimes months or years later, her pelvis is perfectly clear. The pain then disappears!

CLINICAL ASSESSMENT

These women usually present to their GPs, who can undertake many investigations. Urgent referral to a gynaecologist is usually not needed. The advantage of a short delay is that many women experience spontaneous resolution with advice from the GP. This policy may prevent unnecessary invasive investigation (laparoscopy).

Relevant History

Presenting Complaint

MAIN SYMPTOM – The nature of the **pain** and its relation to the menstrual cycle plays an important role in the diagnosis. Pain starting prior to menstruation and lasting throughout the period, dull and aching in nature with poor localisation, is suggestive of endometriosis. Radiation of the pain to the back of the legs, which is made worse by standing up and relieved by lying down, is associated with pelvic congestion. However, cyclical pain does not necessarily indicate gynaecological disease, because bowel function and mood vary with the cycle because of the effect of progesterone.

COMMONLY ASSOCIATED SYMPTOMS – **Dyspareunia** is a commonly associated symptom. Again it does not necessarily indicate gynaecological disease. It is a feature of endometriosis and infection but it is also common in IBS and psychosexual disorder. **Immediate postcoital aching** is said to be associated with pelvic congestion, whereas pain several hours after intercourse is felt to be indicative of irritable bowel syndrome.

Vaginal discharge may be indicative of pelvic infection, particularly if associated with soreness or irritation, but, equally, the discharge may simply be normal leucorrhoea which the woman misinterprets as abnormal. A detailed gastrointestinal history is essential. **Intermittent diarrhoea** and **constipation** or **abdominal bloating** associated with relief of symptoms after defaecation suggest irritable bowel syndrome. Constipation can cause a chronic left iliac fossa discomfort with acute episodes of colicky pain.

The **passage of blood per rectum** suggests inflammatory bowel disease or cancer. **Associated urinary symptoms** tend to suggest bladder pathology but may also be related to a pelvic tumour.

EFFECT ON THE PATIENT – It is vital to assess the impact of the pain on the patient's lifestyle and whether it affects her sleep, work, exercise or family life. This will help decide how far investigations and treatment should be taken. Some women simply want to know that there is no serious cause. Others need pain relief.

Gynaecological History

GYNAECOLOGICAL DISEASES – Episodes of acute pelvic infection may have caused chronic inflammation or adhesion formation. The method of diagnosis is essential, as many women get labelled as having pelvic inflammatory disease without proper evidence. The woman may have been shown to have endometriosis in the past.

MENSTRUAL HISTORY – The last menstrual period should be recorded, and if there is associated amenorrhoea in a woman of child bearing potential a pregnancy test should be performed. A detailed menstrual history should look at previous cycles to see if there has been a recent change in regularity, pain, symptoms or loss. Cycle irregularity would tend to indicate PCOD.

FERTILITY REQUIREMENTS – Endometriosis is commonly seen in couples undergoing fertility investigations, so these women may have a history of failure to conceive. Long-term management concerning surgical options will be affected if the woman has no children and wishes to have them.

CONTRACEPTION – Recent insertion of an intrauterine contraceptive device can lead to pelvic pain caused by uterine cramping or pelvic sepsis.

Obstetric History

DELIVERIES – Any recent or traumatic deliveries may have led to a constant perineal/pelvic discomfort which may be psychological in nature. Postnatal depression may present in this way as a cry for help.

Medical History

OPERATIONS – Previous abdominal surgery, especially for inflammatory or infected bowel, may have led to adhesion formation. Women with strange histories and multiple abdominal operations should be carefully investigated before further intervention is considered, as they may have a record of attention-seeking behaviour (Munchausen's syndrome).

MEDICAL CONDITIONS – Previous bowel and urinary tract disease are important.

PSYCHOLOGICAL DISORDERS – A history of mood disturbances, depression or anxiety disorders is common in women presenting with long-term pelvic pain. Care should be taken not to cause offence when enquiring about these. Sensitive matters, especially possible sexual abuse, can be difficult to discuss and should be reserved for those with experience in this field.

Drug History

MEDICATIONS – The type of analgesia required to treat the pain, and whether any are effective, will help gauge the severity of the symptoms. The severity of the pain does not indicate the severity of the pathology. However, sometimes chronic use of opiates such as codeine leads to constipation and worsening of pain as a result of bowel dysfunction.

Social History

AGE – Teenage pelvic pain is possibly due to congenital abnormality.

OCCUPATION – Loss of time off work reflects the severity of the pain. Recent unemployment may be a cause of anxiety and depression.

COMPANIONS – Marital disharmony may be a cause of anxiety, etc.

LIFESTYLE – Reduction in social activity indicates the severity of the pain.

Relevant Clinical Examination

General Examination

GENERAL CONDITION – It should be noted whether the woman looks comfortable and relaxed. Reasonably severe pain will prevent the woman from sitting still. Facial expression should be observed throughout the history taking and examination.

Abdomen

CONTOUR – Abdominal distension may be indicative of bloating and is associated with irritable bowel syndrome or may be due to large pelvic masses.

OLD SCARS – Multiple operations are suspicious unless there is known disease present.

TENDERNESS – 'Ovarian point' tenderness is seen in pelvic congestion; similar signs are seen in IBS. A tender loaded sigmoid colon may indicate constipation. Non-specific generalised tenderness is suggestive of anxiety,

and the woman's face should be observed closely during the examination while attempts are made to distract her.

Pelvic

VULVA/VAGINA/CERVIX – Purulent vaginal or cervical discharge may indicate pelvic infection. Endometriotic deposits may be seen in the posterior fornix.

BIMANUAL EXAMINATION – Thickening at the vaginal vault and uterosacral ligaments with uterine fixation is seen with endometriosis. Ovarian cysts may be palpable. Bulky tender uterus may be due to adenomyosis. Diffuse tenderness can be misleading, and care should be taken to find a definitive point; this may be helped by distracting the woman.

RECTAL EXAMINATION – The rectum can be palpated through the vagina. Faecal loading from constipation is easily felt. Rectal tenderness is a feature of IBS.

Relevant Initial Investigations

Haematology

WCC – May be raised with pelvic infection

Biochemistry Tests

C-REACTIVE PROTEIN – Raises the possibility of PID and inflammatory bowel disease.

Endocrine Tests

URINE β-hCG – Any woman with a recent history of amenorrhoea should have the possibility of a chronic ectopic pregnancy excluded.

LH/FSH – A raised LH/FSH ratio is indicative of polycystic ovarian disease.

Microbiology

BACTERIAL CULTURE – The vagina should be swabbed if there is discharge present. Endocervical swabs should be sent for general bacteriology and chlamydial ELISA. Urine should also be sent for culture and microscopy to exclude infection. Dipstick examination will demonstrate haematuria, which should be investigated further with renal tract ultrasound and cystoscopy to rule out renal tract tumours and stones.

SEROLOGY – Chlamydia serology can be useful to screen for chronic pelvic inflammatory disease.

Diagnostic Imaging

ULTRASOUND – Has a vital role to play not only in the detection of pelvic masses but in the reassurance a normal scan provides initially, avoiding more invasive investigations. Pelvic cysts, fibroids and polycystic ovaries can be visualised using transvaginal scanning (Figure 16.1). Dilated pelvic veins may suggest pelvic congestion syndrome. The kidneys can be examined to look for evidence of urinary tract pathology.

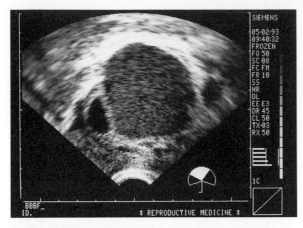

Fig 16.1 *Endometriotic (chocolate) ovarian cyst.*

PLAIN X-RAYS OF SPINE AND HIPS – These may be carried out if orthopaedic problems are suspected, but they are not routinely requested.

AXIAL IMAGING – This has little role to play except in suspicious or difficult cases.

CONTRAST RADIOLOGY – Pelvic venography has been used as a research tool to diagnose pelvic congestion syndrome but it is rarely used in clinical practice.

Direct Visualisation

LAPAROSCOPY – This has been the gold standard investigation in the past, but because of the large number of normal investigations, some feel that it should only be used if the pain is of over 6 months' duration, if pelvic

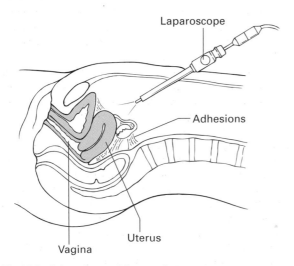

Fig 16.2 *Pelvic adhesions following infection.*

pathology is strongly suspected, or if the woman cannot be reassured by a negative ultrasound. It is used to look for evidence of PID, adhesions (Figure 16.2) and endometriosis. The difficulty is that the findings may not be the cause of the pain. Endometriosis, for example, is extremely common, and about 30% of asymptomatic women undergoing laparoscopic sterilisation have easily identifiable deposits. It should also be stated that for some women the reassurance gained from a negative laparoscopy means that it is not a wasted examination.

DETAILS OF INDIVIDUAL CONDITIONS

1. Endometriosis

Background

DEFINITION – The presence of endometrial-like tissue outside the uterine cavity and myometrium (endometrial tissue within the myometrium is known as adenomyosis). The incidence of symptomatic endometriosis is difficult to determine, but it is believed to affect around 10% of the female population. Tissue is generally seen on the internal genitalia but may be found on bowel, bladder and at distant sites such as lung and brain. Endometriosis is reasonably common in episiotomy and caesarean section scars.

AETIOLOGY – Several theories exist as to the cause, with all of them probably playing a part.

Endometrial implantation – retrograde menstrual flow with vascular and lymphatic passage – is a popular theory but does not adequately explain why all women do not suffer from this condition, as most women experience retrograde menstruation. Implantation certainly seems likely to be the cause of scar endometriosis.

Activation or metaplasia of **embryonic rests** has also been suggested, with cells lining the peritoneal cavity undergoing metaplasia to endometrial cells possibly related to incessant ovulation because of reduced family size.

Immunological theory states that an alteration of cell and humoral mediated immune response exists in some women, explaining why they develop endometriosis from implantation and others do not. There are associated risk factors: mainly, a family history, prolonged menstrual cycle (> 27 days), prolonged menses (> 7 days) and genital outflow obstruction. It seems likely that all of these theories play a part. Some workers have suggested a two-stage theory which proposes that virtually all women have microscopic deposits of endometriosis within the pelvic peritoneum and that symptoms only arise in those who develop an immunological reaction to the tissue.

MAKING THE DIAGNOSIS – Laparoscopy with or without biopsy is the definitive method. Additional tests should be undertaken to rule out other causes. Imaging studies are used to look for evidence of bowel or urinary tract involvement if this is suspected (see Table 16.1).

MAIN COMPLICATIONS – The majority of women are probably **asymptomatic**. **Subfertility** is one of the main problems, with endometriosis being found in about 20% of women undergoing investigation. In the absence of severe scarring and tubal damage, the relationship between endometriosis and subfertility is poorly understood. It is not even clear whether endometriosis causes the subfertility or the other way around. **Chronic pelvic pain**, with or without painful periods, or **dyspareunia** account for the majority of other presentations, although in some women with clinically proven disease there are no symptoms present. **Endometriotic cysts** may develop, especially on the ovary, which are filled with old blood; hence they are known as chocolate cysts. **Bowel obstruction** and **ureteric damage** may occur in severe cases. **Recurrent (cyclical) haemoptysis** is a feature of lung endometriosis.

SCREENING/PREVENTION – None known.

Treatment Options

ADVICE – In asymptomatic women in whom fertility is not required, reassurance and explanation should be provided.

CHANGE OF LIFESTYLE/DIET – Even though obesity and smoking have not been proven associations, there is evidence that weight loss and stopping smoking may help.

DRUG THERAPY – Drug therapy is useful for symptomatic, small-volume disease but it does not improve fertility and will not eradicate chocolate cysts. There are a wide variety of agents used, and choice depends on individual needs.

Prostaglandin synthetase inhibitors such as mefenamic acid reduce prostaglandin production and have been shown to help with pelvic and menstrual pain.

Hormone therapy relies on the fact that endometrial deposits possess oestrogen, progestogen and androgen receptors. Such treatments are likely to affect active disease only, and old scarring will not necessarily improve. The **combined oral contraceptive pill** has proven successful in reducing symptoms, particularly in young women requiring contraception. It is said to induce a state of pseudo-pregnancy. **Progestogens** act directly on the deposits, inducing atrophy. They also inhibit ovarian function and lower oestrogen concentrations. Used continuously they may induce premenstrual symptoms and irregular bleeding but they are as effective as any other therapy and are inexpensive.

Danazol, a synthetic steroid, acts directly on androgen and oestrogen receptors and in higher doses acts centrally, inhibiting pituitary gonadotrophin production and inducing oestrogen-deficiency. It has proven effective but it has unpleasant side effects (weight gain, hirsutism, acne, deepening of the voice).

Gonadotrophin-releasing hormone analogues **(GnRHa)** desensitise the pituitary to native GnRH and thereby suppress production of FSH and so ovarian activity. The hypo-oestrogenic state which follows promotes regression of active deposits. This is one of the most effective methods of reducing symptoms from endometrial deposits, but its use is limited by the risk of bone loss osteoporosis and by cost. It is a useful **preparatory agent** before surgery for severe, large-

Table 16.1	Diagnosing endometriosis
Making the diagnosis	**Endometriosis**
History	Chronic pelvic pain / dyspareunia
	Aching pain prior to and during menses
	Inability to conceive
Examination	Apyrexial
	Pelvic tenderness
	Adnexal mass, uterine fixation with uterosacral ligament thickening
Investigations	
– Ultrasound	Can be used to detect ovarian 'chocolate' cysts, but small deposits cannot be seen
	If ureteric disease is suspected, a renal ultrasound should be performed
– Barium studies/ colonoscopy	If bowel involvement is suspected
– Laparoscopy	Direct visualisation of powder burn (black), haemorrhagic (red), vesicular (white) deposits
	Biopsies can be taken if there is uncertainty
– Histology	Tissue from pelvic biopsies
– Microbiology/WCC	Negative/normal

volume disease. Overall, progestogens make good first-line therapy and GnRHa should be reserved for severe or refractory disease.

SURGERY – The aim of surgery is either to restore the normal pelvic anatomy or to remove or destroy the endometrial deposits. Destruction can be performed laparoscopically using either laser ablation or electro-diathermy coagulation. More major reconstructive surgery is still performed abdominally by many surgeons. Hysterectomy with bilateral oophorectomy remains the only hope of relief from symptoms for some women.

FERTILITY THERAPY – The association between subfertility and endometriosis is poorly understood. Surgery can be used for tubal disease, but medical and surgical therapy for small-volume disease does not appear to increase the chance of conception. After just 1 to 2 years of failure to conceive, the chance of spontaneous conception is still moderately good (30% in 12 months), but for longer periods of subfertility the chance gets ever smaller and assisted conception techniques should be offered.

OVERVIEW – There is no one satisfactory treatment option, and those that are available should be reserved for women with severe or symptomatic disease. The treatment should be tailored to the symptoms experienced and the fertility requirements of the woman. Drug therapy is used first unless there are endometriotic cysts present. Surgery should be confined to those women with refractory disease, large endo-metriotic cysts or tubal disease requiring reconstruction for fertility.

Follow-up

SHORT TERM – Careful follow-up of women is important, especially if they are on medical treatment. If fertility is required, referral to an appropriate specialist unit should take place.

2. Pelvic Congestion Syndrome

Background

DEFINITION – Dilatation and engorgement of the pelvic veins leading to variable pelvic pain in the absence of pathological causes.

AETIOLOGY – Unknown, but the symptoms are felt to relate to the cyclical engorgement of pelvic veins. There may be an association with anorgasmia and also with poly-cystic ovarian disease, but these are not well understood.

MAKING THE DIAGNOSIS – See Table 16.2.

MAIN COMPLICATIONS – Chronic pelvic pain, deep dyspareunia and postcoital ache which radiates to the back and thighs. The symptoms are exacerbated by standing and relieved by lying down.

SCREENING TESTS – None available.

Table 16.2 Diagnosing pelvic congestion syndrome	
Making the diagnosis	Pelvic congestion syndrome
History	Deep dyspareunia with postcoital aching
	Exacerbated on standing, radiating to back and legs and relieved by lying
Examination	Apyrexial
	Variable abdominal signs, often non-tender
Investigations	
– Ultrasound	Visualisation of dilated pelvic veins and polycystic ovaries
	Exclusion of other pathology
– Laparoscopy	Dilated/engorged veins seen, otherwise normal
– Microbiology	Negative

Treatment Options

ADVICE – Ultrasound findings alone may be enough to reassure the woman there is no serious pathology. If the pain is persistent for > 6 months duration, laparoscopy may be required. The syndrome is said to be self-limiting.

CHANGE OF LIFESTYLE/DIET – Nothing specific unless associated with stress.

DRUG THERAPY – **Progestogens** (medroxyprogesterone acetate) have been shown to benefit women, especially in association with psychotherapy, but symptoms return on stopping hormone treatment. **Non-steroidal anti-inflammatory agents** may help with postcoital pain.

OVERVIEW – Reassurance and psychotherapy probably play the most important role in treatment, with medication being reserved for those with severe persistent symptoms.

Follow-up

SHORT TERM – The woman should be seen in the gynaecology clinic to have the results of investigations explained.

LONG TERM – After exclusion of serious pathology the follow-up should be arranged with the GP and/or counsellor.

3. Irritable Bowel Syndrome

Background

DEFINITION – A condition of abdominal pain and bloating associated with intermittent episodes of diarrhoea and constipation with no demonstrable pathology.

Table 16.3 Diagnosing irritable bowel syndrome

Making the diagnosis	Irritable bowel syndrome
History	Abdominal pain and bloating.
	Relief after defaecation
	Intermittent diarrhoea and
	constipation
	Dyspareunia several hours
	after intercourse
	Symptoms often cyclical in
	women
Examination	Apyrexial
	Variable abdominal signs, often
	non-tender
	Rectal tenderness
Investigations	By definition all negative

AETIOLOGY – Unknown but felt to have a psychological element. Alterations in gut flora may play a part also.

MAKING THE DIAGNOSIS – See Table 16.3.

MAIN COMPLICATIONS – Pelvic pain and bloating with bouts of diarrhoea and constipation. Can have a major effect on quality of life. About half of suffers still have symptoms at 5 years.

SCREENING TESTS/PREVENTION – None proven but it is suggested that a normal diet and avoidance of excessive stress may prevent problems.

Treatment Options

ADVICE – A careful explanation is important emphasising the benign nature of the condition.

CHANGE OF LIFESTYLE/DIET – Moderate-fibre diet, increased fluid input, weight loss and exercise will help. Hypnotherapy has been shown to relieve symptoms.

DRUG THERAPY – Artificial fibre can be provided (fybogel), but too much may worsen symptoms.

Antispasmodics such as mebeverine and peppermint oil have achieved some degree of success in the short term, but there is little proof of effect from clinical trials. The same is true of sedatives such as diazepam.

OVERVIEW – A careful explanation is helpful to provide reassurance. Changes in lifestyle should be attempted before medical intervention.

Follow-up

SHORT AND LONG TERM – The woman should be seen in the gynaecology clinic to have the results of investigations explained. Care is then continued by the GP and/or a gastroenterologist.

4. Pelvic Inflammatory Disease

See Chapter 15.

GOLDEN POINTS

1. A systematic and sympathetic approach is essential.

2. Non-gynaecological pathology is commoner than pelvic pathology.

3. A careful bowel history is particularly important.

4. If there are no suspicious features and simple tests are negative, reassurance should be given.

5. Laparoscopy should be undertaken if the history is highly suspicious or if symptoms persist.

6. Referral to a chronic pain clinic is appropriate if organic disease has been ruled out but pain persists.

7. Psychological factors play a major role, and counselling should be considered.

17 Pelvic mass

CLINICAL SIGNIFICANCE

Pelvic mass is an uncommon reason for referral to a gynaecology clinic but an important one nevertheless because it may be the first evidence of a malignant ovarian tumour.

Carcinoma of the ovary is the commonest cause of death due to gynaecological malignancy in this country, killing nearly four thousand women each year in England and Wales, equivalent to all other gynaecological cancers combined. The position of the ovaries within the peritoneal cavity means that symptoms are rare when the tumour is small, and dissemination occurs early such that two-thirds of women present with disease outside the pelvis.

DIFFERENTIAL DIAGNOSIS

MAIN CATEGORY		DIAGNOSIS
Gynaecological		
1. **Ovary**	*Physiological*	Follicular cyst Corpus luteal cysts
	Metaplastic	Endometriotic (chocolate) cyst
	Benign neoplasia	Epithelial tumours Germ cell tumours Sex-chord stromal tumours
	Borderline tumours	

	*Malignant
	  tumours*
		Epithelial cancers
		Germ cell tumours
		Sex-chord stromal
		  tumours
		Secondary deposit

2. **Fallopian
  tube**
	Non- neoplastic	Pyosalpinx/abscess
		Ectopic pregnancy
		Tuberculosis (very
		  rare)

	*Malignant
	  tumour*
		Primary carcinoma
		  (very rare)

3. **Uterus**	*Non-neoplastic-*	Haematometra Fibroids

	*Malignant
	  tumours*
		Carcinoma of
		  endometrium
		Uterine sarcomas
		  (very rare)

Non-gynaecological		

1. **Gastro-
  intestinal**
	Non-neoplastic	Diverticular
		  abscess
		Abscess secondary
		  to Crohn's disease
		Appendix abscess
		Constipation
		Volvulus

	Malignant tumours	Large-bowel cancer

2. **Genito-
  urinary**
	Non-neoplastic
	*Malignant
	  tumours*
		Retention of urine
		Pelvic kidney
		Bladder tumour

The main focus of this chapter is those women who present with a pelvic mass alone. Acute pelvic pain is considered in Chapter 15.

The majority of pelvic masses are the result of benign disease – most commonly, ovarian tumours such as cystic teratomas, or uterine tumours such as fibroids.

Pregnancy presents rarely as a pelvic mass but should always be kept in mind as a possibility in women in the reproductive years.

Non-gynaecological problems are relatively rare but are easily forgotten by gynaecologists. It is particularly important to remember retention of urine, which may require emergency treatment.

Symptoms are often spartan and in many cases the diagnosis can only be determined by laparotomy. Even the findings at laparotomy may be misleading, with actinomyces and lymphomas all mimicking epithelial cancers. Histopathological confirmation is therefore essential if operative management is deemed impossible.

CLINICAL ASSESSMENT

Some women present with acute symptoms if there is severe pelvic infection or there is torsion or rupture of an ovarian cyst, but for many the onset of symptoms is very gradual. Indeed, in a significant proportion of cases, large masses are an incidental finding at a routine examination for cervical cytology.

Relevant History

Presenting Complaint

MAIN SYMPTOM – **Abdominal swelling** and **vague discomfort** are the commonest symptoms. The speed of onset and severity say little about the cause. **Dyspepsia** is said to be the commonest first symptom in women with ovarian cancer. **Pain** of gradual onset is an ominous symptom which may indicate malignant disease. Acute pain is more in keeping with infection, torsion or haemorrhage into an ovarian cyst. Colicky pain is suggestive of large or small bowel diseases.

COMMONLY ASSOCIATED SYMPTOMS – A careful **menstrual history** should be taken. **Primary amenorrhoea** should raise the possibility of a congenital malformation of the genital tract leading to haematocolpos. A history of **heavy regular periods** is consistent with fibroids. Ovarian masses identified after the **menopause** are more likely malignancy. **Urinary frequency** may be indicative of bladder pathology but is more usually due to pressure from an extrinsic mass. In contrast, **haematuria** is more specific for urinary tract disease. **Blood in the faeces**, **variable bowel habit** and **tenesmus** point towards

bowel disease such as ulcerative colitis, diverticulitis or large bowel cancer. **Lethargy, anorexia** and **rapid weight loss** are suggestive of malignancy.

Gynaecological History

GYNAECOLOGICAL DISEASES – A recent history of pelvic infection tends to suggest that a pelvic abscess is more likely. Similarly, a recent history of severe endometriosis points towards 'chocolate' cyst formation.

CERVICAL CYTOLOGY – Important to be up to date in case the woman needs a hysterectomy.

FERTILITY REQUIREMENTS – Any surgery performed might be influenced by the woman's wishes about future pregnancy.

CONTRACEPTION – Consideration should be given to removal of an IUCD if there is evidence of pelvic infection.

Obstetric History

DELIVERY – A very recent pregnancy increases the chance that the mass is due to retention of urine or pelvic infection.

Medical History

OPERATIONS – Previous abdominal surgery or radiotherapy for malignant disease. Always ask if they have had their appendix removed.

MEDICAL CONDITIONS – Inflammatory bowel disease increases the risk of abdominal abscesses but also of bowel tumours (ulcerative colitis).

Drug History

MEDICATIONS – Physiological cysts are more common in women undergoing ovulation induction with clomiphene. Women receiving exogenous gonadotrophins therapy are more likely to develop theca-lutein cysts.

Social History

AGE – The older the woman, the more likely it is that any ovarian lesion is malignant; less than 3% of malignant ovarian tumours present under the age of 30, and after 50 years the risk of malignancy greatly increases.

COMPANIONS – It is important to consider the home circumstances for those who require radical surgery for malignancy.

LIFESTYLE – The quality of life of very elderly women should be considered before radical surgery is undertaken.

Relevant Clinical Examination

General Examination

GENERAL CONDITION – Wasting (cachexia) is typical of advanced malignant disease but may also be found in chronic bowel diseases such as ulcerative colitis. Hirsutism and virilisation are features of testosterone-secreting ovarian tumours. Leg swelling and oedema may be due to pressure on the pelvic veins.

JAUNDICE – Yellow discoloration may be found in women with extensive liver metastases.

LYMPH NODES – Supraclavicular nodes may be enlarged with abdominal and pelvic malignancies.

BREASTS – A breast lump may represent a breast primary tumour with secondary spread to the abdomen.

BONES – Focal tenderness may represent metastases.

Cardiorespiratory System

Examine the chest for evidence of pleural effusions secondary to malignant disease.

Abdomen

CONTOUR – Pulsation may be indicative of an aortic / iliac artery aneurysm. The umbilicus is a rare site for metastasis from intra-abdominal tumours.

TENDERNESS – Is there evidence of peritonism or is it the mass itself that is tender? Suprapubic tenderness with a history of difficult micturation may be due to acute retention of urine.

MASSES – The size, shape, regularity, consistency and mobility should be assessed. Moderately large, smooth, mobile masses arising from the pelvis tend to be benign ovarian masses or fibroids. Hard, irregular, fixed lesions are more likely to be ovarian malignancy.

LYMPH NODES – Inguinal lymphadenopathy may be found in women with pelvic malignancy.

FREE FLUID – Shifting dullness should be tested by percussion. Ascites in association with a pelvic mass is a sinister sign but may more rarely accompany some benign ovarian tumours (Meig's syndrome).

BOWEL SOUNDS – Auscultate if there is any suspicion of intestinal obstruction.

Pelvic

VULVA/VAGINA/CERVIX – A purulent vaginal loss is a common feature of pelvic infection but also of endometrial cancer. Rarely, faeces or urine may be seen passing through a fistula. In postmenopausal women, bleeding is always a suspicious sign, and consideration should be given to endometrial sampling.

BIMANUAL EXAMINATION – Bimanual examination will allow more information to be gathered. It is easier to tell if the mass is coming from the pelvis, its size, shape, consistency and mobility. Nodules and fixation are found in malignant disease but also with severe endometriosis. If the uterus can be felt separately, fibroids are unlikely, though they may occasionally be pedunculated. Acute pelvic tenderness, especially if unilateral, could be due to infection and abscess formation or a cystic accident.

RECTAL EXAMINATION – May reveal evidence of a primary rectal cancer or direct invasion from an ovarian tumour.

Relevant Initial Investigations

Haematology

Hb – Normochromic/normocytic anaemia is a common feature of advanced malignant disease. Iron deficiency anaemia may accompany bowel disease and menorrhagia.

WCC – The neutrophil count tends to be raised in women with pelvic infection, but it is a rather non-specific sign.

PLATELET COUNT – Thrombocytopaenia is a feature of marrow involvement by malignant tumours.

CLOTTING STUDIES – Not routinely performed but undertaken if there is a low platelet count or if there is evidence of secondary deposits within the liver.

Biochemistry

SERUM U+Es – If the mass is large and renal involvement is suspected.

SERUM LFTs – May find elevated transaminase levels with hepatic metastases, and hypoalbuminaemia often accompanies malignant ascites.

SERUM C-REACTIVE PROTEIN – A very high concentration is suggestive of an infective cause.

Endocrine Tests

OESTRADIOL – Marker for oestrogen-secreting tumours such as the granulosa cell tumour.

β–hCG AND αFP – Tumour markers for germ cell tumours such as yolk sac tumour and ovarian choriocarcinoma.

CA125 – Raised in epithelial ovarian cancers but also with infection and endometriosis. Is taken as a baseline in case an ovarian cancer is found at laparotomy.

Microbiology

BACTERIAL CULTURE – If pelvic infection is suspected, swabs should be taken from the urethra, cervix and vagina for conventional and chlamydial bacteriology. If retention of urine is confirmed, urine should be sent for microscopy and culture.

Diagnostic Imaging

Diagnostic imaging is important for women with pelvic masses but its value is limited. Ultimately, for many women, the only means of accurate diagnosis is laparotomy and histopathology.

PLAIN FILMS – Chest x-ray – used to screen for lung and rib metastases if malignant disease is strongly suspected. **Plain abdominal x-ray** is generally unhelpful and is only indicated if there is a suspicion of intestinal obstruction.

CONTRAST RADIOLOGY – Barium studies are indicated only if a primary lesion of the large bowel is likely on clinical grounds or if symptoms suggest involvement from a malignant ovarian lesion. IVP should only be performed if there is evidence of urinary tract obstruction at ultrasound.

ABDOMINO-PELVIC ULTRASOUND – Ultrasound is not entirely reliable for diagnosis but it does give some idea of the likely cause. Malignant ovarian tumours tend to be heterogeneous with cystic and solid areas (Figure 17.1), and ascites is a common feature as well. Unilateral, unilocular cysts with no solid areas tend to be benign. Fibroids are nearly always solid and are defined by their continuity with the uterus/cervix. Ultrasound is particularly useful for examining the liver for metastases and the renal tract for evidence of obstruction.

AXIAL IMAGING – Usually adds little to the findings at ultrasound and is not routinely performed.

Cytology

PLEURAL EFFUSION – If there is evidence of an effusion, an aspirate should be analysed for evidence of malignant cells.

Histopathology

ENDOMETRIAL – An endometrial aspirate should be taken if there is suspicion of endometrial pathology.

Direct visualisation

LAPAROSCOPY – This is contraindicated with large pelvic masses because of the risk of rupture.

DETAILS OF COMMON CONDITIONS

This section is confined to the management of ovarian lesions. Details on uterine fibroids can be found in

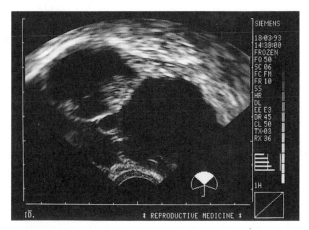

Fig 17.1   *Ovarian carcinoma.*

Chapter 7, and the management of pelvic abscess is discussed in Chapter 15.

The initial management of ovarian masses largely depends on the findings at ultrasound scan (simple cyst vs complex mass), the fertility needs of the woman (completed family vs incomplete family), and the age of the woman. Consider these three scenarios:

1. A young nulliparous woman with an asymptomatic simple cyst of diameter 6 cm or less can initially be managed conservatively.

2. In a young nulliparous woman with a complex cyst, a staging laparotomy is performed to make the diagnosis. Confirmatory histology is usually awaited before definitive surgery.

3. In a postmenopausal woman with a large complex mass and ascites, a staging laparotomy is undertaken and definitive surgery is performed with removal of the uterus, both ovaries, omentum and all tumour deposits.

1. Physiological Ovarian Cysts

Background

DEFINITION – **Follicular cysts** may be multiple, particularly in women undergoing ovulation induction, but the majority are unilateral, unilocular simple cysts lined by granulosa cells. **Luteal cysts** are similar but often have evidence of blood within the cavity.

AETIOLOGY – The cause is largely unknown. **Follicular cysts** are more common with infertility treatment with clomiphene and exogenous gonadotrophin therapy which increase the number of developing follicles in a cycle. Theca-lutein cysts are sensitive to chorionic gonadotrophins and therefore are found in association with molar pregnancies.

MAIN COMPLICATIONS – **Pain** is the commonest feature in these cysts usually due to rupture, torsion or internal haemorrhage, but many are asymptomatic. They may be bilateral and cause pressure symptoms. Follicular cysts may lead to unopposed oestrogen stimulation, leading to **erratic menstruation**.

MAKING THE DIAGNOSIS – These cysts are usually detected on ultrasound and may be seen at laparoscopy. Histology is the only real way of ensuring identification of the type of cysts but this is not necessary in all cases.

PREVENTION – They may recur repeatedly in a small number of women; the combined oral contraceptive pill will help to prevent further recurrences.

Treatment Options

ADVICE – This is all that is required for most women. A follow-up scan should be arranged for 12 weeks to confirm that the cyst has resolved.

DRUG THERAPY – Analgesia with **diclofenac** is helpful for acute pain. Ovarian suppression with the **combined OCP** will help for those cysts that do not disappear.

SURGERY – If there are no adverse features clinically or at scan, surgery should be avoided whenever possible. For cysts > 6 cm there is the risk of torsion, and ovarian cystectomy (conserving the ovary) should be considered if < 40 years and oophorectomy if > 40 years. There is no benefit to be gained from routine aspiration under ultrasound control for cysts less than 7 cm.

OVERVIEW – Most simple cysts disappear spontaneously, and surgery should be avoided for all but the largest which are at risk of torsion and those that persist beyond 6 months.

2. Benign Epithelial Tumours

Background

DEFINITION – **Serous cystadenomas** are usually unilocular cysts, often with papilliferous processes on the inner surface. **Mucinous cystadenomas** are typically large, unilateral, multilocular cysts with a smooth inner capsule. **Brenner cell tumours** are solid fibrotic tumours with islands of transitional epithelial. **Endometrioid cystadenomas** are similar to the chocolate cysts from endometriosis.

AETIOLOGY – Unknown.

MAKING THE DIAGNOSIS – These cysts are usually detected on ultrasound and may be seen at laparoscopy, but histology is the only real way of ensuring identification of the type of cysts.

MAIN COMPLICATIONS – Any cyst may undergo torsion causing ovarian necrosis, and rupture. These tumours are generally not considered to be premalignant, but a small proportion of tumours will undergo malignant transformation. **Mucinous cystadenomas** have the potential to become extremely large (> 60 kg) and cause pressure on pelvic veins and thrombosis. If **benign mucinous tumours rupture**, cells may attach to the mesentery and secrete mucin (**pseudomyxoma peritonei**).

Treatment Options

ADVICE – After removal the woman can be reassured that the risk of recurrence is low.

DRUG THERAPY – Not needed.

SURGERY – Oophorectomy if the family is complete, and ovarian cystectomy if it is not, is all that is required. However, because the diagnosis is not known before laparotomy, many more elderly women undergo pelvic clearance. The contralateral ovary should be examined very carefully to make sure there are no small lesions.

OVERVIEW – Most benign epithelial tumours are unilateral, and simple surgery is curative.

3. Ovarian Epithelial Carcinoma

Background

DEFINITION – Ovarian carcinomas are mostly epithelial in origin. **Serous** cystadenocarcinomas have a cystic and solid appearance and are bilateral in up to 90% of women. **Mucinous** are typically multilocular, thin walled cysts with smooth external surface. **Endometrioid** are cystic and often unilocular, filled with a thick brown fluid. **Clear cell** carcinomas are thick walled unilocular filled with bloodstained fluid and solid areas and are bilateral in 10%.

AETIOLOGY – Associated with nulliparity, early menarche and late menopause. These are all thought to be due to increased number of ovulation cycles. In 1% of cases there is a genetic predisposition related to the BRCA-1 gene. There is some evidence to suggest that ovulation induction may increase the chance of ovarian cancer.

MAKING THE DIAGNOSIS – These tumours may be palpated on examination, being fixed and hard. Ultrasound demonstrates the cyst or tumour, but the diagnosis and staging can only be confirmed after laparotomy and histological examination.

MAIN COMPLICATIONS – **Local** – abdominal distension secondary to ascites, pain, small bowel obstruction. **General** – cachexia, dyspnoea secondary to pleural effusions, and thromboembolism.

STAGING – See Table 17.1.

SCREENING/PREVENTION – There is ongoing research into the use of transvaginal ultrasound and tumour markers (CA125) but they are of unproven value at present. Most research is being focused on those women with a strong family history of cancer. The OCP reduces the risk of ovarian cancer by up to 40% depending on duration of use. Prophylactic oophorectomy may be performed for women undergoing hysterectomy and for women with a strong family history.

Treatment Options

ADVICE – Women should be told of the possible extent of surgery, including stoma formation.

SURGERY – Laparotomy is required for diagnosis and therapy. In the majority of cases a midline incision should be made, providing clear access to the pelvis and abdominal organs. On entering the peritoneum, washings should be taken for cytology. The ovarian cyst should be inspected and surgically removed along with both ovaries, the uterus and Fallopian tubes. The abdomen should be inspected for seedlings onto the omentum and under the diaphragm. An omental biopsy should be

Table 17.1 FIGO staging of ovarian cancer

Stage		
1		**Growth limited to the ovaries**
	1a	– one ovary (no ascites, and capsule intact)
	1b	– both ovaries (no ascites, and capsule intact)
	1c	– 1a or 1b and rupture of capsule or ascites
2		**Growth involving ovary with pelvic extension**
	2a	– metastases to uterus or tubes
	2b	– extension to other pelvic organs
	2c	– 2a or 2b and extension with capsule ruptured or ascites
3		**Ovarian tumour and deposits outside pelvis**
	3a	– within true pelvis microscopic seeding
	3b	– macroscopic metastases on peritoneum < 2 cm
	3c	– abdominal implants > 2 cm or positive nodes
4		**Growth involving ovary with distant metastases**

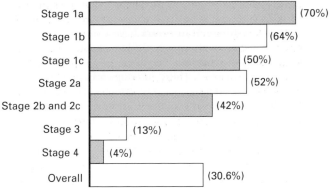

Fig 17.2 *5-year survival for ovarian carcinoma (epithelial).*

taken to allow histological analysis for microscopic seedlings. In large adherent tumours, debulking (cytoreductive surgery) should be performed to remove as much of the tumour as possible to increase the results from further treatment. These women should have bowel preparation preoperatively, especially for large tumours, as bowel resection is possible.

ADJUVANT THERAPY – Stage 1 disease with the capsule intact does not require further treatment. Additional treatment should be considered for all other stages.

DRUG THERAPY – Chemotherapy plays a major role following surgery. Stage 1 disease (within capsule) does not require further treatment. **Single-agent chemotherapy** uses either alkylating agents or heavy-metal compounds. Alkylating agents (cyclophosphamide) have been used for decades, and response rate can be almost 50%. The heavy metal compounds (cisplatin and the newer carboplatin) have proved more successful for Stage 3 and Stage 4 epithelial carcinoma. Cisplatin can be associated with quite severe vomiting and renal damage and occasional neuropathy. Carboplatin has fewer of these side effects but may induce marrow suppression. **Combination chemotherapy** has been tried, but as yet there is no positive proof that it confers benefit to the woman.

RADIOTHERAPY – This has little place in the treatment of advanced disease.

OVERVIEW – Surgery forms the mainstay for both diagnosis and treatment and staging. Chemotherapy, particularly the heavy-metal compounds, is favoured for Stage 2, 3 and 4 disease after surgical debulking. Radiotherapy may be chosen for palliation. The prognosis for ovarian cancer has not changed substantially in the last 20 years (Figure 17.2).

Follow-up

SHORT TERM – Initial follow-up is made to discuss staging and organise further treatment if required. This may take place before hospital discharge.

LONG TERM – Long-term monitoring takes place initially every 3 months to assess progress. Specialist clinics should have a multidisciplinary team involving gynaecologist, oncologist and nurse specialists. Screening using tumour markers (CA125) and examination with ultrasound is recommended if there is suspicion of recurrence. Women are usually followed up for 5 years.

4. Sex-chord Stromal Tumours

Background

DEFINITION – Derived from gonadal stromal tissues. Many are hormonally active, secreting oestrogens, progesterone or androgens. **Granulosa cell tumours** are usually oestrogen-secreting tumours. Some also produce inhibin. **Theca cell tumours** are oestrogen- and progesterone-secreting tumours of theca cell origin. They are soft, often with a yellow cut-surface. **Fibromas** are tumours of stromal origin similar to thecomas. They are typically hard, mobile and lobulated with a white cut-surface. **Sertoli–Leyding cell tumours** have a variety of cells in their structure, with many producing androgens and occasionally oestrogens.

MAIN COMPLICATIONS – These tumours may be benign or malignant. In addition, to any effects of the tumour itself, there may be effects due to hormone production, including amenorrhoea, menorrhagia and virilisation. Rarely, an endometrial cancer may develop in response to unopposed oestrogenisation.

PROGNOSIS – They represent 6% of ovarian tumours occurring at any age of life. **Granulosa cell** are mostly malignant but slow growing. **Theca cell** can produce oestrogen to have systemic effects such as precocious puberty, postmenopausal and erratic bleeding, endometrial hyperplasia and carcinoma. **Fibromas** present around 50 years of age, usually benign and unilateral. **Sertoli–Leydig** are of low-grade malignancy.

Treatment Options

Although they may metastasise, most tumours are slow growing, and surgery is usually curative. The extent of surgery depends on the age and fertility requirements of the woman.

SURGERY – Laparotomy is required for diagnosis and therapy. Sex-steroids or inhibin can be used as tumour markers to monitor tumour activity after surgery.

5. Benign and Malignant Germ Cell Tumours

Background

DEFINITION – **Teratomas** are tumours of embryonic origin lined by stratified squamous epithelium and containing a variety of neuro-cutaneous elements (hair, teeth, cartilage, thyroid and neural tissue). **Choriocarcinoma** and **yolk sac tumours** are of extra-embryonic origin. **Dysgerminoma** are from undifferentiated germ cells. Serum **hCG** is a marker for choriocarcinoma, and **AFP** a marker for yolk sac tumours.

Treatment Options

ADVICE – **Teratomas** are the most common tumour in women under 30 years of age. Dermoid cysts (immature teratoma) tend to be unilateral, seldom over 15 cm in diameter, and are rarely malignant. They are usually symptomless but can undergo torsion. Solid tumours, otherwise known as mature teratomas, tend to be malignant and have a poor prognosis. **Choriocarcinoma** and

yolk sac tumour tend to be aggressive tumours, but with chemotherapy the prognosis is improving. **Dysgerminoma** is a rare tumour but chemo- and radiosensitive.

DRUG THERAPY – Women who develop regular symptomatic functional cysts may benefit from the OCP, which should stop ovulation and follicle development.

SURGERY – The tumours tend to occur in younger women, and only the tumour should be removed. This may be performed laparoscopically or, alternatively, by abdominally removing the cyst and leaving as much of the ovary as possible. Women over the age of 50 should have them removed. Tumour markers can be used to monitor tumour activity after surgery: hCG for choriocarcinomas and AFP for yolk sac tumours.

OVERVIEW – Management depends on the age of the woman and stage of the disease. Women over the age of 35 should have an oophorectomy, under 35 with a cyst > 10 cm should have an examination under anaesthetic followed by cystectomy or oophorectomy. If the cyst is under 10 cm and benign looking, repeat the scan in 3 months and review. The problem with surgery is the risk of removing a healthy ovary.

GOLDEN POINTS

1. Remember non-gynaecological causes, especially bowel tumours and diverticular disease.

2. Always examine the breasts for occult tumours, as breast cancer commonly metastasises to ovary.

3. Ultrasonography has limited ability to distinguish between different types of pelvic mass.

4. Ovarian cancer is the commonest cause of death from gynaecological tumours. Primary ovarian cancers generally present at an advanced stage, and the 5 year survival is poor.

5. Ovarian cancer screening has not been shown to reduce the age-specific mortality.

6. Laparotomy for ovarian cancer should include a detailed examination of the entire abdominal cavity to stage ovarian tumours.

18 Recurrent miscarriage

CLINICAL SIGNIFICANCE

Miscarriage can be defined as the spontaneous expulsion of a pregnancy or extraction of a failing pregnancy (delayed miscarriage). Recurrent miscarriage defined strictly is three or more consecutive losses of intrauterine pregnancies. The vast majority of losses are in the first trimester, but a much smaller proportion of women have recurrent midtrimester miscarriages. Some authorities add that the pregnancies should be by the same male partner and that there should be no successful pregnancies. These definitions serve a scientific need of clinical researchers. Most clinicians would recognise three or more miscarriages.

The incidence of miscarriage in recognised pregnancies is 15%, and most of these are due to sporadic, non-recurring causes. The frequency of three consecutive losses is 1%, which is twice as common as one would expect by chance alone. It suggests that about half of couples with recurrent miscarriage have simply had bad luck on three occasions, and this is supported by the negative results of investigations.

Many couples have an increased chance of loss in the next pregnancy, and some of the underlying causes have important implications for the mother and/or fetus if the next pregnancy continues to term. In addition, early miscarriage poses a great emotional challenge to many couples, and recurrent pregnancy loss only serves to multiply the anguish several fold. Human reproduction is surrounded by many myths and superstitions, and there is a very real risk of self-blame and feelings of guilt.

DIFFERENTIAL DIAGNOSIS

MAIN CATEGORY	DIAGNOSIS
1. *Idiopathic*	Chance alone Unidentifiable cause
2. *Maternal age*	
3. *Genetic*	Parental translocations
4. *Thrombophilic defects*	Antiphospholipid syndrome Factor V Leiden mutation Other rare congenital thrombophilias
5. *Anatomical disorders*	Congenital uterine abnormalities Intrauterine adhesions Uterine fibroids Cervical incompetence
6. *Endocrine*	Polycystic ovarian disease Poorly controlled diabetes
7. *Infection*	Bacterial vaginosis (second trimester) Syphilis
8. *Systemic maternal disease*	Chronic renal failure Cyanotic heart disease
9. *Drug therapy*	Warfarin

Far many years endocrine disorders such as hypothyroidism, occult diabetes and luteal phase deficiency were thought to be associated with early pregnancy loss but recent studies have refuted this. Similarly, some research workers felt that there was an association between the human lymphocyte antigen (HLA) types of the parents and miscarriage, but further study has failed to confirm this hypothesis. Because infection can cause sporadic early miscarriage, much research has focused on the possible role of micro-organisms. Bacterial vaginosis, group B Streptococcus and Chlamydia probably play a part in recurrent **midtrimester** losses, but most of the putative infective agents of first-trimester miscarriage such as toxoplasmosis and brucellosis have been discounted.

CLINICAL ASSESSMENT

Due to the frequency of early miscarriage, it is generally accepted that investigation should only take place after three successive confirmed miscarriages. Many clinicians would consider investigation after just two (or even one) **midtrimester** loss.

Organisation of Care

The plan of management of recurrent miscarriage is similar to that of subfertility. Ideally the couple should be seen together, but any need for individual confidentially must be recognised and respected. In addition, the following should be done.

- Organise a dedicated clinic.
- See as a couple but respect individual needs for confidentiality.
- Systematically investigate for proven causes.
- Explain background miscarriage rate.
- Explain specific prognosis without and with therapy.
- Attempt to allay fears and myths without dismissing them.
- Describe treatments and side effects.
- Give general pregnancy advice about rubella vaccination, folic acid, smoking and diet.
- Consider special pregnancy issues, e.g. chance of trisomy 21 if high maternal age.
- Consider need for emotional support and counselling.
- Offer support in next pregnancy.

It is essential to remember that unproven therapies may carry unknown risk to fertility and to future pregnancies. Diethyl-stilboestrol (DES), a synthetic non-steroidal oestrogen, was used in the 1960s for women with recurrent pregnancy loss. Female and male fetuses exposed to DES developed genitourinary malformations, and a significant proportion of the female fetuses have since developed the otherwise rare clear-cell cancer of the cervix.

Relevant History

Presenting Complaint
MAIN SYMPTOM – Full details should be taken of the dates, duration and outcome of all pregnancies of both partners. This enquiry should include questioning into how the pregnancies were proven: a positive pregnancy test or identification of products of conception. Particular attention should be taken of any complications such as infection and any surgical procedures such as uterine evacuation which may lead to Aschermann's syndrome.

Any investigations of the fetuses should be collated, particularly those miscarried in the second trimester. Later miscarriages may reflect cervical incompetence or bacterial vaginosis. Such losses are associated with few contractions or little or no pain.

COMMONLY ASSOCIATED PROBLEMS – Menstrual disorder may reflect PCOD or fibroids. Vaginal discharge may be a feature of bacterial vaginosis or Chlamydia infection.

EFFECT ON COUPLE – These couples are often very anxious, especially if they have not previously had a healthy pregnancy. There is a real chance of severe grief reactions, acute anxiety and marital disharmony. These problems should be considered in parallel with the investigation of the miscarriages.

Gynaecological History
GYNAECOLOGICAL DISEASE – There may be a known history of fibroids which might be distorting the endometrial cavity. Previous surgery to the cervix might have led to weakness of the cervix (incompetence) and late miscarriage.

CONTRACEPTION – Severe infection associated with an IUCD raises the possibility of intrauterine adhesions. Very rarely it is possible that an IUCD has been inserted and then forgotten.

FERTILITY REQUIREMENTS – Couples who have already had children may find recurrent miscarriages so distressing that they request contraception or even sterilisation to prevent it from happening again. Great care should be taken when counselling such women, and the decision should not be rushed.

Medical History
MEDICAL CONDITIONS – Chronic autoimmune diseases such as systemic lupus have been linked with early miscarriage. Poorly controlled diabetes is also associated with a higher spontaneous miscarriage rate. A history of thromboembolism may be part of an antiphospholipid syndrome or another thrombophilic defect. Cyanotic heart disease and chronic renal disease are rare causes of recurrent pregnancy failure.

SURGERY – Previous surgery to the endometrium may have caused scarring.

PSYCHOLOGICAL DISORDERS – Anxiety often accompanies recurrent miscarriage but probably reflects a secondary effect, and stress has not been clearly shown to be a cause of miscarriage.

Drug History

MEDICATIONS – Drug teratogenesis is a very uncommon but nevertheless a potentially important cause of miscarriage. Warfarin is probably the drug which would most commonly lead to recurrent pregnancy failure. Previous radiotherapy and chemotherapy are **not** associated with an increased chance of miscarriage.

SMOKING AND ALCOHOL – There is an association between cigarette smoking and early pregnancy loss but the association is weak. Extreme alcohol intake has a small effect, but modest alcohol intake is thought to be safe. Other recreational drugs are likely to increase the risk of miscarriage.

Social History

AGE – The risk of pregnancy loss increases with maternal age, and this alone may be the cause of recurrent pregnancy failure. In addition, the prognosis for women with an identifiable cause such as thrombophilia varies with age.

OCCUPATION – Exposure to organophosphates has been suggested as a cause of miscarriage, but further information is still needed. VDU operators are not at increased chance of miscarriage as initially thought.

LIFESTYLE – There is no evidence to suggest active lifestyle increases the likelihood of repeat miscarriages. The belief that bed rest reduces the risk of miscarriage has not been supported by studies for the vast majority of women, and it may increase the chance of thromboembolism.

Family History

PCOD – A family history of maturity-onset diabetes is a marker for PCOD, which is often occult in women with recurrent miscarriage.

COAGULOPATHIES – There may be a family history of venous thrombosis which has never been investigated.

CHROMOSOMAL ABNORMALITIES – There may be a history of babies born with malformations or dysmorphic features, that has never been investigated.

Relevant Clinical Examination

General Examination

GENERAL CONDITION – Anxiety or depression may be evident.

BODY-MASS INDEX – Obesity may be a sign of polycystic ovarian disease.

Abdomen

CONTOUR – Look for masses arising from the pelvis such as large fibroids.

PALPATION – Usually will be soft and non-tender. Chronic pelvic infection usually leads to diffuse tenderness.

Pelvic

PERINEUM – Previously unrecognised congenital anatomical abnormalities may be evident.

VULVA/VAGINA/CERVIX – Congenital abnormalities such as septae in the lower genitourinary tract may be visualised and may indicate further abnormalities in the uterus, for example.

BIMANUAL EXAMINATION – An enlarged uterus due to fibroids can be obvious, but submucosal fibroids are difficult to detect and are more likely to cause problems. Congenital uterine abnormalities such as bicornate uterus are generally not identifiable.

Relevant Initial Investigations

Haematology

Hb – Anaemia may arise from recurrent haemorrhage.

PLATELET COUNT – When checking for thrombophilic disease especially antiphospholipid syndrome.

CLOTTING STUDIES – Detailed investigation in specialist laboratory to test for lupus anticoagulant, factor V Leiden and deficiencies of antithrombin III, factor XII and the anticoagulants Protein C and S.

IMMUNOLOGICAL – Anticardiolipin, anti-dsDNA and anti-thyroid antibodies have been found more commonly in women who suffer recurrent miscarriages.

Chromosomes

BLOOD KARYOTYPING – Blood should be tested in both parents, as a balanced chromosomal rearrangement is the most common genetic abnormality associated with miscarriage.

Endocrine Tests

TSH – No proven evidence that thyroid disease leads to recurrent miscarriages.

LH/FSH – Measured on blood taken on day 8 of two or three menstrual cycles. A raised level of LH or ratio of LH to FSH is diagnostic of PCOD, which is commonly found in women with recurring pregnancy loss.

Microbiology

BACTERIAL CULTURE – If vaginal infection is suspected, appropriate swabs should be sent for culture; there is some evidence implicating bacterial vaginosis in particular.

CHLAMYDIAL SEROLOGY – To look for evidence of chronic infection.

RUBELLA SEROLOGY – Non-immune women should be offered vaccination.

Diagnostic Imaging

TRANSVAGINAL ULTRASOUND – Transvaginal ultrasound provides excellent visualisation of the uterus and ovaries. It may allow the demonstration of bicornate uterus and tumours such as fibroids. Examination of ovarian architecture may show PCO morphology.

Endosocopy

OUTPATIENT HYSTEROSCOPY – Demonstrates clearly the endometrial cavity, revealing adhesions, malformations, polyps and submucosal fibroids. This will confirm the suspected diagnosis after ultrasound. An operating hysteroscope can be used to remove polyps or small fibroids.

LAPAROSCOPY – Inspection of the uterine contour is necessary if a uterine malformation is found, to decide if the abnormality can be corrected by hysteroscopy or not.

DETAILS OF COMMON CONDITIONS

Counselling skills are an important part of the management of couples with recurrent miscarriage. There is a need for support with regard to previous losses, but it is also important to avoid generating guilt and discord when one partner has a medical condition.

For couples with idiopathic recurrent miscarriage or maternal age-related effects, all that is available is advice about the chance of success in future pregnancy and psychological support which some researchers have suggested will improve the chance of a good outcome of pregnancy. For all women over 40 years the miscarriage rate is about 50%. For younger women with three miscarriages and no obvious cause, the chance of success is about 60%.

1. Chromosomal Rearrangements

Background

DEFINITION – **Parental chromosomal rearrangement** occurs in up to 5% of parents who suffer recurrent miscarriages. Robertsonian translocation occurs when two chromosomes join, giving a total number of 45, one chromosome counting as two. The outcome depends on which chromosomes are involved. Reciprocal translocation occurs when a portion of one chromosome joins with another, resulting in two abnormal chromosomes but a total number of 46. **Recurrent fetal aneuploidy** occurs when there is an abnormal number of chromosomes (trisomy or monosomy). This usually arises during meiosis. It may be due to mosaicism in the maternal ovaries or paternal testis but is probably more commonly simply chance repetition of sporadic events.

AETIOLOGY – The most common is a balanced reciprocal or Robertsonian translocation.

MAKING THE DIAGNOSIS – There may be a family history of babies born with congenital problems, but usually there is simply a history of recurrent miscarriage sometimes interspersed by successful pregnancies. Regardless, all couples with recurrent miscarriage should be tested by a blood lymphocyte karyotype analysis. As yet, **germ line mosaicism** cannot be tested for. There is little point in testing the products of conception, as sporadic genetic faults such as trisomy are a common cause of sporadic miscarriage, and abnormal results may confuse the couple.

MAIN COMPLICATIONS – The affected partner will have no problems because he/she will have a normal amount of genetic material. It is only during meiosis of reproduction when the genetic material is sorted that the arrangement becomes unbalanced. Miscarriage occurs or there may be fetal malformation in an ongoing pregnancy.

SCREENING/PREVENTION – Screening is usually not performed until multiple losses have occurred, unless there is a family history. There is no method of primary prevention for apparently normal women and men.

Treatment Options

GENETIC COUNSELLING – Genetic counselling should be provided by properly trained health professionals. Clear explanation of the nature of the genetic defect and the chance of problems in future pregnancies is given. This includes details of the chance of an ongoing pregnancy with a genetically abnormal fetus and of prenatal diagnostic tests. There is no true treatment, but donor sperm can be used if the paternal genotype is abnormal. This is not acceptable to many couples, however the chances of a repeat problem are very low, and this should be made clear.

The genetics team will offer to arrange investigation of other blood relatives.

OVERVIEW – The management of these couples is difficult. There is no direct treatment, only the offer of advice and support from the clinical genetics team. Prenatal screening should be offered for future pregnancies.

2. Thrombophilic Defects

Background

DEFINITION – Abnormalities occurring in part of the clotting cascade and associated elements. Accounts for about 20% of cases of recurrent miscarriage. The antiphospholipid syndrome accounts for the large majority of these.

AETIOLOGY – **Antiphospholipid syndrome** associates thrombosis with pregnancy loss in the presence of antiphospholipid antibody (aPL). aPLs are implicated in damage of the developing placenta by thrombosi within small vessels. **Factor V Leiden mutation (activated protein C resistance)** has recently been implicated in recurrent miscarriage, especially in the second trimester. Other abnormalities of the coagulation system have been found in higher frequencies also, including deficiencies of antithrombin III, and proteins C and S.

MAKING THE DIAGNOSIS – These congenital and acquired coagulation disorders should be tested for in all women through a specialist haematology laboratory.

MAIN COMPLICATIONS – Venous, and less commonly arterial, thrombosis with or without recurrent fetal loss are the main complications associated with these conditions.

SCREENING/PREVENTION – Thromboprophylaxis during subsequent pregnancies helps to prevent maternal thrombosis. Occasionally, life-long anticoagulation is necessary. If an hereditary coagulopathy is identified, other blood relatives should be offered testing.

Treatment Options

ADVICE – Risks to the mother (thrombosis and pre-eclamspia) and fetus (miscarriage and intrauterine growth retardation) must be discussed and considered. The exact advice varies with the nature of the coagulation disorder and the maternal history. It should be remembered that there is a reasonable chance of success without therapy (at least 40%).

DRUG THERAPY – Prophylaxis during subsequent pregnancies is being thoroughly researched. Most work has been done in women with the antiphospholipid syndrome. **Low-dose aspirin** (LDA), **heparin** and **corticosteroids** have all been used, but many of the studies are of poor quality. Corticosteroids have been shown not to be of benefit and to carry significant risk to the mother. LDA has been shown to improve the chance of a live birth. Low-dose heparin probably increases this effect and decreases the risk of maternal thrombosis. LDA is very safe but carries the risk of haematemesis, worsening of asthma, and allergy. Heparin requires daily injections and may cause osteoporosis with fractures in a very small proportion of cases. **Warfarin** is generally advised against because it is teratogenic and it causes fetal bleeding.

These treatments are currently being evaluated for the treatment of **activated protein C resistance**.

OVERVIEW – It is clear that the antiphospholipid syndrome and factor V Leiden do require treatment in subsequent pregnancies, although the data are not conclusive.

3. *Congenital and Acquired Uterine Abnormalities*

Background

DEFINITION – Any anatomical defects that leads to failure to maintain a pregnancy. Uterine abnormalities account for about 5% of cases of recurrent miscarriage.

AETIOLOGY – Congenital uterine abnormalities occur because of a failure of the Mullerian ducts to fuse correctly (Figure 18.1). Uterine fibroids are smooth muscle tumours of unknown cause. Intrauterine adhesions may develop secondary to severe infection and/or surgery to the uterine cavity, causing necrosis and scarring. Severe adhesions obliterate the endometrial cavity and cause amenorrhoea and infertility rather than recurrent miscarriage.

MAKING THE DIAGNOSIS – Ultrasound is used to diagnose uterine pathology and congenital abnormalities. Hysteroscopy (with laparoscopy) is necessary to provide confirmation and to demonstrate smaller lesions such as intrauterine adhesions or small septa at the fundus which will not be evident at scan.

MAIN COMPLICATIONS – Congenital defects from failure of fusion of the Mullerian ducts cause a range of abnormalities ranging from extra septate membranes to uterine malformation. Uterine malformations range from complete failure of fusion, leading to duplication of the reproductive tract (uterus didelphys), to partial fusion (uterus bicornis), failure of reabsorption (septate uterus) and failure of canalisation (vaginal agenesis). They are often associated with renal tract abnormalities

SCREENING/PREVENTION – The women should be offered a renal ultrasound to screen for associated urinary tract malformations.

Treatment Options

ADVICE – It is difficult to define in individual women what the role of uterine abnormalities is in causing miscarriage, because many women with malformations and fibroids have normal reproductive function. Careful counselling is essential before surgery is contemplated because of the risk of making the outcome of pregnancy worse and also because of the risk of emergency hysterectomy during surgery.

SURGERY – Unicornate uteri cannot be surgically corrected but they may carry an increased chance of cervical incompetence, and cervical cerclage should be considered (see below). Hysteroscopic techniques, which can be used to divide septae and adhesions, have the best results, open surgical procedures being more likely to cause tubal scarring. Fibroids can be removed hysteroscopically if they are small enough.

OVERVIEW – Surgical procedures can be used to correct some anatomical abnormalities, but surgery may lead to damage of pelvic anatomy.

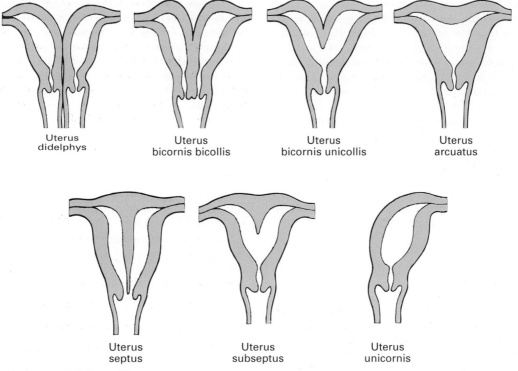

Uterus
didelphys

Uterus
bicornis bicollis

Uterus
bicornis unicollis

Uterus
arcuatus

Uterus
septus

Uterus
subseptus

Uterus
unicornis

Fig 18.1 *Uterine congenital abnormalities.*

4. Cervical Incompetence

Background

DEFINITION – Weakness of uterine cervix resulting in passive dilatation of cervix during second or third trimester.

AETIOLOGY – It may rarely be congenital in women with inherited disorders of connective tissue, and in those with uterine malformations (see above). Most causes appear to arise after cervical dilatation or cone biopsy.

MAKING THE DIAGNOSIS – Suspicion is raised by the typical history. The classical story is of sudden loss of normally formed fresh fetus in midtrimester. Controlled trials suggest that cervical incompetence has been overdiagnosed in the past, with only a third of women previously diagnosed actually suffering this problem. The presentation may be indistinguishable from that of miscarriage associated with bacterial vaginosis and group B Streptococcus colonisation, and of miscarriage due to congenital uterine malformations. Formal bacteriology is essential and the uterine cavity should be investigated (see above). Serial transvaginal ultrasonography during pregnancy can be used to identify early dilatation at the level of the internal os. This allows many women to avoid unnecessary cerclage.

MAIN COMPLICATIONS – Painless second trimester miscarriage or preterm delivery. Preterm prelabour rupture of membranes.

SCREENING/PREVENTION – Avoid trauma to cervix during surgery. Use cervical ripeners (softeners) before termination of pregnancy.

Treatment Options

ADVICE – The prospects for future pregnancies are good (80% chance of success) if only one pregnancy has been lost, and some women will choose careful observation in preference to treatment.

CHANGE OF LIFESTYLE/DIET – None.

DRUG THERAPY – Antibiotics should be used if there is strong suspicion of bacterial vaginosis.

SURGERY – Purse-string suture of the cervix (Figure 18.2) is thought to delay delivery by at least 7 weeks. Cerclage carries risks of infection and cervical laceration.

OVERVIEW – Cervical incompetence is a rare cause of recurrent midtrimester miscarriage. It is difficult to diagnose, and many women with a suggestive history will have a normal pregnancy outcome next time without treatment. It needs to be distinguished from bacterial vaginosis. For women with a very suspicious history, cervical cerclage can be used.

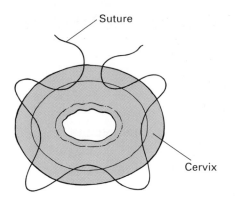

Fig 18.2 *Cervical cerclage.*

5. Polycystic Ovarian Disease

See also Chapter 20.

Brief Background

PCOD is the commonest cause of recurrent miscarriage, accounting for about 40% of cases. The exact mechanism is poorly understood. It is clear that most pregnant women with PCOD have successful pregnancies. The prognosis for future pregnancies for those with repeated miscarriages is likely to be quite good, but data

are awaited. Attempts to improve the outcome using GnRH analogues to suppress endogenous LH levels and endogenous FSH to induce ovulation have been met with failure. Laparoscopic ovarian electrodiathermy is associated with a normal miscarriage rate when used for anovulatory infertile women with PCOD, suggesting it may also be useful for those with recurrent miscarriage, but it carries risk of ovarian damage and even of ovarian failure. Further studies are awaited.

GOLDEN POINTS

1. Systematic investigation after three miscarriages.

2. Give prognosis with and without treatment.

3. Expain risks of treatment carefully.

4. Give general pregnancy advice.

5. Consider wider health issues for mother.

6. Consider emotional needs in parallel.

7. Offer detailed support in future pregnancy.

19 Failure to conceive

CLINICAL SIGNIFICANCE

About 15% of apparently normal couples having regular unprotected intercourse fail to conceive within 12 months. At least one in six couples seek help with difficulty conceiving at some stage.

Child rearing is a main focus of many relationships, and the distress caused by subfertility can lead to severe psychological upset and even marital breakdown.

Successful treatment is now available for most causes of subfertility, but many of the newer assisted conception techniques are not available on the NHS. The lack of resources causes additional distress for some couples and financial hardship for many more.

DIFFERENTIAL DIAGNOSIS

MAIN CATEGORY	DIAGNOSIS
Idiopathic	Unexplained infertility (minimal endometriosis)
Female factors	
1. *Anovulation*	Primary ovarian failure (premature menopause) Secondary ovarian failure Polycystic ovarian disease General endocrine disorders
2. *Tubal damage*	Infection Endometriosis Previous abdominal surgery
3. *Cervical factors*	Mucus hostility (acidified mucus) Mucus antisperm antibodies Absence of mucus secondary to cone biopsy
4. *Uterine factors*	Submucosal fibroids Intrauterine adhesions
5. *Sexual dysfunction*	Vaginismus Dyspareunia
Male factors	
1. *Azoospermia*	Congenital absence of vas Obstruction of vas deferens Hypogonadotrophic hypogonadism Hypergonadotrophic hypogonadism
2. *Sperm dysfunction*	Inflammatory disease Seminal antisperm antibodies Idiopathic Genetic (Kartagener's syndrome)
3. *Erectile impotence*	Vascular disease Neurological disease Psychosomatic disorder

Investigation and treatment of oligo-amenorrhoea is dealt with in Chapter 20.

Female factors are the most common, being found in nearly 50% of cases, whereas male factors are present in about 30%. For about 20% of couples there is more than one factor involved, emphasising the need for the couple to be investigated jointly.

For over 25% of couples there will be no cause found for the subfertility, and this can be more difficult to contend with psychologically even though they tend to be the group with the highest success with assisted reproduction.

CLINICAL ASSESSMENT

Organisation of Care

Unless there is an obvious impediment to conception, such as amenorrhoea, couples are generally encouraged to try to conceive for 12 to 18 months before investigation.

The general practitioner plays an important role in the initial assessment of these couples. General advice can be given, such as rubella vaccination and folic acid therapy. In addition, basic fertility tests can be arranged before referral to the specialist clinic. The GP will also play an important role in the support of the couple during investigation and treatment.

The scheme of specialist management is as follows.

• Organise dedicated reproductive medicine clinic with specialist doctors, nurses and counsellors.
• See as a couple, but respect individual needs for confidentiality.
• Explain about timing of intercourse.
• Undertake systematic investigation for proven causes.
• Explain specific prognosis for category of subfertility, without and with therapy.
• Describe treatments, side effects and complications.
• Give general pregnancy advice about rubella vaccination, folic acid, smoking and diet.
• Consider special pregnancy issues, e.g. chance of trisomy 21 if high maternal age.
• Consider need for emotional support and counselling.
• Arrange for follow-up if treatment fails, to consider wider health issues.

Relevant History – Female

Presenting Complaint

MAIN SYMPTOM – A failure to conceive after unprotected intercourse. The duration should be noted, as this determines prognosis in certain cases. A full **coital history** should be taken, including the timing of the intercourse with the menstrual cycle. Women with regular 28 day menstrual cycles ovulate on about day 14. The fertile days are days 11 to 14. Couples may have moved or been seen elsewhere, so any previous investigations and results should be elicited to avoid expensive, time-wasting repetition.

COMMONLY ASSOCIATED SYMPTOMS – Painful intercourse (**dyspareunia**) might be a sign of pelvic disease (PID or endometriosis) or psychological problems (vaginismus). Recurrent pain may lead to sexual dysfunction, regardless of the cause, and intercourse can become infrequent and ineffective.

EFFECT ON COUPLE – One or both members of the couple may be very distressed by the failure to conceive. This may lead to individual grief, marital disharmony, psychosexual disorder, etc. The couple should be seen together, but each may have individual confidential issues which must be respected.

Gynaecological History

GYNAECOLOGICAL DISEASE – The woman may have known gynaecological/pelvic disease and may have been advised to seek referral when considering starting a family. **Tubal disease** accounts for 15% of cases and is commonly caused by severe pelvic inflammatory disease. **Endometriosis** is associated with subfertility, and previous surgery such as **ovarian cystectomy** may have induced pelvic adhesions.

MENSTRUAL HISTORY – A **regular menstrual cycle** increases the likelihood of ovulation taking place, and some women even report a light midcycle bleed. A history of irregular or infrequent menses raises the possibility of ovarian dysfunction, commonly PCOD. **Amenorrhoea** may be due to pregnancy or anovulation.

CERVICAL CYTOLOGY – Treatment to the cervix for premalignant disease may cause scarring and stenosis of the os. Check for smear status.

CONTRACEPTION – Post-pill amenorrhoea does not actually exist, and therefore a woman should not have her investigations delayed because she has stopped the pill for 12 months. The IUCD is associated with pelvic infection which may have been subacute and gone undetected.

Obstetric History

Previous children is a good prognostic sign for spontaneous and assisted conception.

OBSTETRIC COMPLICATIONS – Puerperal infection leading to tubal damage may occur after a normal or assisted delivery.

Medical History

MEDICAL CONDITIONS – General health is important for fertility, and some treatments may be contraindicated with severe maternal disease (e.g. Eisenmenger's complex). HIV has implications for handling of gametes and for health of offspring.

SURGERY – Adhesions or scar formation leading to tubo-ovarian damage can be caused by previous pelvic surgery.

PSYCHOLOGICAL DISORDERS – The investigations and treatments offered for the infertile couple are demanding and can create or exacerbate pre-existing psychological problems.

Drug History

MEDICATIONS – May need to alter if drug is teratogenic.

SMOKING AND ALCOHOL – Advice on stopping smoking and drinking should be provided if pregnancy is being contemplated.

Social History

AGE – The chances of conception decrease with age, and women over the age of 35 should not have any delay in referral as the investigations and treatments available do take time to set up.

OCCUPATION – May determine whether assisted conception can be afforded or not.

LIFESTYLE – There is a responsibility to the potential offspring of any treatment, and many subfertility units have an ethical policy. Issues such as current drug abuse and a history of child sex abuse are taken into account.

Relevant Clinical Examination – Female

General Examination

GENERAL CONDITION – Hirsutism and thyroid state.

BODY-MASS INDEX – Severe weight loss leads to anovulation due to disruption to the hypothalamic/pituitary axis. Obesity can be associated with polycystic ovarian syndrome, and extreme morbid obesity may even prevent effective coitus.

Abdomen

OLD SCARS – Previous abdominal, especially subumbilical, surgical scars may be from a laparoscopy either in the diagnosis of pelvic disease or from previous infertility investigations.

PALPATION – Routine abdominal inspection and palpation are carried out to look for pelvic swellings from tumours or tenderness from infection.

Pelvic

PERINEUM/VULVA/VAGINA/CERVIX – To exclude anatomical or congenital anomalies that may prevent normal intercourse.

BIMANUAL EXAMINATION – Carried out to detect pelvic tumours such as ovarian cysts or an enlarged uterus due to fibroids or uterine abnormalities. Tenderness is a feature of PID and endometriosis.

Relevant Initial Investigations – Female

Investigations for oligo-amenorrhoea are described in Chapter 20.

Tests for Ovulation

SERUM PROGESTERONE – Traditionally, a serum progesterone concentration is measured in the midluteal phase of women who are menstruating. This is initially performed in two consecutive cycles. A concentration greater than 30 nmol/l suggests that ovulation is taking place. However, it is extremely rare to find that women with regular menstruation have persistent cycle dysfunction, and about 20% of cycles are dysfunctional in fertile women. Some authorities have suggested that women with regular menstruation do not warrant testing, therefore.

MUCUS TESTING (BILLING'S METHOD) – Self-testing for the presence of fertile mucus just before midcycle is highly suggestive that good ovulation takes place. It also helps couples to predict when to have intercourse.

BASAL BODY TEMPERATURE – There is a midcycle rise in temperature of 0.5 to 1°C caused by the increase in luteal phase progesterone. It has been used to diagnose ovulation but is very inaccurate. In addition, it is of little value for the timing of intercourse, because ovulation is over by the time the temperature has risen. It has been abandoned by most units.

ENDOMETRIAL – Endometrial biopsies were previously used to assess the endometrial response to progesterone in the luteal phase, but this practice has now been abandoned.

Other Endocrine Tests

TSH – Occult hypothyroidism is said to be more common in subfertility.

LH/FSH – A **raised serum FSH concentration** in the early follicular phase is suggestive of incipient ovarian failure (the menopause). This may be of value when deciding the speed at which investigations should be performed and for predicting the outcome of fertility treatment. A **raised LH/FSH ratio** in the early follicular phase is indicative of PCOD. **Urinary LH assays** can be bought over the counter to help couples time intercourse. This can lead to pressure on the male, however, and male psychosexual problems may follow.

Microbiology

BACTERIAL CULTURE – Swabs can be taken if there is a history of STDs or pelvic infection. Serum screening for HIV and Hepatitis B virus is performed when assisted conception is considered.

RUBELLA SEROLOGY – If negative, the woman should be offered vaccination to prevent congenital rubella syndrome.

CHLAMYDIAL SEROLOGY – A positive immunofluorescence test (IFT) may indicate old pelvic infection or be more suggestive of current infection (positive complement fixation test (CFT)). The test has two uses. First, any woman with positive serology should have antibiotic prophylaxis before hysteroscopy and laparoscopy. Second, serology predicts tubal disease, and, if the result is positive, consideration should be given to expediting the investigations for tubal disease.

HEPATITIS SEROLOGY – Serum screening for hepatitis B virus is performed when assisted conception is considered.

Tests of Pelvic Anatomy

ULTRASOUND – Transvaginal scanning is now seen as routine in the investigation of an infertile couple, providing accurate information on ovarian and uterine pathology. It is less useful for tubal disease, but hydrosalpinges may be evident.

CONTRAST RADIOLOGY – Hysterosalpingography (Figure 19.1) involves injection of contrast medium through the cervix, across the uterine cavity and into the fallopian tubes. The abdomen is screened fluoroscopically during this, and x-rays are taken. Uterine lesions and tubal blockage can be identified. It is uncomfortable. False positives may occur because of tubal spasm.

HYSTEROSCOPY – Can be used to confirm uterine lesions seen on transvaginal ultrasound.

LAPAROSCOPY AND DYE HYDROTUBATION – Nowadays nearly routinely performed for the subfertile couple. Because of the invasive nature of this investigation it is usually left until 2 years if all other tests are negative. Expedited if chlamydial serology is positive or if there is a history

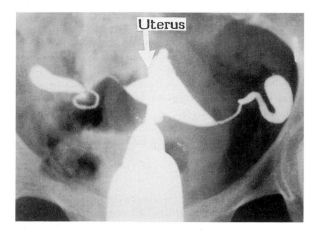

Fig 19.1 *Hysterosalpingogram demonstrating hydrosalpinx.*

of previous infection or previous surgery. It allows clear visualisation of the uterus, Fallopian tubes and ovaries, revealing adhesions, endometriosis and tubal disease. Injection of indigo carmine dye through the cervix reveals patency of the Fallopian tubes.

Tests of Cervical Mucus Receptivity

POSTCOITAL TEST (PCT) – Cervical mucus quality can be tested as part of postcoital and crossed-penetration tests (see below).

IMMUNE TESTS – To check for mucus antisperm antibodies in women with abnormal PCT and crossed-penetration test.

MUCUS pH – Mucus acidity is a cause of mucus hostility.

Relevant History – Male

Presenting Complaint

MAIN SYMPTOM – Usually no outward symptom suggestive of a problem.

COMMONLY ASSOCIATED SYMPTOMS – There may be an erectile problem, but this is rarely volunteered and will have to be elicited sympathetically. Care should be taken to discover the frequency and timing of intercourse.

EFFECT ON PATIENT – Psychological disturbance and upset is not limited to the woman. The man may have a grief reaction or feelings of inadequacy. Psychosexual erectile impotence is not an uncommon consequence of subfertility, particularly during investigations requiring intercourse/ejaculation.

Parental History

FATHERHOOD – The man may have already had children with another partner. It is a good prognostic sign but does not mean that male factor testing can be overlooked.

Medical History

MEDICAL CONDITIONS – A history of sexually transmitted disease, especially epididymal or prostatic infection, can cause scarring of the ducts, preventing sperm release. History of maldescent of testis may indicate cause of azoospermia. HIV has implications for handling of gametes and for health of offspring.

SURGERY – Hernia and testicular surgery may have damaged a testis. Any bladder neck or prostatic surgery may induce retrograde ejaculation.

PSYCHOLOGICAL DISORDERS – A failure to conceive may have been the cover used to present with psychosexual problems (impotence, premature ejaculation).

Drug History

MEDICATIONS – Chemotherapy for malignant disease, sulphasalazine, and antihypertensives may lead to a low sperm count or ejaculatory problems.

SMOKING AND ALCOHOL – Both are linked to a low sperm count and reduced fertilisation rates when used in excess.

Social History

OCCUPATION – Exposure to toxic chemicals is known to reduce the sperm count. Sedentary jobs that require sitting, such as truck driving, lead to a regular increase in testicular temperature resulting in low sperm counts.

LIFESTYLE – Sedentary lifestyle and tight clothing raise testicular temperature and reduce sperm counts.

Relevant Clinical Examination – Male

Male examination is rarely helpful. It could be argued that it should be reserved for men with azoospermia or sperm dysfunction.

General Examination

GENERAL DEMEANOUR – Secondary sexual characteristics.
BODY-MASS INDEX – Obesity.

Abdomen

CONTOUR – For tumours.
OLD SCARS – Previous major abdominal surgery may have damaged the autonomic supply to the genitals, leading to impotence or ejaculatory failure.
PALPATION – Check inguinal canal for maldescended testes if not in scrotum.

Pelvic

SCROTUM AND TESTICLES – Make sure both testicles are present, checking their consistency and excluding any tumours. Both vas deferens should be palpated to feel for their presence and for thickening and hardening. Varicocoeles (dilated veins) can be demonstrated on standing but they are not relevant to subfertility treatment.

RECTAL EXAMINATION – The prostate may be enlarged or extremely tender if infection is present.

Relevant Initial Investigations – Male

There are three questions to be answered:

1. Is the man able to ejaculate?
2. Does the ejaculate contain sperm?
3. Are the sperm functionally normal?

In the past there has been a great emphasis on sperm numbers, but sperm function is a much more important factor. Ask yourself, would you rather scrum down against Wyggeston Boys 3rd XV or the Leicester Tigers 1st XV.

Seminal Analysis

SPERM COUNT – This is essentially to see if a man can ejaculate and, if so, if he produces sperm. Unless there is very severe oligozoospermia (less than 5 million sperm per ml), the sperm count is of little predictive value. Microscopic assessment of sperm motility is also of little value.

Tests of Sperm Function

POSTCOITAL TEST – The PCT is primarily a test of sperm function. It does assess mucus quality as well, but mucus problems are very much rarer than sperm dysfunction. The tests comprises microscopy of cervical mucus taken 12–18 h after sexual intercourse. The test is timed to the fertile part of the ovarian cycle to ensure good mucus quality. If there are problems with timing, mucus production can be stimulated by oral oestrogen. The mucus is assessed to check that it looks to be of good quality (plentiful, clear and ductile). At microscopy, the number of sperm per high-power film that are moving forwards is noted. Five progressing sperm per high-power film is highly predictive of good sperm function.

CROSSED-PENETRATION TEST – If the PCT is negative or abnormal, the next step is to undertake a crossed-penetration test (XPT). This involves a 4-way cross-over testing of patient mucus and sperm, and donated mucus or sperm. This helps to determine whether the PCT abnormality was the result of a sperm function problems or mucus hostility, or both.

LABORATORY SPERM FUNCTION TESTING – A wide range of laboratory tests have been devised. Some to replace the PCT (computerised seminal analysis, Hamster egg penetration test), some to complement it (crossed-penetration test), and some for specific disorders (acrosome staining, etc.).

IMMUNE TESTING – To check for seminal antisperm antibodies. The mixed antiglobulin reaction (MAR test) is used as a screening test. Other, more sophisticated tests are available to determine the quantity and type of antibody in semen (e.g. immunobead test).

Microbiology

BACTERIAL CULTURE – Cultures should be taken of the ejaculate if chronic infection is suspected.

HEPATITIS SEROLOGY – Serum screening for hepatitis B virus is performed when assisted conception is considered.

DETAILS OF COMMON CONDITIONS

I. Tubal Disease

Background

DEFINITION – Any condition leading to blockage or reduced mobility of the Fallopian tube or preventing the sperm reaching and fertilising the ovum.

AETIOLOGY – The majority of tubal damage is secondary

to either infection or severe endometriosis. Pelvic surgery, especially following ectopic pregnancy or ruptured bowel, also leads to adhesion formation.

MAKING THE DIAGNOSIS – See Table 19.1.

MAIN COMPLICATIONS – The **failure to conceive** can be due to either tubal blockage or ovarian scarring which interferes with ovulation. **Chronic pelvic pain** and dyspareunia commonly feature in these cases and may themselves interfere with intercourse, preventing fertilisation. **Ectopic pregnancy**.

SCREENING/PREVENTION – Avoid IUCDs in young women with no children. Treat PID promptly. Screen and treat infection before termination of pregnancy. Give antibiotics prior to hysterosalpingography and tubal surgery.

Treatment Options

ADVICE – The chance of spontaneous pregnancy is generally very low (10% over 2 years). The main choice is between tubal surgery and assisted conception (in-vitro fertilisation + embryo transfer). Tubal surgery is a single act of motivation associated with a normal chance of multiple pregnancy, but it involves major surgery, and the chance of success is just 20% overall. IVF requires great motivation, and there is a high chance of multiple pregnancy, but the success rate is 25% per cycle of treatment.

SURGERY – Tubal surgery is offered for mild to moderate disease. Salpingostomy involves surgical opening of the tubal ostia, allowing access for the ovum to enter and meet with the ascending sperm. The blockage can be surgically excised and the exposed ends re-anastamosed. Both of these techniques have similar success rates of around 20%, but much lower with severe disease.

OVERVIEW – Treatment is usually required, and advances in assisted conception have meant surgical techniques are less successful, but it is available on the NHS, making it a cheaper option for the woman. Ectopic pregnancy is much higher in women who have had surgery for tubal disease.

Follow-up

SHORT TERM – These women should be seen regularly to monitor progress and allow further treatments if the surgery fails. If a period is missed, the woman should have early tests and ultrasound confirmation that any pregnancy is in the uterine cavity, to exclude ectopic pregnancy.

LONG TERM – If surgery is unsuccessful, the woman should be offered assisted conception.

2. *Minimal Endometriosis*

See also Chapter 16.

Brief Background

Endometriosis is thought to be found more commonly in women with subfertility than in fertile controls. The **relationship between subfertility and endometriosis** is easy to understand in women with endometriosis distorting pelvic anatomy. For the majority of women, the volume of endometriotic tissue is very small, however, and then the relationship between the condition and subfertility is more difficult to understand. It might be that subfertility (lack of pregnancy) leads to endometriosis, that endometriosis causes subfertility, a combination of both, or, finally, that there is a condition which both causes subfertility and endometriosis. The exact relationship remains unclear despite extensive research. Current research is looking into follicular dysfunction in endometriosis. For those with severe endometriosis with tubal/ovarian damage, microsurgery is often helpful. For couples in whom endometriosis is the only factor, there is a modest chance of spontaneous conception without treatment, but conventional treat-

Table 19.1 Diagnosing tubal subfertility	
Making the diagnosis	Tubal disease
History	Failure to conceive after 12 months
	Pelvic pain / dyspareunia
	Pelvic inflammatory disease / STDs
	Previous surgery (e.g. ectopic, appendicitis)
Examination	Pelvic tenderness
	Adnexal mass, uterine fixation or uterosacral ligament thickening
Investigations	
– Serology	Positive chlamydial serology highly predictive
– Ultrasound	Hydrosalpinx or endometriotic cysts may be seen
– Hysterosalpingogram	Blockage seen on hysterosalpingogram
– Laparoscopy	Distension of the Fallopian tubes and failure for dye to be passed when introduced cervically
	Pelvic adhesions or endometriosis

ments (hormone suppression), normally used for physical symptoms of minimal endometriosis, such as pelvic pain, do not increase the chance of natural conception. If the couple have prolonged subfertility then assisted conception (intrauterine insemination or GIFT) appears to offer the best chance of success.

3. Mucus Hostility

Brief Background
Mucus acts as a receptor of sperm into the cervix. Mucus abnormality may prevent sperm entering and/or passing through the mucus. It is detected by stepwise investigation of negative PCT, using XPT, immunobead testing to look for mucus antisperm antibodies, etc. Treatment depends on the exact nature of the mucus disorder. **Acid mucus** => alkaline douching; **mucus antisperm antibodies** => IVF; **non-specific mucus disorder** => exogenous oestrogen therapy to increase endogenous oestradiol production and improve mucus quality; **absent mucus secondary to cervical surgery** => intrauterine insemination.

4. Ovulatory Disorders

See Chapter 20.

5. Unexplained Subfertility

Background
DEFINITION – No cause found for infertility.
AETIOLOGY – Some such couples may have failed to conceive by chance alone, but most probably have an unidentifiable factor preventing conception.
MAIN COMPLICATIONS – The lack of any substantive explanation is very frustrating for many couples.
MAKING THE DIAGNOSIS – A diagnosis of exclusion.

Treatment Options
ADVICE – It is not uncommon for these couples to conceive while under investigation or awaiting treatment. If the duration of subfertility is short and the woman is young, the chance of spontaneous conception is moderate (30% over 2 years).
DRUG THERAPY – Clomiphene (anti-oestrogen) has a small effect on the conception rate.
ASSISTED CONCEPTION – Assisted conception may be necessary for these couples and has a high success rate. GIFT gives the best chance of success (30%) per treatment cycle.

Follow-up
SHORT TERM – After careful explanation these couples may opt for assisted conception, requiring close follow-up.

LONG TERM – If the couple decide initially not to have treatment but change their minds, they can be referred back.

6. Sperm Dysfunction

Background
DEFINITION – Abnormalities of sperm motility, morphology or survival.
AETIOLOGY – A variety of causes, many poorly defined as yet. There is a congenital form due to autosomal recessive abnormality of cilial function (Kartagener's syndrome), and acquired forms secondary to testicular infection or trauma. Most forms are idiopathic.
MAKING THE DIAGNOSIS – Suspicion raised by negative or abnormal PCT. Detailed investigation of sperm function attempts to identify the cause and severity of the problem.
SCREENING/PREVENTION – Prevention or early treatment of STDs. Early correction of maldescent of testes.

Treatment Options
ADVICE – Important to emphasise that sperm dysfunction is a form of subfertility and not sterility. If couple are not advised of this, the male partner may become suspicious of the woman's fidelity if she does conceive.
CHANGE OF LIFESTYLE/DIET – There are some general factors which have a small effect on sperm function. Although they may not themselves cause subfertility, they may play a critical part in men who have sperm dysfunction. The general factors include raised testicular temperature – which occurs in sitting jobs, e.g. long-distance driving, and wearing tight clothing – smoking and alcohol. Alterations of these habits may lead to a small improvement.
DRUG THERAPY – **High-dose corticosteroids** have been advocated by some for men with seminal antisperm antibodies, but they carry risks of osteoporotic bone fractures. **Antioxidants** such as vitamin E have been used for sperm dysfunction associated with testicular inflammation, but definitive data are awaited. **Hormone therapies** have been tried but with no success.
SURGERY – Not relevant. Correction of varicocoeles has now been discredited.
ASSISTED CONCEPTION – The big advance in the treatment of couples childless because of sperm dysfunction has been the development of assisted conception techniques. Mild sperm dysfunction can be treated by sperm washing and standard IVF. For more severe forms with very low sperm numbers and/or highly abnormal sperm motility, microinjection techniques have to be used **(intracytoplasmic sperm injection** (ICSI – see Figure 19.2). Donor insemination remains an option.

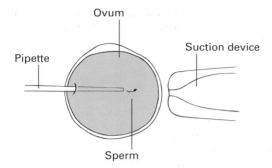

Fig 19.2 *Intracytoplasmic sperm injection.*

OVERVIEW – Sperm dysfunction is one of the commonest causes of subfertility. In the majority of cases the cause cannot be identified. For most couples, assisted conception offers the most realistic chance of success, but it is costly and availability is limited.

7. Obstructive Azoospermia

Brief Background

This is the commonest reason for azoospermia, but it is still rare. Main cause of blockage is infection, but cystic fibrosis is a rare factor. Even rarer is congenital absence of vas deferens. Diagnosis is suggested by azoospermia with normal endocrine investigation (FSH, LH and testosterone). Confirmation is by exploration of testis. Surgical correction is possible, but seminal antisperm antibodies and conception rate can be disappointing. If blockage cannot be reversed, one can aspirate sperm or spermatids (immature sperm) and perform ICSI. Insemination with donated sperm remains an option.

8. Azoospermia – Hypogonadotrophic Hypogonadism

Brief Background

Testicular failure secondary to hypothalamic or pituitary failure. Testis is essentially normal. Causes include hyperprolactinaemia, hypothalamic/pituitary surgery or radiotherapy, and Kallmann syndrome (absence of GnRH). Very rare. Diagnosed by low levels of LH, FSH and testosterone. Additional tests include serum prolactin and cranial radiology. In contrast to female counterpart (secondary ovarian failure), induction of spermatogenesis and androgenesis is relatively simple with twice weekly injections of hCG which acts like LH. Success rate is high.

9. Azoospermia – Hypergonadotrophic Hypogonadism

Brief Background

Primary testicular (end-organ) failure resulting from genetic defects (e.g. Klinefelter's syndrome – 47XXY), radiotherapy and chemotherapy, or severe trauma. Very rare. Diagnosed by persistent elevation of serum FSH (i.e. male equivalent of menopause). No therapy available but may get late spontaneous recovery (more than 5 years) after radiotherapy and chemotherapy. Couple may wish to apply for fostering or adoption, but insemination with donated sperm is also an option. Male partner may need androgen replacement therapy if there is failure of both spermatogenic and androgenic parts of the testis.

Men about to undergo chemotherapy or radiotherapy should be allowed to have sperm freeze-stored.

10. Erectile Impotence

Background

DEFINITION – The inability to achieve penile erection for adequate intercourse.

AETIOLOGY – Vascular disease leads to poor blood flow and nerve damage, seen more often in men who smoke and those with diabetes. Psychosexual problems can lead to erectile dysfunction.

Treatment Options

ADVICE – Erection occurs when the penile cavernous bodies fill up with blood, which is under the control of the parasympathetic nervous system. By altering lifestyle the prognosis can be excellent.

CHANGE OF LIFESTYLE/DIET – Good diabetic control will reduce the risk of impotence occurring, as will relaxation and removal of stress along with improved diet. Cessation of smoking and reduction of alcohol intake are also important.

DRUG THERAPY – The injection of vasoactive drugs into the cavernosum leads to vasodilation and erection for several hours. They work best for those with neurogenic and psychological dysfunction as opposed to vascular disease. The men are taught to inject themselves but should present if the erection lasts more than 6 hours.

MECHANICAL DEVICES – Pumps may help to develop erection, and devices are also available that restrict blood flow at the base of the penis after an erection has been achieved.

ELECTRO-EJACULATION – Can be used for men with spinal injuries.

PSYCHOSEXUAL THERAPY – For men with psychogenic problems.

ASSISTED CONCEPTION – Can use artificial insemination of partners or donor semen.

OVERVIEW – Very rare and requires very specialist knowledge. Need to take care not to damage esteem of the man.

SPECIAL SECTION – ASSISTED CONCEPTION

Background

Initial fertility treatments for tubal disease aimed to restore tubal patency, but it was soon evident that although tubal anatomy could be corrected in many women, tubal function could not. Several researchers aimed to achieve fertilisation of collected oocytes in the laboratory (**in-vitro fertilisation, IVF**, or test-tube fertilisation) and then return the developing embryo(s) into the mother's womb through the cervix (**embryo transfer, ET**). IVF + ET was finally achieved about twenty years ago. Since then the treatment regimens for IVF + ET have been steadily improved (see Table 19.2), and newer methods of assisted conception have been introduced for different categories of subfertility (Table 19.3).

Table 19.2   Stepwise explanation of method of IVF + ET

Technique	Reason
Full investigation and counselling	
Pituitary desensitisation with GnRHa	Achieve complete control of ovary
Induce multiple follicular growth with FSH (superovulation)	Able to collect more oocytes per cycle
Monitor cycle with USS and oestradiol	Able to determine when oocytes mature
Administer hCG (and stop FSH)	Acts like LH and induces final oocyte maturation
Collect oocytes and prepare sperm sample	Allows fertilisation to occur in vitro
Determine quality of embryos	Enables choice of best three
Return embryos to uterus via cervix	Allows implantation and pregnancy
Support luteal phase	Prevents early pregnancy loss
Scan pregnancy at 42 days	To rule out ectopic pregnancy

Table 19.3   Different assisted conception techniques and the indications

Technique	Main indication(s)
IVF + ET	Tubal infertility
	Female antisperm antibodies
GIFT	Unexplained infertility
	Minimal endometriosis
Superovulation + IUI	Low-tech version of GIFT
IVF with ovum donation	Ovarian failure
	Maternal autosomal dominant condition
IVF with preimplantation diagnosis	Autosomal recessive condition
IVF with ICSI	Severe sperm dysfunction
	Absent/blocked vas deferens
Embryo cryopreservation	To store spare embryos
	To limit chance of multiple pregnancy

1. **GIFT** (gamete intrafallopian transfer) is very similar to IVF + ET except that, instead of the oocytes and sperm being mixed in the laboratory, they are placed in a fine catheter and placed immediately in the Fallopian tube. This has the advantage of not requiring oocyte culture in vitro and, by luck, appears to give a better chance of conception (see Table 19.4). It is unsuitable for tubal subfertility but is ideal for prolonged unexplained subfertility and minimal endometriosis.

2. **IUI** (intrauterine insemination) involves preparation of sperm and injection (flushing) of the sample into the uterus with a fine catheter. It is combined with superovulation to increase oocyte numbers. It has modest success compared with GIFT but has the advantage of not requiring oocyte collection and of lower cost.

3. **Ovum donation** was developed for women with absent or failed ovaries. The artificial cycles of the donor and recipients are synchronised. The oocytes are collected from the donor, fertilised in vitro, and the embryos are transferred to the recipient. Some units do GIFT with the donor oocytes instead of IVF.

4. **Embryo cryopreservation** was developed to allow spare embryos to be stored and used at a later date in a natural cycle. It therefore helps to maximise the chance of success from a single oocyte retrieval. It has the additional benefit of allowing fewer embryos

Table 19.4 Success rates from assisted conception (women under 40 years)

Category	Conception rate (/treatment cycle)	Birth rate (/treatment cycle)
Female subfertility and unexplained (normal sperm function)		
IVF + ET	25%	21%
GIFT	36%	30%
Male subfertility		
IVF + ET alone	15%	11%
IVF + ICSI + ET	20%	N/A

Table 19.5 Problems of assisted conception

Problem	Adverse outcome
High cost	Financial hardship/loss of house, etc.
Lowish chance of success	Risk of emotional upset
Surgical procedure	Risk of haemorrhage and infection
High chance of multiple pregnancy	Risk of preterm delivery/perinatal deaths
	Social problems/financial hardship
	Impact on neonatal services
Risk of tubal implantation	Risk of ectopic/heterotopic[a] pregnancy
Ovarian hyperstimulation syndrome	Risk of severe illness, including thromboembolism
	Risk of death (rare)

[a]Pregnancy with one or more embryos in the uterus and one in the Fallopian tube.

to be transferred initially (because those not used can be stored) and thereby limiting the chance of multiple pregnancy.

5. **ICSI** (intracytoplasmic sperm injection), the latest development, does involve IVF but, instead of allowing natural fertilisation to occur in the laboratory, a single sperm head is injected directly into the oocyte. This is a treatment for severe sperm disorders and obstructive azoospermia.

The techniques have also been applied to couples with genetic problems. IVF allows use of donated oocytes to avoid maternal autosomal dominant conditions, and IVF + ET allows preimplantation diagnosis of autosomal recessive disorders such as cystic fibrosis for women who could not contemplate termination of pregnancy.

Although the success of these techniques has undoubtedly transformed the management of subfertility and the lives of many couples to the good, they are not without their problems (see Table 19.5). It is essential that all issues are discussed in detail with the couple before treatment goes ahead.

Multiple pregnancy is in many ways the most difficult problem because of the initial expectancy of success which is often followed by miscarriage, perinatal death or long-term health problems in childhood. The chance of cerebral palsy for instance is increased 18-fold for triplet fetuses (see Table 19.6). But this does not tell the whole truth; the severity of cerebral palsy varies greatly, and parents and child may be very happy with a member affected by mild (and even severe) mental and physical problems.

SPECIAL SECTION – END-STAGE COUNSELLING

Brief Background

For couples who have tried all available treatments with-

Table 19.6 Cerebral palsy rates and multiple pregnancy

Pregnancy	Relative risk for a fetus	Relative risk for the pregnancy
Singleton	1	1
Twin	5	10
Triplet	18	54

out achieving conception, there is a time for them to decide to cease all therapy. Psychologically, it is probably better for the couple to make that decision whenever possible, but it is the duty of the doctor to raise the issue; some couples are afraid of offending the doctor because of all the efforts of the subfertility team. For some couples it comes as a relief, tinged with sadness of course, to make the decision. After years of trying, the despair of childlessness may be less painful than the continuing small hope of conception. And some more elderly couples may eventually decide that they feel too old to have a family and request sterilisation.

Once the decision is made, certain other issues may arise.

• Explain the residual (small) chance of natural conception and the need for contraception/sterilisation.

- Offer treatment of symptomatic conditions, e.g. endometriosis.
- Consider wider health issues, e.g. risk of osteoporosis in amenorrhoea.
- Discuss the need for personal counselling to come to terms with the lack of children.

GOLDEN POINTS

1. The couple should be seen and investigated together at specialist subfertility unit.

2. Appropriate investigations should be performed, starting with the least invasive, but with a plan to complete within 6 months.

3. Subfertility is a very distressing problem requiring detailed explanation and psychological support.

4. Pre-pregnancy advice should be given.

5. Confirmed pregnancies should be screened to exclude ectopic implantation.

6. Wider health issues and contraception should be considered if all available treatment fails.

7. Psychological morbidity is common, and personal counselling should be made available.

20 Absent or infrequent periods

CLINICAL SIGNIFICANCE

The combined prevalence of amenorrhoea (absent periods) and oligomenorrhoea (infrequent periods) is about 1%. For many it is a temporary, self-limiting condition but for others it is a sign of an inherited disorder or of irreversible ovarian failure (a premature menopause).

For the woman, failure to menstruate regularly provokes anxiety over her femininity and over her ability to conceive.

The clinical significance revolves around underlying endocrine, anatomical or psychological causes. It is crucial to ascertain whether normal menstruation has ever taken place for at least 6 months when primary amenorrhoea is diagnosed. Failure to menstruate for 6 months in a woman who has previously menstruated is classified as secondary amenorrhoea. Infrequent menstruation (oligomenorrhoea) is menstruation every 6 weeks to 6 months. Psychological causes and weight loss both account for a third of all cases referred to gynaecologists.

DIFFERENTIAL DIAGNOSIS

MAIN CATEGORY	DIAGNOSIS
Physiological	Pregnancy Lactation Natural menopause
Pathological 1. *Primary ovarian failure*	Karyotypic abnormalities (Turner's syndrome) Pure gonadal dysgenesis Idiopathic / premature menopause Ovarian surgery / radiotherapy / chemotherapy Antiovarian antibodies Resistant ovary syndrome
2. *Secondary ovarian failure*	Hyperprolactinaemia Stress / weight-loss / excess exercise Kallmann syndrome Hypothalamic / pituitary tumours Hypothalamo-pituitary radiotherapy or surgery
3. *Polycystic ovarian disease*	Secondary to insulin resistance Secondary to adrenal hyperandrogenaemia
4. *General endocrine disease*	Thyroid dysfunction Acromegaly Cushing's disease Ovarian and adrenal tumours
5. *Anatomical*	Congenital absence of uterus (including; testicular feminisation) Congenital imperforate hymen – haematocolpos Acquired – cervical stenosis Acquired – Aschermann's syndrome

This chapter is concerned with oligo-amenorrhoea in adult women. Delayed menarche/puberty is cared for by paediatric endocrinologists, and the reader is referred to a paediatric text for information on this topic.

Some authorities distinguish between amenorrhoea (absence of periods for 6 months) and oligomenorrhoea (infrequent periods more than 42 days apart). This is a little arbitrary because one day a woman may have amenorrhoea and the next day have a small bleed and then be classified as oligomenorrhoea. Both can be caused by the majority of conditions listed above, but the frequency distributions do differ. The large majority (90%) of cases of oligomenorrhoea are the result of PCOD, whereas amenorrhoea is more likely to be caused by hypothalamo-pituitary disease and primary ovarian failure.

If one imagines that the hypothalamus, pituitary and ovary are a rider, whip and horse, respectively, there is an easy way of remembering the five pathological categories.

1. Primary ovarian failure – dead horse
2. Secondary ovarian failure – riderless horse
3. Polycystic ovarian disease – wild horse
4. General endocrine diseases – wild animal (that upsets the rider and horse)
5. Anatomical conditions – no stable (for the horse to keep her young).

There are numerous causes of oligo-amenorrhoea but the commonest are PCOD (55%), hypothalamic dysfunction secondary to stress and exercise (15%), hyperprolactinaemia (10%) and premature menopause (7%). All other causes are very rare.

WIDER HEALTH ISSUES

The ovarian cycle is dependent upon general health, and conversely, a woman's general health is dependent upon ovarian function. As well as disease such as hypothyroidism or pituitary tumours leading to ovarian disorder, functional disorders of the hypothalamic–pituitary–ovarian axis may result in long-term health problems which are less obvious than the gynaecological consequences of anovulation but to which attention should be paid to prevent problems. The various long-term health risks are given in Table 20.1.

CLINICAL ASSESSMENT

Rapid Emergency Assessment

Amenorrhoea per se is not an emergency, but certain underlying conditions may require urgent admission for

Table 20.1 Wider health issues secondary to functional ovarian disorders	
Functional disorder	Health problems
Primary ovarian failure	Symptoms of oestrogen deficiency (menopausal-type symptoms)
	Increased chance of osteoporosis
	?Increased chance of cardiovascular disease
Secondary ovarian failure	Symptoms of oestrogen deficiency (menopausal-type symptoms)
	Increased chance of osteoporosis
	?Increased chance of cardiovascular disease
Polycystic ovarian disease	Symptoms of androgen excess (hirsutism)
	Syndrome X (hypertension, NIDDM, etc.)
	Endometrial cancer

assessment and treatment. Examples include severe anorexia nervosa and Addison's disease.

Organisation of Care

Most women present to their GP, who is able to exclude pregnancy, advise on need for contraception, and arrange baseline tests. Women with hyperprolactinaemia or thyroid disease should be seen by a general endocrinologist. Women with eating disorders require psychotherapy. Women with premature menopause and PCOD are usually seen by a gynaecological endocrinologist.

The diagnosis of cause is largely based on the hormonal findings, and the history and examination are rarely helpful. There are certain important points which can only be assessed by questioning and physical examination.

The first task is to determine the physiological or pathological group (categorisation) and then to define the underlying cause (diagnosis). The scheme of management is:

• endocrine evaluation by GP, including pregnancy test (categorisation and diagnosis)
• referral to appropriate specialist for advice and management

- history and examination
- discussion about fertility and subfertility
- infertility treatment if the woman and partner wish to conceive
- consideration of wider health issues if they do not want to conceive.

Relevant History

Presenting Complaint

MAIN SYMPTOM – **Cessation of menstruation** for 6 months in a previously menstruating woman, or no menstruation by the age of 16 years, is the minimum period for amenorrhoea. Oligomenorrhoea is usually defined as cycles greater than 42 days. In girls who have not menstruated there may be regular cramping abdominal pains and bloating which may be related to an imperforate hymen (**cryptomenorrhoea**). A full menstrual history should be taken, and it should be established whether a normal cycle ever existed. Problems arising from menarche are most usually related to PCOD.

COMMONLY ASSOCIATED SYMPTOMS – Weight-loss accounts for a large proportion of cases of amenorrhoea, usually occurring after loss of 10 kg. **Weight gain** or **hirsutism** in the presence of absent or irregular periods points to polycystic ovarian syndrome. **Anosmia** (absence of olfaction) is a feature of Kallmann syndrome (congenital absence of GnRH secretion). **Headaches** and **visual disturbance** may be features of cranial tumours such as a craniopharyngioma or prolactinoma.

EFFECT ON PATIENT – There are numerous **concerns over sexuality**, especially in younger women. A failure to develop secondary sex characteristics may lead to peer pressure and bullying at school. **Fertility** is often a major concern, and this should be taken into consideration when deciding on the investigations and treatment offered.

Gynaecological History

GYNAECOLOGICAL DISEASE – Pelvic irradiation or chemotherapy may lead to ovarian failure. Uterine surgery may have led to endometrial adhesions or cervical stenosis.

CONTRACEPTION – Occasionally the woman will not have mentioned she is on the OCP or that she has received a progestogen implant. There is no evidence to support the idea of a period of amenorrhoea after stopping the combined OCP. If these women have no periods for 6 months, they should be investigated fully.

FERTILITY REQUIREMENTS – If subfertility is also a problem, thorough investigation and appropriate referral should be undertaken.

Obstetric History

DELIVERY – Previous pregnancies confirm a normal genital tract and appropriate chromosome makeup. Recent pregnancy (and lactation) is relevant because ovulation may not resume for some months.

OBSTETRIC COMPLICATIONS – Cervical trauma or endometrial infection may rarely lead to amenorrhoea. Severe postpartum haemorrhage with profound hypotension can rarely cause pituitary infarction and varying degrees of hypopituitarism (Sheehan's syndrome).

Medical History

MEDICAL CONDITIONS – Uncontrolled thyroid disease. Severe renal dysfunction. Malignancy treated with cytotoxics or pelvic/abdominal radiotherapy.

SURGERY – Difficult conservative surgery of the ovaries may lead to ovarian failure. The commonest would be surgery for endometriosis.

PSYCHOLOGICAL DISORDERS – Psychological disturbance has long been known to affect the hypothalamus, leading to cessation of menstruation. Leaving home for the first time is a reasonably common temporary cause of amenorrhoea.

Drug History

MEDICATIONS – Cytotoxics or radiotherapy. Anabolic steroids.

Social History

OCCUPATION – Busy and stressful jobs.

DEPENDANTS – There may be illness in other family members, leading to stress.

LIFESTYLE – As mentioned, weight-loss has an important role to play, as does the stress of daily living and extreme, high-impact exercise.

Relevant Clinical Examination

General Examination

GENERAL CONDITION – The woman should be observed for signs of acute thyroid disease. The woman may display features of anorexia nervosa: emaciation, pallor and lanugo hair. Hirsutism tends to suggest PCOD or androgen-secreting tumour. Webbed neck, wide spaced nipples, short stature and failure of secondary sexual development are features of Turner's syndrome. Stigmata of acromegaly, Cushing's disease and Addison's should be examined for quickly.

BODY-MASS INDEX – Weight and height should be measured to check BMI. A value less than 19 kg/m^2 is suggestive of weight-loss-related amenorrhoea.

BREASTS – In general there is no value in examining the breasts. Galactorrhoea is not predictive of prolactin state, and indeed squeezing the breast can falsely elevate the serum concentration. The breasts should be examined before prescribing any endocrine therapy.

BLOOD PRESSURE - Hypertension is a common feature of PCOD.

VISUAL FIELDS AND OPTIC FUNDI - To look for atrophy of optic discs in women with headaches.

Abdomen

CONTOUR - A blockage of the cervix or absent vagina preventing blood from escaping may lead to enlargement of the uterus seen as abdominal swelling. Hormone-secreting tumours give rise to ascites.

OLD SCARS - Scars from previous pelvic surgery may explain a premature menopause.

PALPATION - Feel for ovarian masses or haematocolpos. Gonads may be palpable in the inguinal canal in testicular feminisation syndrome.

Pelvic

PERINEUM/VULVA - Careful inspection should take place, especially with primary amenorrhoea. A bluish membrane covering the introitus may be an imperforate hymen. There may be palpable testes in the vulva associated with testicular feminisation. Pubic hair should be seen by the age of 12 years.

VAGINA - Although rare, an absent vagina and cervix do occur even in girls who have otherwise experienced normal puberty.

CERVIX - Signs of stenosis or abnormalities may indicate genital tract defects.

BIMANUAL EXAMINATION - Enlarged or abnormal uterus. Ovarian tumours.

Relevant Initial Investigations

The investigation is in three stages:

1. ruling out pregnancy
2. defining pathological category
3. undertaking additional tests to define exact diagnosis.

Ruling out pregnancy - Even women with an overt pathological condition such as PCOD may have conceived. It is essential to exclude pregnancy in all cases, particularly before prescribing medications such as clomiphene which may have adverse effects on a developing fetus.

Categorisation - Of the five categories (see above), only three are common. Endocrine disorders and anatomical lesions are rare. Anatomical lesions are indicated by a history suggestive of cryptomenorrhoea or of recent uterine surgery. Thyroid function (TSH measurement) is assessed to screen for thyroid disease. Oestradiol and

Table 20.2 Discrimination of functional categories of anovulation

Category	Serum FSH	Progestogen challenge
Primary ovarian failure	Elevated	Negative
Secondary ovarian failure	Non-elevated	Negative
Polycystic ovarian disease	Non-elevated	Positive

testosterone measurement and a transvaginal ovarian scan are used to screen for hormone-secreting tumours. The rarer diseases such as acromegaly are not tested for routinely, but only if there are stigmata suggestive of an endocrine syndrome.

For the remaining three (functional) categories of oligo-amenorrhoea, which account for 95% of cases, just two tests will help to discriminate between them: **serum FSH concentration** and **progestogen challenge** (Table 20.2). The progestogen challenge is an assessment of oestrogenisation (of the endometrium). It is better than measuring serum oestradiol for this purpose because it summates all the effects of a variety of oestrogens. Progestogen is given for 5 days, and the menstrual response is noted. Bleeding indicates oestrogenisation, and no response indicates oestrogen deficiency. This categorisation is a very good guide, but it is not perfectly accurate. It is, of course, important to take into account the clinical history and physical examination. A small proportion of women with severe PCOD are oestrogen deficient, and some women with eating disorders are oestrogenised.

DIAGNOSIS – DETAILS OF FIVE CATEGORIES OF OLIGO-AMENORRHOEA

1. Primary Ovarian Failure

Read also Chapter 23.

Background

DEFINITION - Lack of functioning ovarian tissue (congenital absence or iatrogenic destruction) or end-organ resistance to FSH. Also known as hypergonadotrophic hypogonadism.

AETIOLOGY - There are various causes (see differential diagnosis).

MAKING THE DIAGNOSIS - Categorisation is made by finding persistent elevation of serum FSH concentration (FSH level greater than the elevation of serum LH concentration) in women with amenorrhoea and occasionally oligomenorrhoea. The women also have oestrogen deficiency (negative progestogen challenge).

ADDITIONAL INVESTIGATIONS – **Karyotype** – 45X (Turner's syndrome), unbalanced translocations, 47XXX (triple X syndrome), and 46XY (gonadal dysgenesis). **Autoimmune profile** – for antiovarian antibodies. **Thyroid function** – increased chance of thyroid disease in women with antiovarian antibodies. **Laparoscopy** – used to see if there is ovarian tissue and rule out possibility of streak ovaries. Those with streak ovaries can be certain that there is not even a small chance of fertility. Ovarian biopsy is said to be unhelpful.

MAIN COMPLICATIONS – Infertility, unwanted pregnancy (resistant ovary syndrome), symptoms of oestrogen deficiency, osteoporosis, and possibly increased risk of cardiovascular disease. There is a risk of gonadal tumours for women with 46XY karyotype (gonadal dysgenesis). There is a high incidence of auto-immune thyroid disease in women with antiovarian antibodies.

PROGNOSIS – For the vast majority of cases the ovarian failure is permanent, but a small proportion of women with idiopathic primary ovarian failure flip in and out of normal ovarian activity. This has not been properly explained.

SCREENING/PREVENTION – HRT to prevent menopausal-type problems. Removal of gonads in women with 46XY karyotype.

Treatment Options

ADVICE – Patients need special counselling about per-manent fertility. Also, there is a small chance of sponta-neous resumption of ovulation. For most women the only chance of pregnancy is to have assisted conception with donated oocytes, but availability is limited. Other women will wish to pursue adoption and fostering.

CHANGE OF LIFESTYLE/DIET – Nil relevant.

DRUG THERAPY – **Oestrogen deficiency** – oestrogen-based HRT. **Subfertility** – this is largely an irreversible state. There are data to suggest that high-dose sex-steroid therapy/exogenous gonadotrophin therapy increase the chance of ovulation. This is akin to flogging the dead horse, but it is not known how this works.

SURGERY – Laparoscopic gonadectomy for women with 46XY karyotype.

OVERVIEW – Generally irreversible form of end-organ resistance. A small proportion spontaneously resume ovarian activity. The primary aim of the doctor is to enable the woman to come to terms with sterility and to give advice about wider health issues.

Follow-up

SHORT TERM – To check on compliance with HRT.

LONG TERM – To give advice about changes in infertility treatments.

2. *Secondary Ovarian Failure*

Background

DEFINITION – Ovarian inactivity secondary to hypothalamic and pituitary conditions. The ovary is essentially normal. Also known as hypogonadotrophic hypogonadism.

AETIOLOGY – Numerous causes of hypothalamic and pituitary ovarian dysfunction and failure.

MAKING THE DIAGNOSIS – Categorisation is made by presence of non-elevated FSH concentration and oestrogen deficiency (negative progestogen challenge). The underlying cause is then suggested by a variety of factors, including history of weight-loss or excessive exercise, low BMI, serum prolactin and cranial radiology.

ADDITIONAL INVESTIGATIONS – **Serum prolactin** – to screen for hyperprolactinaemia. **Cranial radiology** – CAT or MRI imaging provides a clearer view of the pituitary fossa. Used to test for hypothalamic and pituitary tumours in women with hyperprolactinaemia or unexplained headaches/visual disturbance. **Tests for hypopituitarism** – If there is a large pituitary tumour. **Haemoglobin and serum biochemistry** – to test for chronic renal failure if history is suggestive. To test for anaemia and electrolyte derangement in women with serum eating disorders.

MAIN COMPLICATIONS – Subfertility, unwanted pregnancy, osteoporosis, and problems from the underlying cause (e.g. eating disorder or pituitary tumour).

SCREENING/PREVENTION – HRT to prevent osteoporosis.

Treatment Options

ADVICE – Give advice about improving diet and reducing exercise. Discuss wider health issues.

CHANGE OF LIFESTYLE/DIET – See above.

DRUG THERAPY – **Oestrogen deficiency** – oestrogen-based HRT to prevent osteoporosis, etc. **Subfertility** – depends on cause, weight loss related => diet and psy-chotherapy; hyperprolactinaemia => dopamine agonist therapy (cabergoline or bromocriptine); Kallmann syndrome => pulsatile GnRH therapy or exogenous gonadotrophins; idiopathic => therapeutic trials of clomiphene therapy, pulsatile GnRH or exogenous gonadotrophins.

SURGERY – For hypothalamic or pituitary tumours.

OVERVIEW – Common cause of anovulation. The ovary is essentially normal but is quiet because of lack of stimulation by hypothalamo-pituitary unit. Many forms are reversible. The outcome of fertility treatment is very good.

3. Polycystic Ovarian Disease (PCOD)

See also sections in Chapters 18 and 21.

Background

DEFINITION – Ovarian disorder typified by continuing oestrogenisation, raised serum concentrations of LH and enlarged ovaries with an expanded stromal compartment surrounded by numerous small follicles. Also known as Stein–Leventhal syndrome and polycystic ovary syndrome. The big difference between PCOD and other forms of anovulation is that oestrogen is still produced in reasonable quantities and the endometrium remains oestrogenised.

AETIOLOGY – Most cases probably result from inherited or acquired forms of insulin resistance. Insulin is a gonadotrophic agent working in concert with FSH and LH, and the hyperinsulinaemia which results from insulin resistance promotes ovarian disorder. Adrenal hyperandrogenism probably plays a role in a small proportion of cases.

MAKING THE DIAGNOSIS – Categorisation is made by presence of non-elevated serum FSH and positive progestogen challenge.

ADDITIONAL INVESTIGATIONS – **Serum LH** – an elevated LH concentration is highly indicative of PCOD if additional evidence is needed (though it is usually not). It should be remembered that the majority of women have a normal serum LH concentration on a single reading. **Transvaginal ultrasound** can be used to examine ovarian morphology (Figure 20.1) but it is not a reliable method of diagnosing PCOD for a variety of reasons and should be reserved for complex cases. **Glucose tolerance testing** – for women in pregnancy to screen for gestational diabetes. **Endometrial sampling** – for women with prolonged amenorrhoea or oligomenorrhoea.

MAIN COMPLICATIONS – Oligo-amenorrhoea, dysfunctional uterine bleeding, endometrial cancer, unwanted pregnancy, subfertility, hirsutism, recurrent miscarriage, syndrome X (Box 20.1) and possibly ovarian tumours.

Box 20.1 Features of syndrome X (insulin resistance)

- Mild essential hypertension
- Hyperinsulinaemia/mild glucose intolerance
- Hypertriglyceridaemia
- Central adiposity
- Increased chance of cardiovascular death

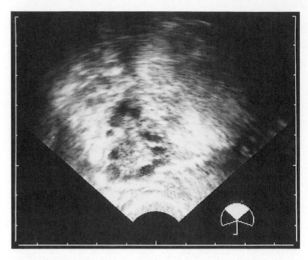

Fig 20.1 *TVS demonstrating circumferential ovarian cysts associated with PCOD.*

SCREENING/PREVENTION – Maintenance of normal body-weight may prevent expression of the insulin resistance. Advice on diet, smoking and exercise may prove to be important for these women because of cardiovascular risk, but further information is awaited. For women with infrequent or absent periods, there is an increased risk of endometrial cancer because of unopposed oestrogenisation. Progestogen should be given to induce regular withdrawal bleeds.

Treatment Options

ADVICE – Consider discussion about wider health issues.

CHANGE OF LIFESTYLE/DIET – Maintain normal body weight. Avoid additional cardiovascular risk factors such as smoking and take good exercise.

DRUG THERAPY – **Subfertility** – antioestrogen therapy (clomiphene) is the first agent. Laparoscopic ovarian surgery – for women who do not respond to clomiphene. **Hirsutism** – cosmetic remedies. Ethinyloestradiol and cyproterone acetate. **Menstrual-disorder** and **endometrial protection** – combined OCP or cyclical progestogen. **Recurrent miscarriage** – laparoscopic ovarian surgery.

SURGERY – Hysterectomy may be needed for menstrual disorder.

OVERVIEW – The commonest cause of anovulatory infertility, recurrent miscarriage and hirsutism. Range of presentation is extremely wide. Most women have virtually no outward signs of the condition. Diagnosis depends on clinical situation. Wider health issues include syndrome X and endometrial cancer.

4. *General Endocrine Disorders*

Background

DEFINITION – Generalised endocrine disorder such as oestrogen- and androgen-secreting tumours, acromegaly, Cushing's disease, Addison's disease and thyroid dysfunction.

AETIOLOGY – The whole of the endocrine system is interlaced, and dysfunction in any part may influence the hypothalamic–pituitary–ovarian axis.

MAIN COMPLICATIONS – Those of the underlying disorder.

SCREENING/PREVENTION – Nil relevant.

MAKING THE DIAGNOSIS – All women with oligo-amenorrhoea should undergo thyroid testing which may show no outward signs. All women should be tested for androgen- and oestrogen-secreting tumours (serum oestradiol, serum testosterone and transvaginal ultrasound). A high index of suspicion should be maintained for rarer endocrinopathies, and diagnostic tests instituted if appropriate. For other details consult a general endocrinology text.

5. *Anatomical Defects*

Background

DEFINITION – Abnormalities of the genital tract, preventing release of menstrual debris. One exception is the testicular feminisation syndrome in which there is a female phenotype with absence of uterus and 46XY karyotype. This is the result of an abnormality of the androgen receptor, which prevents masculinisation of the male fetus.

AETIOLOGY – A variety of congenital and acquired anatomical defects of the vagina or uterus.

MAIN COMPLICATIONS – Retention of menstrual blood (haematocolpos or haematometra – see Figure 20.2).

Infertility (all causes) and recurrent miscarriage (Aschermann's syndrome).

SCREENING/PREVENTION – Care during evacuation of uterus especially in the presence of infection.

MAKING THE DIAGNOSIS – Very rare, and tests are not routinely undertaken. Should be suggested by the history: primary amenorrhoea with cyclical pain (congenital causes) or secondary amenorrhoea after cervical or uterine surgery.

ADDITIONAL INVESTIGATIONS – If haematocolpos is suspected, transabdominal scanning will help to identify any pelvic mass, but ultimately an **examination under anaesthetic (with possible laparoscopy)** will be needed. If Aschermann's syndrome is suspected, **direct visualisation** with hysteroscopy is needed.

Treatment Options

ADVICE – Need for surgery but prognosis is poor for acquired lesions.

CHANGE OF LIFESTYLE/DIET – Nil relevant.

DRUG THERAPY – Oestrogen therapy after surgery to help development of endometrium in women with intra-uterine adhesions.

SURGERY – Opening of imperforate hymen. Dilatation of stenosed cervix. Hysteroscopic division of adhesions.

OVERVIEW – Very rare, and diagnosis depends on careful history. Surgery is the mainstay of treatment.

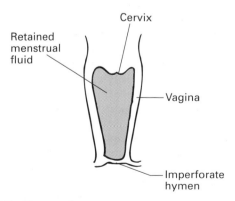

Fig 20.2 *Haematocolpos.*

Labels: Cervix, Retained menstrual fluid, Vagina, Imperforate hymen

---

GOLDEN POINTS

1. Always exclude pregnancy, particularly before prescribing any medication.

2. Consider wider health issues such as osteoporosis and endometrial cancer.

3. Explain that the woman may not be infertile, and need for contraception should be considered if sexually active.

4. Explain that for most causes of anovulation, subfertility can be treated successfully.

5. Before inducing ovulation, carefully explain chance of multiple pregnancy.

6. There is no such thing as post-pill amenorrhoea; look for true cause.

2

21 Abnormal hair growth

CLINICAL SIGNIFICANCE

Abnormal hair growth or hirsutism is excessive growth of male pattern hair. Even relatively mild hair growth can cause great distress to women.

Many women complaining of excessive facial or body hair simply have normal variations in growth. True hirsutism is most often related to polycystic ovarian disease, but non-gynaecological endocrine disease and androgen-secreting tumours must be borne in mind.

DIFFERENTIAL DIAGNOSIS

MAIN CATEGORY	DIAGNOSIS
1. *Ovarian*	Polycystic ovarian disease (and hyperthecosis) Androgen-secreting tumours
2. *General endocrine*	Cushing's syndrome Acromegaly Androgen-secreting adrenal tumours Maturity-onset adrenal hyperplasia
3. *Iatrogenic*	Anabolic steroids (self-prescribed) Corticosteroids Danazol Androgen implants Progestogens
4. *Miscellaneous*	Pregnancy The postmenopause
5. *Idiopathic*	Normal familial variation Normal racial variation

Hirsutism is excessive growth of hormone-dependent hair. It is distinct from hypertrichosis, or excessive general hair, which is sometimes seen with rare genetic syndromes and also during phenytoin therapy. Lanugo, or fine downy hair similar to that seen in new-born babies, is found in women with eating disorders.

Most women who present to their GP complain of increased hair growth which lies within the normal limits and represents slightly thicker or darker than average hair due to familial or racial tendencies. Although this can be considered a normal variant by clinicians, it may be wholly unacceptable to the woman, and her complaint should not be dismissed lightly.

Polycystic ovarian disease is the commonest cause of hirsutism, accounting for more than 90% of cases before the menopause. Mild hirsutism after the menopause usually reflects oestrogen deficiency rather than androgen excess. Severe hirsutism of rapid onset is suggestive of an androgen-secreting tumour, particularly if accompanied by other signs of virilisation such as deepening of the voice, temporal hair loss, or enlargement of the clitoris.

CLINICAL ASSESSMENT

The primary role of the clinician is to rule out the possibility of hormonally active tumours and non-gynaecological endocrine disorders such as Cushing's syndrome and acromegaly. Tumours should be routinely screened for by serum testosterone measurement, but Cushing's and acromegaly are only tested for if there are other stigmata. It is important to maintain clinical suspicion, therefore.

It is also important to consider the possibility of drug-related hirsutism and self-administered anabolic steroids in particular. The information may not be volunteered to the gynaecologist.

In women with definite true hirsutism but no obvious cause, a presumptive diagnosis of PCOD is made. There is no need to distinguish between PCOD and maturity-onset congenital adrenal hyperplasia.

Relevant History

Presenting Complaint

MAIN SYMPTOM – The speed of hair growth helps to determine the potential diagnosis. A gradual onset over years is most likely to be familial variation or PCOD, whereas a rapid onset over a few months is more likely to be caused by increased androgen production from a tumour.

COMMONLY ASSOCIATED SYMPTOMS – Other features of hyperandrogenism may be present, such as acne, greasy skin (seborrhoea) and male pattern baldness. Deepening of the voice is a particularly worrying symptom both because it is often a reflection of an underlying tumour and also because it is sometimes irreversible.

EFFECT ON PATIENT – Loss of confidence is very common. It is also important to try to gain some understanding of what concerns the woman. For some it is simply the appearance, but others are worried about future fertility, and some may have a negative fantasy that they are turning into a man.

Gynaecological History

GYNAECOLOGICAL DISEASE – The woman may already be known to have a history of polycystic ovarian disease (PCOD) with menstrual disorder or anovulatory infertility.

MENSTRUAL HISTORY – Infrequent, absent or irregular periods from menarche, associated with slow onset hirsutism, is typical of PCOD, but a normal menstrual cycle does not rule out the possibility. Postmenopausal women usually have a gradual onset of mild hirsutism.

CONTRACEPTION – The combined oral contraceptive pill with androgenic progestogens may worsen acne and abnormal hair growth. The progestogen-only contraception may inhibit ovulation and lower oestrogen levels, altering the oestrogen/androgen ratio. If certain anti-androgen treatments are prescribed, full contraception is advised, to avoid the potential risk of teratogenesis.

FERTILITY REQUIREMENTS – Medical treatment can be teratogenic, so pregnancy should be avoided during therapy.

Obstetric History

OBSTETRIC COMPLICATIONS – Infertility and recurrent miscarriage are features of PCOD. Hirsutism may start in pregnancy. This is likely to disappear spontaneously, provided it is not related to an androgen-secreting tumour.

Medical History

MEDICAL CONDITIONS – Acromegaly and Cushing's disease may already have been diagnosed. Epilepsy treated with phenytoin is a cause of hypertrichosis.

Drug History

MEDICATIONS – In addition to questions about oral medication such as corticosteroids, danazol and phenytoin, it is also important to enquire about testosterone implants which are used to treat loss of libido in the menopause.

Social History

AGE – Prior to puberty, hirsutism and virilisation are extremely rare and are then due to congenital adrenal hyperplasia or tumours of the adrenal gland or ovary.

Relevant Clinical Examination

It should remembered that many women will have prepared themselves carefully before attending the clinic and that their appearance may not reflect the true severity of their symptom.

General Examination

GENERAL CONDITION – **Hair** – assess the pattern, looking for distribution and thickness of hair present. The face, chest, abdomen, back and legs should all be examined carefully (Figure 21.1). There are systems for scoring hair growth, but these tend not to be used in everyday practice. Simple descriptions usually suffice, but clinical photographs provide an excellent method of recording the baseline state. **Skin** – the presence of acne should be recorded. Pigmented velvety patches (acanthosis nigricans) on the skin flexures and neck are a feature of PCOD. **Voice** – listen to the voice carefully for evidence of deepening. **Stigmata** – examine for signs of Cushing's syndrome and acromegaly.

BODY-MASS INDEX – Obesity also reduces self-esteem in some women. Moreover, weight-loss is an important component of treatment in obese women with PCOD.

BREASTS – It is important to examine the breasts if sex-steroid therapy is to be used. Atrophy may reflect oestrogen deficiency.

Abdomen

CONTOUR – Distension from adrenal and ovarian tumours is rare, as they tend to be very small.

Pelvic

VULVA/VAGINA – Clitoromegaly indicates more severe virilisation.

BIMANUAL EXAMINATION – To exclude ovarian tumours.

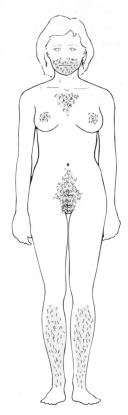

Fig 21.1 *Male pattern hair growth.*

Relevant Initial Investigations

Traditionally, clinicians have undertaken extensive endocrine testing. This is largely unnecessary, detailed hormonal assessment only being required if the woman also has amenorrhoea (see Chapter 20).

Endocrine Tests

TESTOSTERONE – Testosterone is used solely to screen for androgen-secreting tumours. A serum concentration greater than 5 mmol/l should initiate a search for adrenal and ovarian tumours.

LH/FSH – Can be used to confirm PCOD, but in practice the diagnosis is made by the exclusion of others.

Diagnostic Imaging

PELVIC ULTRASOUND – Transvaginal scanning will demonstrate polycystic ovaries but it is not necessary for this purpose. Androgen-secreting ovarian tumours tend to be small (about 2 cm) and must be looked for carefully. Colour-flow Doppler may help with the detection of small ovarian tumours.

AXIAL IMAGING – MRI is used to examine the adrenal gland

for tumours if the testosterone concentration is very high, but this is indicated in a very small proportion of cases.

DETAILS OF COMMON CONDITIONS

1. Idiopathic hirsutism

Background

DEFINITION – Subjectively increased growth in women with regular menstruation and no evidence of organic disease. It is probably occult PCOD (see below).

2. Polycystic Ovarian Disease (PCOD)

Background

DEFINITION – PCOD is a variable syndrome which may result from a range of endocrine disorders.

AETIOLOGY – The commonest cause is probably insulin resistance/hyperinsulinaemia, which in many cases is probably inherited. The high levels of insulin stimulate androgen production by the ovarian stromal tissues, and disorders of ovarian function generally. Adrenal hyperandrogenaemia is an important factor in a small proportion of women. Worldwide, PCOD is the commonest endocrinopathy, with as many as 20% of women having polycystic ovaries.

MAIN COMPLICATIONS – The classical syndrome described by Stein and Leventhal, including anovulation, hirsutism and obesity, is quite rare (<2% of the female population), but many women have occult forms of the disease. It may lead to menstrual disorders, anovulatory infertility, recurrent miscarriage and hirsutism. In later life, there is a higher chance of Type 2 diabetes and cardiovascular disease related to the insulin resistance.

MAKING THE DIAGNOSIS – There is no single test for PCOD. A combination of morphological and endocrine tests should be used together with the clinical findings. In women with true hirsutism, however, the primary aim of diagnosis is to rule out other causes, and PCOD can be assumed with some confidence if nothing else is identified. See Table 21.1.

SCREENING/PREVENTION – There is no known method of prevention, though maintenance of a normal bodyweight with a balanced diet may limit the degree of ovarian disorder. Because PCOD is a marker for insulin resistance, and therefore cardiovascular disease, such women should be given advice about diet, smoking and exercise.

Treatment Options

ADVICE – PCOD cannot be cured, but rather symptoms can only be controlled. Mild hirsutism does not necessarily require treatment. Some women are content to be reassured by the absence of life-threatening disease.

Table 21.1	Diagnosing PCOD
Making the diagnosis	PCOD
History	Oligo/amenorrhoea Subfertility
Examination	Obesity / hirsutism / acanthosis nigricans
Investigations	
– Endocrine	The best endocrine test in part depends on the method of presentation In menstruating women, a raised LH:FSH ratio is indicative of PCOD Normal levels of LH and testosterone do not rule out the diagnosis, however In women with amenorrhoea, serum LH (and FSH) can be measured, but a positive progestogen challenge, indicating oestrogenisation, is also indicative of PCOD
– Ultrasound	TVS may demonstrate enlarged thickened ovaries with typical cysts

CHANGE OF LIFESTYLE/DIET – Weight-loss may help improve general appearance and self-esteem in overweight women. Calorie control may also improve the ovarian disorder. If the hair growth is particularly disturbing, simple remedies of bleaching, plucking, waxing and electrolysis should be discussed. Shaving is also an option, but many women find it degrading. Moreover, although the look of the face may improve, the texture of the skin is still very rough.

DRUG THERAPY – If the hirsutism is severe and contraception is required, a combination of **ethinyloestradiol** and **cyproterone acetate** (CPA, a progestogen with anti-androgenic properties) is a good choice. CPA can be given in low dose (as with dianette OCP) or in high dose (25 to 50 mg daily). This combination starts to show effect by 6 months at the earliest and it takes about 18 months to achieve full effect. Side effects are generally those of the **combined OCP**. In addition,

CPA may cause reversible liver dysfunction, and any male fetus exposed in utero may fail to masculinise. Long-term treatment is not recommended, and, at about 24 months, the woman can be converted to a standard combined oral contraceptive pill. **Flutamide**, a non-steroidal antiandrogen, can be used for women in whom the OCP is contraindicated, but gastrointestinal side effects are common and many cannot tolerate it. It too can affect male fetuses. Some American groups are keen on the diuretic **spironolactone** which has anti-androgenic properties, but there has been some suggestion that it is carcinogenic. **Corticosteroids** are only weakly effective and they tend to promote weight gain.

SURGERY – Ovarian electrodiathermy used for women with PCOD and infertility is contraindicated for hirsutism because the effects are short lived.

OVERVIEW – Again, conservative measures may be sufficient for many women. Antiandrogen therapy should be reserved for moderately severe cases. Risks must be discussed carefully.

Information for Patient

This condition is still not fully understood but, if asymptomatic, does not require treatment. The association with insulin resistance and the resulting cardiovascular risk factors should be used to encourage a healthier lifestyle.

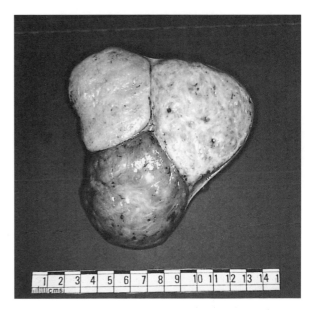

Fig 21.2 *Testosterone-secreting ovarian tumour.*

Follow-up

SHORT TERM – It is advised that liver function tests are checked at one month and then 6 monthly in women who are receiving cyproterone.

LONG TERM – If therapy is not required, long-term follow-up is not necessary, but, if future fertility is required, they should be referred for investigations after 6 months of trying.

3. Androgen-secreting Tumours

Brief Background

Many are benign (Figure 21.2) and simple resection will result in a rapid fall in androgen levels. The hair growth will resolve over the next 18 months.

GOLDEN POINTS

1. PCOD is by far the commonest cause. The diagnosis is assumed if other rare causes are excluded.

2. Serious causes such as androgen-secreting tumours are rare but should be excluded. A very raised testosterone level and other features of virilisation such as deepening voice are worrying signs.

3. Thyroid disorder should be excluded but detailed endocrine testing is not indicated unless there are stigmata for specific endocrinopathies such as Cushing's syndrome and acromegaly.

4. Remember cosmetic remedies are useful in mild cases.

5. Remember pharmacological treatments are not curative, carry risks of serious side effects and take more than 6 months to show effect.

22 Premenstrual syndrome

CLINICAL SIGNIFICANCE

Premenstrual syndrome was first described in 1931. Many theories have been proposed to explain its nature, but, sixty years on, PMS remains extremely difficult to understand, to diagnose and to treat. Research has failed to identify the true nature of the syndrome, and treatment largely remains anecdotal and ineffective.

The symptoms vary widely from physical feelings of abdominal bloating and breast tenderness to severe psychological depression and aggression. Women are much more likely to commit suicide and criminal acts during the few days before menstruation than at any other time in the cycle. Worldwide, research has shown that 3 billion pounds per year is lost to PMS because of absence from work.

The vast majority (about 95%) of women in the United Kingdom experience at least one adverse premenstrual symptom, but about one third of women feel that the premenstrual phase is the best time of the ovarian cycle. Only a minority of women find the symptoms significantly reduce quality of life.

THE SYNDROME

Physical symptoms

1. *Breast heaviness and tenderness*
2. *Abdominal bloating*
3. *Pelvic pain*
4. *Headaches*
5. *Clumsiness*

Psychological symptoms

1. *Low mood*
2. *Irritability*
3. *Lack of ability to concentrate*
4. *Depression*

Premenstrual syndrome is a collection of a wide range of physical and psychological symptoms. By definition, the syndrome is cyclical. There is no diagnostic test, and the differential diagnosis for each symptom should be carefully considered. Alternative serious pathology should be excluded if necessary.

The differential diagnosis is too extensive to list here, because of the wide range of symptoms. It is important to remember that even the symptoms of true organic disease can vary with the menstrual cycle because of the influence of ovarian hormones on physiology and mood.

Important conditions to consider include thyroid disease, diabetes, anaemia, the perimenopause, endometriosis, ovarian tumours, breast tumours, constipation, irritable bowel syndrome, depression and anxiety.

CLINICAL ASSESSMENT

Most women consult the GP, and hospital care is only needed for extreme cases.

Relevant History

Presenting Complaint

MAIN SYMPTOM – The timing, character and severity of the symptoms and their relationship to the menstrual cycle should be carefully documented. Menstrual charting will help with this (Figure 22.1). The symptoms should start prior to the onset of menstruation, usually in the midluteal phase, and stop before it is finished. There are a large number of physical and psychological symptoms associated with PMS. The commonest **psychological symptoms** are irritability, aggression,

Fill in months (e.g. May)	Days of month																														
	1	2	3	4	5	6	7	8	9	10	11	12	13	14	15	16	17	18	19	20	21	22	23	24	25	26	27	28	29	30	31
1st Month JULY					D/T	T	B/T	B/T	B/T	B/T	B/T	T	M	M	M	M														T	B/T
2nd Month AUGUST	B/T	B/T	B/T	B/T/D	B/T	B	B	B	B/M	M	M	M	M															B/T	B/T	B/T	B
3rd Month SEPTEMBER	D/B	T	B/T	B/T	M	M	M	M																							

Key to symptoms
D= Depression   P= Pain — backache or headache T= Tension or irritability   F= Fatigue B= Bloated feeling   M= Menstruation

Fig 22.1 *Menstrual calendar.*

depression and anxiety. The severity of these can vary widely. The commonest **physical symptoms** include breast pain, headache, sweats, flushes, abdominal bloating and pelvic pain. When the pain or discomfort is not cyclical in nature, there is a higher chance that a local pathological problem is present.

COMMONLY ASSOCIATED SYMPTOMS – Unexplained crying, increased tension, poor concentration and clumsiness are reported by some as is weight gain and distorted body image.

EFFECT ON PATIENT – An important factor in assessing these women is quantifying the effect on their quality of life. This can be achieved using general health questionnaires which also help determine any underlying psychological influence and allow progress to be monitored.

Gynaecological History

GYNAECOLOGICAL DISEASE – There may be a history of pelvic infection or endometriosis, and symptoms of these may be confused with PMS.

CONTRACEPTION – The method of contraception should be recorded along with any changes in symptoms that have occurred if it was recently altered.

FERTILITY REQUIREMENTS – In severe cases, hysterectomy may be the method of control of symptoms.

Obstetric History

DELIVERY – A young child may lead to emotional disturbance causing psychological problems. There is an association between PMS and postnatal depression.

Medical History

MEDICAL CONDITIONS – Hypothyroidism and anaemia can cause lethargy and poor concentration but tend not to be cyclical in nature.

SURGERY – Multiple pelvic or abdominal operations causing chronic pelvic discomfort may be mistaken for PMS.

PSYCHOLOGICAL DISORDERS – A history of mood disturbances, depression or anxiety disorders can present in a similar fashion to PMS. Symptoms of true psychological disorders may be cyclical because of the effect of progesterone on mood, but symptoms tend to remain after the end of the period.

Drug History

MEDICATIONS – These women may be on medication for depression or other psychiatric disease.

Social History

AGE – Premenstrual symptoms are uncommon in younger women, usually presenting after their first child. In older women menopausal symptoms can give rise to similar symptoms though these are not cyclical.

LIFESTYLE – It has been described more in middle-class women but this may simply reflect their willingness to present with these symptoms. Change of job or career may create additional stress which precipitates presentation. Lack of leisure time and exercise may prevent a feeling of general wellbeing.

Relevant Clinical Examination

General Examination

GENERAL CONDITION – Look for stigmata of anaemia, hypothyroidism or mood disturbance.

BREASTS – To exclude pathology, particularly if breast symptoms continue throughout the cycle.

Abdomen

CONTOUR – Abdominal distension (bloating) may be due to ascites or a pelvic mass.

TENDERNESS – The abdomen should be soft with no specific tender points.

MASSES – There should be no abdominal masses felt.

Pelvic

VULVA/VAGINA/CERVIX – Examination is only necessary if there is pelvic discomfort.

Relevant Clinical Investigations

Haematology
Hb - Will exclude anaemia if there is clinical suspicion.

Biochemistry
U+Es/CALCIUM/GLUCOSE/LFTs - If there is any suspicion of metabolic disorder.

Endocrine Tests
TSH - Used to exclude hypo/hyperthyroidism if there is a clinical suspicion.

Cytology
CERVICAL - The opportunity should be taken to discuss cervical cytology if a smear is due.

Diagnostic Imaging and Direct Visualisation
ULTRASOUND OR LAPAROSCOPY - Should only be used to exclude clinical suspicion of pelvic pathology in women whose pelvic discomfort is severe.

Background
DEFINITION - A syndrome of psychological, behavioural and somatic symptoms that present prior to menstruation, resolving before the cessation of menstrual bleeding. There should be at least 1 week free of symptoms during the cycle. The symptoms should have been present for 4 out of the last 6 months.

AETIOLOGY - There are numerous theories attempting to explain the reason for PMS. It is clearly related to the ovarian cycle, since it is not present in lactating or menopausal women and since women with severe symptoms can be cured by surgical castration. It seems likely that it is related to progesterone hormone, but no consistent abnormality of secretion has been found. Some researchers hold that it is not an endocrine disorder as such but rather an abnormal behavioural response to normal (physiological) changes during the menstrual cycle. PMS 'symptoms' are common and generally they are well tolerated. Women with severe, intractable symptoms may have lost the ability to cope because of anxiety or occult intercurrent disease such as thyroid dysfunction, anaemia, diabetes, etc.

MAKING THE DIAGNOSIS - See Table 22.1.

MAIN COMPLICATIONS - Suicide, loss of job, marital disharmony, etc.

SCREENING/PREVENTION - Not relevant.

Treatment Options
ADVICE - The exclusion of serious pathology accompanied by reassurance may suffice for some women. Psychotherapy has proven successful in helping some women. Other forms of therapy such as relaxation and stress

Table 22.1 Diagnosing premenstrual syndrome	
Making the diagnosis	Premenstrual syndrome
History	Anxiety, irritability and aggression with associated abdominal bloating and breast tenderness. These symptoms should settle prior to the end of menstruation
Examination	Nothing to find except diffuse mild abdominal tenderness during luteal phase
Investigations	Normal or negative: this is a diagnosis of exclusion

management techniques, hypnosis and acupuncture should be considered.

CHANGE OF LIFESTYLE/DIET - Improvement has been seen in women's quality of life with a better diet and implementation of an exercise regime. There is some anecdotal evidence to suggest that a reduction in caffeine intake is beneficial.

DRUG THERAPY - Many medical therapies have been used, with little scientific proof of their effectiveness. Placebo therapy has also been as effective as many drug therapies. **Diuretics** have been used to avoid fluid retention. **Laxatives** may help prevent bloating due to bowel inactivity in the luteal phase under the influence of progesterone. **Vitamin B$_6$** is a cofactor in the formation of neurotransmitters. There is no evidence of a deficiency of these transmitters or of vitamin B$_6$. Trials suggest that any benefit seen is a placebo effect. High doses have proved toxic to peripheral nerves. **Oil of evening primrose** contains polyunsaturated essential fatty acids which are necessary for the production of certain neurotransmitters. It is reported to help prevent irritability, and there is good evidence that it alleviates breast tenderness. **Bromocriptine** - prolactin suppression with dopamine agonist therapy has been used with success to reduce breast tenderness.

Hormonal therapy using the combined oral contraceptive pill and progestogens has been used, but as yet no clinical trials have shown lasting effectiveness. Suppression of the ovarian cycle will alleviate symptoms, but, until recently, treatment could only be given for short periods of time. Recently there has been a report of **high-dose oestrogen** given by pellets, together with a **levonorgestrel IUCD** to protect the endometrium from hyperplastic change, achieving relief in a high proportion of cases.

GnRH analogues desensitise the pituitary and induce ovarian quiescence, causing down-regulation of pituitary function and thereby suppressing gonadal production of sex steroids. They can only be used for 6 months. **Anti-depressants** should be prescribed if the woman is clinically depressed and psychotherapy has failed.

SURGERY – In severe cases, especially in women who have a completed family, hysterectomy and bilateral oophorectomy may be considered, with continuous oestrogen-only HRT afterwards. They should have undergone a therapeutic trial of medical castration using GnRH analogues together with HRT prior to surgery. The difficulty is that any drug trial is subject to a large placebo effect.

OVERVIEW – It is apparent that no one therapy has proven to be totally effective, and, as the aim of treatment is to improve the woman's symptoms, several forms of therapy may be required before success is achieved. Psychotherapy and counselling should play a major role in treatment plans. Surgery should be reserved for those women who have severe symptoms.

Follow-up

SHORT TERM – It is useful to follow up the results of initial therapy and provide explanations of the results obtained.

LONG TERM – If severe symptoms persist, referral to specialist counselling unit or psychiatrist may be arranged. If radical surgery is planned, referral should be made to a gynaecology clinic.

GOLDEN POINTS

1. PMS is a diagnosis of exclusion. Severe behavioural and systemic diseases should be considered in the differential diagnosis.

2. A clear relationship between symptoms and the menstrual cycle is essential.

3. Underlying psychological problems frequently may coexist.

4. Treatment is often based on the woman's individual symptomatology.

5. There is little scientific evidence to support the use of most recommended medical therapies, and there is a large placebo effect. High-dose oestrogen and the levonorgestrel IUCD may prove to be the most effective.

6. Explanation and counselling play an important role in management.

7. A therapeutic trial of ovarian suppression and HRT should be attempted prior to undertaking surgery.

23 Request for hormone replacement therapy (HRT)

CLINICAL SIGNIFICANCE

The average age for the menopause in this country is 51, and, with increasing life expectancy, most women will spend a third of their life beyond the menopause. About 1% of women will pass through the menopause prematurely, and an ever-growing number of younger women experience the profound endocrine changes of prophylactic oophorectomy performed during hysterectomy.

The menopause is an outward sign of ovarian failure and oestrogen-deficiency which leads to acute and chronic physical and psychological symptoms. In addition, the lack of oestrogen *increases the chance of morbidity and mortality from cardiovascular disease and osteoporosis.*

Androgen deficiency may also play a part in menopausal symptoms such as lethargy and loss of sexual desire, particularly for those women who undergo bilateral oophorectomy.

Symptoms and disease can be prevented by use of hormone replacement therapy. Attention in the media has increased public awareness, and requests for advice about the menopause and HRT form an ever-increasing part of the workload for GPs and gynaecologists.

THE MENOPAUSE

The menopause simply denotes the last period. The climacteric is the period of time surrounding the menopause; the climacteric is, to the menopause, what puberty is to the menarche.

It was previously believed that once the ovary had failed it could not resume activity, but it is now clear that, for some women in the perimenopause, ovarian function fluctuates widely between complete inactivity and normal ovulation. This is important to recognise, because it means that some women move in and out of fertility and infertility. Contraception should therefore be used for 2 years beyond the last period if the woman is less than 50 years and for 1 year if she is more than 50 years.

The menopause is generally easy to define clinically in most individuals, but it can be diagnosed by measuring LH and FSH in blood if there is any confusion. The menopause is indicated by elevated levels of both hormones, but the concentration of FSH is greater than that of LH.

CLINICAL ASSESSMENT

Organisation of Care

Most advice is now given by GPs. Specialist menopausal clinics should be run in gynaecology units for complicated problems.

Women may present complaining of physical or psychological symptoms or because they wish to take HRT to prevent osteoporosis or cardiovascular disease. Many other women present with other problems, and opportunities should be taken as they arise to discuss the menopause. Posters in health centres will help to encourage women to talk to their GP or practice nurse if they wish.

Relevant History

Presenting Complaint

It is important to remember when assessing complaints in perimenopausal women that symptoms from pathological disease may mimic the climacteric. For instance, flushes may be due to carcinoid tumours or thyroid disease, and bladder symptoms may be due to infection or tumours. Psychological symptoms are particularly difficult to unravel, as depression and anxiety are common problems in midlife, irrespective of the menopause, because of changing jobs and of children in adolescence. Equally, low mood genuinely appears to be a feature of oestrogen deficiency, and, indirectly, menopausal symptoms such as flushes and menorrhagia may promote low self-esteem and reactive depression.

MAIN SYMPTOMS – 80% of women will be symptomatic, experiencing either vasomotor or psychological symptoms. For a large proportion the symptoms of the climacteric start before the menopause proper. Many women will tolerate their symptoms with ease and not seek advice from a doctor or specialist nurse. Others will suffer in silence for years.

Acute vasomotor symptoms – hot flushes are experienced by up to 75% of women, and in one third of women the flushes start before the menopause. These may be short, lasting just seconds or much longer with successive flushes merging. They are often associated with palpitations, dizziness and sweating. Night sweats are common, with the women often describing insomnia and exhaustion. Some women sweat so much they have to change their bedclothes. Vascular headaches are also common.

Chronic symptoms of oestrogen deficiency – thinning of the skin with bruising and hair loss are commonly noticed as is mild facial hirsutism. Many women are also troubled by aching joints, and bladder symptoms such as frequency and urgency are common because of atrophy within the urinary tract. Vaginal dryness and superficial dyspareunia are a feature of genital tract atrophy, but many women feel embarrassed to mention these symptoms.

Psychological symptoms are often harder to ascribe to the menopause directly, but women often describe irritability, low mood, lethargy, forgetfulness and emotional lability.

Reduced libido is also common and may be due to declining androgen levels but may also be simply related to other problems such as difficulties at work or with the family.

COMMONLY ASSOCIATED SYMPTOMS – Menstrual irregularity often occurs, with the periods becoming chaotic and heavy just before the menopause. This is because unopposed oestrogen stimulation from the failure to ovulate results in a thickened and hypertrophied endometrium which is shed erratically. Any irregular bleeding in the perimenopausal years should raise the possibility of genital tract cancer.

EFFECT ON PATIENT – The changes associated with the menopause are not just those described above; there are many things occurring in a woman's life during the climacteric: children leaving home, moving house, change of career, altered body image, and death of elderly parents. Symptoms such as hot flushes reduce a woman's ability to cope with these life events.

Gynaecological History

GYNAECOLOGICAL DISEASE – Surgical removal of the ovaries will also create an instant menopausal state. Some women do not get proper advice about HRT at the time of prophylactic oophorectomy, and others are wrongly advised that they cannot have HRT after surgery for ovarian and cervical cancer.

MENSTRUAL HISTORY – The age at menopause is important, as different forms of HRT can be used according to the length of time since the last period. Irregular vaginal bleeding must be investigated to exclude genital tract malignancy before HRT is commenced.

CERVICAL CYTOLOGY – This is often a good opportunity to ask if a cervical smear test is due.

CONTRACEPTION – It is a good time to review contraception. Advice should be given about the chance of conception, which is very low but not nil.

Medical History

MEDICAL CONDITIONS – There are few medical contraindications to HRT, but a detailed medical history will allow an open discussion about the fears of interaction. Exceptions include liver disease, venous thrombosis and uterine bleeding of unknown cause. Breast and endometrial cancer are relative contraindications but only in the short term. Diabetes, hypertension and angina are not contraindications to HRT provided there is careful supervision.

SURGERY – Surgery for malignant disease, especially breast or endometrial carcinoma, needs to be taken into consideration when discussing possible HRT therapy.

PSYCHOLOGICAL DISORDERS – Confusion may exist between psychological disease and menopausal symptoms (see above).

Drug History

MEDICATIONS – Prolonged corticosteroid therapy increases the risk of osteoporosis. Tamoxifen therapy for breast carcinoma is a form of HRT and will help reduce the risk of osteoporosis and cardiovascular disease.

ALLERGIES – Allergies to medical adhesives may affect those women who may wish to use oestrogen patches.

SMOKING AND ALCOHOL – Smoking and excessive alcohol consumption have been implicated in the development of osteoporosis and cardiovascular disease.

Social History

AGE – Premature ovarian failure (< 40 years) increases all the long-term risks of the menopause. Consideration should be given to investigation for a specific disease, if the menopause starts before 35 years (see Chapter 20).

LIFESTYLE – Lack of exercise and a sedentary lifestyle increases the risk of osteoporosis and cardiovascular disease.

Relevant Clinical Examination

General Examination

GENERAL CONDITION – There may be evidence of thyroid

disease. The woman's mood may also be apparent from speech and manner. Atrophic changes such as thinning and bruising of the skin can be observed.

BODY-MASS INDEX – Obesity is associated with increased risk of cardiovascular disease but it can protect against osteoporosis. Once the ovaries stop producing oestrogen the peripheral fat becomes a major source, therefore thin women are at increased risk of developing osteoporosis.

Cardiorespiratory System

A comprehensive evaluation of the cardiovascular and respiratory system is not necessary unless there are symptoms, but blood pressure must be measured and controlled if markedly raised.

Breast

SCREENING – This provides an ideal opportunity to discuss breast screening and mammography with women over the age of 50. The breast should be examined before prescribing hormone therapy.

Pelvic

Pelvic examination is not absolutely necessary unless there are specific symptoms, but it is useful to exclude large fibroids.

PERINEUM/VULVA/VAGINA – The skin may become thin and dry, causing breakdown and bleeding. There may be suspicious reddened or raised ulcerated areas which should be biopsied to exclude carcinoma or premalignant skin disease.

CERVIX – With irregular bleeding, exclude tumours or polyps.

BIMANUAL EXAMINATION – The opportunity should be taken to screen for pelvic tumours such as fibroids or ovarian cysts, especially if there is a history of irregular bleeding.

Relevant Initial Investigations

Investigations are unnecessary for most women.

Haematology

Hb – Tiredness, lethargy and mood swings may be a sign of anaemia rather than the menopause.

Endocrine Tests

β-hCG – Women of childbearing age with amenorrhoea should have pregnancy excluded.

TSH – Thyroid disease is common in the 50s and 60s, and it may mimic menopausal symptoms.

FSH/LH – An elevated FSH concentration, greater than that of LH, confirms the menopause, but this test is rarely needed.

Diagnostic Imaging

PELVIC ULTRASOUND – To exclude pelvic/endometrial pathology for women with irregular bleeding.

BONE DENSITOMETRY – Bone mineral density is a poor guide to fracture risk and should not be used as a guide to HRT. It should only be used for those women with rare metabolic disorders.

Cytology

CERVICAL – A smear should be taken as part of the screening programme.

Histopathology

ENDOMETRIAL – A Pipelle endometrial biopsy should be performed in the presence of irregular perimenopausal or postmenopausal bleeding.

Direct Visualisation

HYSTEROSCOPY – Heavy irregular bleeding that has not been satisfactorily investigated with endometrial sampling and ultrasound should undergo direct visualisation of the endometrium to exclude pathology.

DETAILS OF COMMON REQUESTS

1. Symptoms of Acute and Chronic Oestrogen Deficiency

Background

DEFINITION – The menopause refers to the woman's last menstrual period. Ultimately it denotes the end of the ovarian cycle. Oestradiol levels decline but weak oestrogens, such as oestrone, and androgens are still produced.

AETIOLOGY – The number of ovarian follicles a woman has is determined while she herself is in utero. As they are consumed, it is thought that only the poor quality follicles remain, possibly those with genetic faults. As oestrogen and inhibin levels decline, levels of pituitary gonadotrophins rise, particularly FSH.

MAIN COMPLICATIONS – Symptoms include flushes, vaginal dryness, dyspareunia and loss of libido. In the longer term, there is loss of bone mass and a rise in the incidence of cardiovascular disease.

SCREENING/PREVENTION – There is no method of delaying the natural menopause.

MAKING THE DIAGNOSIS – This is usually very obvious clinically, and investigations are not necessary. However, if the woman is very young, other causes of amenorrhoea should be considered (see Chapter 20). Even in more elderly women, other (pathological) conditions should be considered if the symptoms are atypical or if they do not respond to treatment. See Table 23.1.

Table 23.1 Diagnosing the menopause	
Making the diagnosis	Menopause
History	Amenorrhoea beyond 40 years
	Hot flushes
Examination	No stigmata of systemic disease
Investigations	Generally none needed to confirm menopausal state
– FSH	Serum FSH (and LH) can be measured if there is doubt
– Other tests	Consider need to test for conditions if symptoms are atypical or do not respond

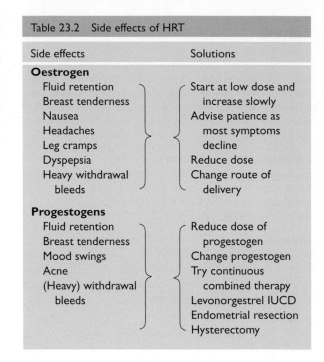

Table 23.2 Side effects of HRT	
Side effects	Solutions
Oestrogen	
Fluid retention	Start at low dose and increase slowly
Breast tenderness	Advise patience as most symptoms decline
Nausea	
Headaches	
Leg cramps	Reduce dose
Dyspepsia	Change route of delivery
Heavy withdrawal bleeds	
Progestogens	
Fluid retention	Reduce dose of progestogen
Breast tenderness	Change progestogen
Mood swings	Try continuous combined therapy
Acne	Levonorgestrel IUCD
(Heavy) withdrawal bleeds	Endometrial resection
	Hysterectomy

Treatment Options

ADVICE – Careful counselling with detailed information and a sympathetic approach should be offered to all women. A decision about treatment of the menopause need not necessarily be made quickly.

CHANGE OF LIFESTYLE/DIET – The acute vasomotor symptoms can be improved by simply reducing alcohol and caffeine intake. Stress reduction programmes prove helpful for some symptoms such as flushing in women who wish to avoid conventional HRT. The women should be encouraged to stop smoking, improve their diet and introduce regular exercise.

DRUG THERAPY – **Clonidine** is an antihypertensive agent which reduces the rate of flushing, but many women find its effect on flushing to be inadequate, and it has no other beneficial effects.

Tranquillisers have been prescribed for many years but their use in the treatment of menopausal symptoms, anxiety and depression probably been detrimental to women.

Hormone replacement therapy generally implies **oestrogen-based therapy** (with or without additional progestogen). Oestrogens control vasomotor symptoms and will reverse many of the tissue changes which result from oestrogen deficiency. They also help to prevent osteoporosis and perhaps cardiovascular disease. Oestrogen can be given orally, transdermally using patches, subcutaneously using slow-release pellets, or topically to the vagina alone by cream, pessary or tablet. Minor side effects (Table 23.2) are common initially, but most are short lived. Major complications are rare, but there is a slight increase in the risk of venous thrombosis in the first year. If unopposed by progestogen in women with an intact

uterus, there is an increased chance of endometrial cancer, but if progestogen is used the chance of endometrial neoplasia is lowered. There may be a small effect on the age-specific incidence of breast cancer but this is not proven. Certainly the incidence of breast carcinoma (1 in 12 women) has not changed dramatically since the introduction of HRT in the 1970s. Contraindications to HRT (Box 23.1) are also rare.

Oral oestrogen is subject to a first-pass effect through the liver converting up to a third into a useless form; it therefore requires higher oral doses to be taken than may be required, and theoretically any adverse effects on liver metabolism may be greater. However, it has the advantage of being convenient to take, easily stopped and inexpensive. Compliance with daily tablets can be variable. **Transdermal oestrogen** allows continuous absorption of oestradiol into the bloodstream, avoiding the first-pass effect of the liver. It is easily applied but occasionally causes allergic reaction at the site of application. The beneficial effect on lipoproteins is not as high as oral preparation, and they are more expensive to use. **Oestrogen implants** have been around for many years and they also have the benefit of continuous delivery by circumventing the first-pass effect of the liver. They are particularly suitable for women without a uterus and are often inserted at the time of hysterectomy with oophorectomy, although a minor surgical procedure is required for insertion after

Box 23.1 Contraindications to HRT

No contraindication	Relative contraindication	Absolute contraindications
Controlled hypertension	Previous PE/DVT	Recent myocardial infarct
Previous myocardial infarct	Gallstones	Current DVT/PE
Previous stroke	Mild liver disease	Active endometrial cancer
Family history of hypertension	Endometriosis	Active breast cancer
Varicose veins	Fibroids	Pregnancy
Obesity	Previous breast cancer	Undiagnosed breast lump
Smoking	Previous endometrial cancer	Undiagnosed vaginal bleeding
Malignant melanoma		Severe active liver disease
Abnormal smear		
Cervical cancer		
Ovarian cancer		
Benign breast disease		

that. Many women like not having to think of their HRT on a daily or weekly basis. They can also be combined with a testosterone implant for women with reduced libido. Being an implant, they are not easily reversed, however, and the effects may take up to 18 months to wear off. Tachyphylaxis may also occur when a woman becomes tolerant of the effects of high-dose oestrogen, and then vasomotor symptoms return early when the oestrogen concentration is quite high. This can be a very difficult situation to manage. **Topical oestrogens** have many advantages, especially with potent local action making them ideal for relieving vaginal dryness and atrophy. There is some systemic absorption if creams are used, but tablets can be used for up to 2 years with no effect on the endometrium. Poor compliance does occur with some preparations, as they can be messy and difficult to apply.

Specific regimens – Unopposed oestrogen therapy can only be used on women who have no endometrium, usually after hysterectomy, because of the risk of endometrial hyperplasia and potential malignant change. This avoids side-effects caused by progestogens. **Combination HRT** – involves the addition of a progestogen. This has a protective effect on the endometrium by altering it from the proliferative into the secretory phase, preventing the development of hyperplasia and neoplasia. Conventionally this was given as continuous oestrogen and cyclical progestogen (**cyclical HRT**) to mimic the ovarian cycle. The disadvantages of progestogen are that it causes systemic (premenstrual) symptoms and some varieties have an adverse effect on blood lipids. In addition, many women are irritated by continuation of menstruation, and the drop-out rate is very high. This can be overcome by

continuous combined HRT in which the oestrogen and progestogen are given throughout the cycle. In the near future, in order to avoid any systemic effects of progestogen, a device may be used which delivers the progestogen directly into the uterus (**levonorgestrel IUCD**). **Progestogen-only HRT** is for women who will not or cannot take oestrogen; progestogen alone will control flushes and give some protection against bone loss.

Tibolone is a synthetic steroid that has both mild oestrogenic and progestogenic properties. It has proven beneficial in controlling vasomotor side effects and, as it does not cause endometrial proliferation, there is no withdrawal bleed. There is also evidence that it has beneficial effects on prevention of bone reabsorption, but its effects on the cardiovascular system are unknown. Tibolone should be reserved for women who are a year from their last period, and if they are switching from conventional HRT they should continue cyclical progestogen until the withdrawal bleeds stop.

Follow-up

SHORT TERM – The women should be reviewed after 3 months to monitor progress and compliance. The continuation rate is low (about 25% at 1 year) and this is often due to misconceptions or medical issues that could be resolved (Box 23.2).

LONG TERM – The women should be seen on an annual basis by the general practitioner or the practice nurse to check for abnormal bleeding, monitor blood pressure and allow breast and cervical screening to take place. Yearly pelvic examination is not necessary.

OVERVIEW – The aim of treatment is to improve the woman's quality of life by resolving acute symptoms.

Box 23.2 Common reasons given for discontinuation

Remediable medical problems	**Misconceptions**	**Other problems**
Periods returned	Unnatural	Media scares
Breast tenderness	Restores fertility	Husband against
Nausea	Causes breast cancer	GP against
Premenstrual symptoms	HRT same as OCP	Friends against
Mild hypertension	Causes weight gain	

This is achieved by balancing the benefits of HRT against the potential risks of therapy. With the wide variety of regimens available today, most women can be successfully helped. Not all women wish to have HRT, however, and choice is important. Non-hormone therapy remains an important form of symptom relief for many.

2. Request for Advice about Long-term Health Problems

Background

DEFINITION/AETIOLOGY – The menopause is associated with oestrogen deficiency in most women. This leads to loss of bone mass (osteoporosis) and changes in vascular biology and lipid concentrations with rises in risk of cardiovascular disease.

Menopausal osteoporosis is a disease of bone resulting in a loss of bone mass and architecture but with normal mineralisation. Peak bone density occurs in the mid-twenties and is maintained until the late-forties, when it starts to reduce slowly (Figure 23.1). After the menopause there is a period of rapid bone loss for up to 10 years before the loss slows again. The risk of developing osteoporosis depends on the peak density of bone mass and the rate of loss, which is subject to a number of environmental factors. Risk factors include an early menopause, low body weight, calcium-poor diet, sedentary lifestyle, history of amenorrhoea, and prolonged corticosteroid therapy. Osteoporosis increases the risk of fracture, particularly of the wrist, hip and vertebrae, and by the age of 80 years the majority of women will have sustained at least one fracture, though many of these would have occurred silently. **Colles' wrist fracture** is 12 times more common in women than in men. Women are twice as likely to **fracture their hip** than men, and by the age of 90 over a third will have done so. This has huge implications on the NHS as well as their life expectancy, with nearly 30% of women dying within a year of fracturing their hip. **Vertebral crush fractures** typically involve T8–L4, causing loss of height and spinal deformity. Oestrogen replacement therapy has been shown to reduce the rate of bone loss and in high doses actually increase bone density. At any age the risk of fracture is a function of bone mass (strength) and the risk of falling. Attempts to prevent falls may play a greater part in preventing fractures than attempts to prevent bone loss, particularly in women with established osteoporosis.

Cardiovascular disease in women increases in incidence after the menopause to equal that of men

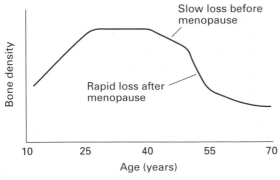

Fig 23.1 *Phases of bone formation and loss.*

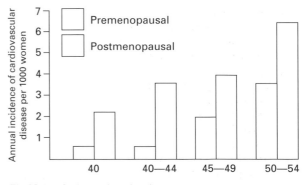

Fig 23.2 *Cardiovascular risk with age.*

(Figure 23.2). This pattern suggests that the reduction of oestrogen causes the change. This has been supported by several studies using surrogate markers. In postmenopausal women there is an alteration in the lipoprotein makeup, with an increase in LDL-cholesterol and reduction in HDL-cholesterol, and vascular biology also changes. Both of these effects can be reversed by oestrogen. There are data to suggest that long-term oestrogen therapy has a protective effect, but this has not been conclusively shown. Of course, there are several other factors which increase a woman's risk of developing cardiovascular disease (Box 23.3).

MAKING THE DIAGNOSIS – See above. Risk assessment for an individual woman is difficult, but other factors (see Box 23.3) may help the physician to tailor advice for a specific person.

MAIN COMPLICATIONS – Increased chance of bone fractures and of myocardial infarction and stroke. Long-term oestrogen deficiency may also increase the chance of uterovaginal prolapse, rectal prolapse and dysfunction, varicose ulcers and senile dementia.

SCREENING/PREVENTION – Basically, healthy living before the menopause with a calcium-rich, low-fat diet and good amounts of physical activity. Avoid smoking and excessive alcohol intake. Any periods of pathological amenorrhoea should be investigated and oestrogen replacement given.

Treatment Options

ADVICE – It is important to remember that it is easier to prevent bone loss than to replace it. The treatment of asymptomatic women is still controversial, but therapy should certainly be advocated for women who are at risk of osteoporosis and cardiovascular disease who have had premature ovarian failure or early menopause,

especially after surgery or chemotherapy. Ultimately, the choice is with the woman.

CHANGE OF LIFESTYLE/DIET – Avoid smoking and excessive alcohol intake, and take regular exercise. Attempts to prevent fractures by **reducing the rate of falls** can be simple and cheap. Moderate exercise improves balance and muscle tone. Careful placement of furniture and carpets, and the use of walking aids, can avert trips and falls. Withdrawal of hypnotic agents such as benzodiazepines prevents daytime drowsiness, and avoidance of excessive treatment of hypertension will prevent dizziness.

DRUG THERAPY FOR OSTEOPOROSIS – **Hormone replacement therapy** – the mainstay of pharmacological prophylaxis of osteoporosis.

Calcium – a calcium rich diet is probably important for the formation of bone in early life but has been shown to be of no value in the prevention of osteoporosis after the menopause.

Fluoride – this has been shown to increase bone mass, but the quality of bone is poor and the fracture rate increases.

Cyclical bisphosphonate therapy (with calcium) – has recently been shown to increase bone mass and prevent fractures. It is expensive at present but is important for women with established osteoporosis who refuse HRT. Further long-term results are awaited.

Vitamin D and calcium – recent evidence suggests that a combination of these prevents bone loss but it will have no effect on cardiovascular disease. It is a useful alternative for very elderly women who wish to avoid hormone therapy.

Calcitonin – a peptide hormone produced from the thyroid gland also reduces the amount of bone loss, but unfortunately the cost is very high.

Box 23.3 Risk factors

Osteoporosis
- Chronic corticosteroid therapy
- Late menarche early menopause (< 45 years)
- Prolonged immobilisation
- Age
- Family history of bone disease
- Caucasian/oriental
- Low body weight
- Nulliparity
- Smoking
- Excessive alcohol intake
- Prolonged amenorrhoea

Cardiovascular disease
- Hypertension
- Elevated plasma cholesterol (especially LDL)
- Elevated plasma triglyceride
- Family history of heart disease
- Smoking
- Diabetes
- Obesity
- Poor diet and exercise
- Excessive alcohol intake

DRUG THERAPY FOR CARDIOVASCULAR DISEASE – It is beyond the range of this text to review and discuss the prevention of cardiovascular disease in detail, but control of hypertension and blood lipids has an important role to play alongside HRT.

OVERVIEW – Cardiovascular disease is the major killer of elderly women, and menopausal osteoporosis is a common cause of morbidity. Attempts at prevention may have a major impact on the health of elderly women.

GOLDEN POINTS

1. Healthy living in early life promotes health in old age.

2. Lifestyle changes in old age may have as much effect on health promotion as HRT, particularly in elderly women.

3. Consider the possibility that systemic disease is the cause of menopausal symptoms if atypical or if HRT is of no benefit.

4. If the uterus is intact, progestogen therapy should be part of HRT (minimum of 12 days) to prevent endometrial cancer.

24 Request for contraception

CLINICAL SIGNIFICANCE

With falling age-specific death rates, the world population has dramatically increased over the last hundred years, making contraception a global issue.

For the individual, contraception has proved to be a liberating force for women throughout the world, allowing spacing of pregnancies, limitation of family size, and sexual freedom. Ironically, the sexual revolution that followed the introduction of the oral contraceptive in the 1960s has been associated with increasing numbers of unplanned teenage pregnancies and rising rates of pelvic infection. For many other women, contraception has brought novel medical problems.

METHODS OF CONTRACEPTION

MAIN CATEGORY	METHOD
1. *Hormonal*	Combined oral contraceptive pill (COCP)
	Progestogen-only pill (PoP)
	Injectable progestogen
	Progestogen implants
2. *Intrauterine devices*	Copper-releasing IUCD
	Progestogen-releasing IUCD
3. *Barrier (with spermicidal creams)*	Condom
	Female condom
	Cervical cap
	Diaphragm
4. *Non-medical methods*	Rhythm method
	Cervical mucus testing
	Withdrawal (coitus interruptus)
	Ovulation testing
	Lactation
5. *Emergency (postcoital) contraception*	Hormonal (morning after pill) 72hrs
	IUCD
6. *Sterilisation*	Female
	Male

This chapter is concerned with reversible contraception. Sterilisation is considered in Chapter 25.

Contraception is a personal choice made with or without medical or nursing guidance. Many factors play a part including religious and cultural beliefs, media reporting, advice from friends and previous experiences. It is possible for a doctor to feel that medical issues are paramount, but, if a couple are given a form of contraception with which they do not feel happy, compliance will be compromised and pregnancy may follow.

When advising about contraception it is helpful to be aware of the cultural needs of different racial/religious groups. It should not be assumed that an individual will abide by these, but it is helpful to discuss particular problems which may occur beforehand. Examples include the need to avoid irregular vaginal bleeding

(common with progestogen-only contraception) in some Islamic women who cannot prepare food on days that they bleed, and the reluctance of some Roman Catholic women to use IUCDs because they are classified by some as abortifacients.

Breast feeding is not particularly effective when compared with modern contraception, but in underdeveloped countries it has a major role in spacing of pregnancies and limitation of family size. Reduction in breast feeding rates because of marketing by formula feed manufacturers can have an adverse effect on family and population dynamics in the third world.

When judging the success of contraceptive methods, the Pearl index is used which expresses failures in terms of the number of pregnancies per 100 woman years of usage. Of the reversible contraceptives, the oral hormonal methods have been the most effective, but the new progestogen-releasing IUCD shows a further improvement and offers yet more choice to women.

CLINICAL ASSESSMENT

Organisation of Care

Contraception demands personal knowledge, and education is the key to uptake and effective compliance. This should be undertaken in schools and colleges at several stages. Information leaflets should also be freely available and on display at health centres and in antenatal clinics, etc.

Discussion of sexual matters is difficult for many women and men, and ideally there should be a range of options including general practice surgeries and specialist family planning clinics (FPCs). Current Government policy is to disinvest in generic FPCs for all and concentrate these resources on the young. Older men and women are now encouraged to access care at the local health centres.

Some authorities have argued that contraception would be more widely used if most methods (except IUCDs) were available over-the-counter at local pharmacies. This policy has yet to be adopted in the United Kingdom but it is used in certain European countries. In the third world, some success has been achieved by training non-medical village members to learn about counselling and administration of methods such as progestogen implants, thereby giving poor women access to modern contraception.

The clinic needs to create a convivial, relaxed atmosphere. It should be well stocked with contraceptive devices and leaflets. There needs to be equipment for cardiac resuscitation for the insertion of IUCDs.

Legal Issues

Many girls below the age of consent (16 years) seek advice about contraception from doctors. They have a right to advice and care without parental consent. The decision lies with the attending doctor who has the right to support the privacy of the patient and may prescribe contraception providing they feel she understands how to use the method prescribed and the implications of it. However, it is often useful to advise the girl to discuss matters with a parent if possible.

Relevant History

Presenting Issue

MAIN ISSUE - **Prevention of pregnancy** means different things to different women and men at different times in their lives. Some simply wish to space out their family but would not be concerned too greatly if conception did

occur, whereas for others it is essential to keep the chance of pregnancy to a minimum. It is important to gain some idea of the specific needs of the individual/couple. Often a good way to start off the consultation is to ask which form of contraception she/he was thinking of using.

COMMONLY ASSOCIATED ISSUES - **Menstrual problems** such a heavy bleeding may lead the woman to request a change of method to control her cycle. **Infections**, especially viral (HIV, hepatitis), have a high media profile, and the use of condoms will reduce their spread as more people become aware of this. **Previous contraception failure** often colours the views of both partners.

EFFECT ON PATIENT - For some individuals, the issue is not only one of which type of contraception to choose but also of whether to enter into a sexual relationship at all. This particularly applies to young women in their first relationship. It is important to be open to discuss sexual matters as well as contraception.

Gynaecological History

GYNAECOLOGICAL DISEASE - A history of pelvic inflammatory disease or ectopic pregnancy would make the non-hormonal IUCD less desirable because of the risk of recurrent problems.

MENSTRUAL HISTORY - A full menstrual history should be taken and any irregularities investigated as appropriate. The IUCD would not be advised in women with heavy, irregular or painful menses. The combined OCP is an ideal choice for many women, providing both effective contraceptive cover and good cycle regulation. Amenorrhoea must be investigated before prescription of the OCP. An IUCD must be inserted during a period to avoid damage to a pregnancy.

CERVICAL CYTOLOGY - If a cervical smear is due, it should be offered to the woman.

CONTRACEPTION - Any previous methods used should be noted along with problems that were associated with them.

FERTILITY REQUIREMENTS - The future fertility requirements are important. If they have completed their family a more permanent method such as sterilisation can be offered. If they plan to start a family soon a barrier method may be more appropriate.

Obstetric History

DELIVERY - Once a woman has had a child it becomes easier to insert an IUCD, although the new hormone-releasing IUCD can be used in nulliparous women. If the woman has had a recent delivery and is still breast feeding, the progesterone-only pill provides excellent contraception.

OBSTETRIC COMPLICATIONS - A history of multiple caesarean sections carries an increased risk of an IUCD perforating through into the abdominal cavity.

Medical History

MEDICAL CONDITIONS – Venous thrombosis, pulmonary embolism, severe hypertension, severe liver disease, etc., are contraindications for the combined oral contraceptive pill. Epileptics should be cautious as their medication may interfere with the OCP. Women with cardiac defects require antibiotic cover for insertion of an IUCD. Physical handicap may make use of barrier methods difficult.

SURGERY – Previous cervical surgery may make IUCD insertion difficult because of stenosis.

PSYCHOLOGICAL DISORDERS – Psychosexual problems or cultural beliefs may mean that the woman is unwilling to be examined or touch her genitals, making barrier methods inappropriate.

ALLERGIES – Women or their partners may be allergic to some spermicidal creams and condoms, so any plastic or rubber allergies should be enquired about. Copper allergy is a contraindication to a copper-containing IUCD.

Drug History

MEDICATIONS – Certain medications alter the metabolism of the OCP, leading to contraceptive failure. Antibiotics effect the gut flora and therefore absorption. Enzyme-inducing drugs such as anticonvulsants, rifampicin and spironolactone increase the metabolism of oestrogen and progesterone. Conversely, the OCP interferes with the action of warfarin and tricyclic medications.

SMOKING AND ALCOHOL – Smoking is associated with an increased risk of thromboembolism, especially when using the oral contraceptive pill.

Social History

AGE – A woman's age is very important. Young girls may be less reliable users of the OCP. For more elderly women it should be emphasised that hormone replacement therapy does not provide contraception. It is often said that elderly women know less of contraception than their daughters. Knowledge should not be assumed for this age group, and detailed counselling must be made available.

LIFESTYLE – Cultural differences prevent some women from using modern methods of contraception, but there are still traditional techniques such as the rhythm method, withdrawal and breast feeding which are not as effective but still provide some protection against conception.

Relevant Clinical Examination

Examination is not required for all women.

General Examination

GENERAL CONDITION – Raised blood pressure is a contraindication for the OCP because of the increased risk of thrombosis. Anaemia from excessive menstruation may be helped by hormonal preparations.

BODY-MASS INDEX – Obesity is associated with increased risk of thrombosis using the OCP. Changes in body weight may cause difficulty when fitting vaginal diaphragms or cervical caps.

Abdomen

PALPATION – Provides an opportunity to screen for abdominal or pelvic tumours.

Pelvic

Genital tract examination is not necessary for most forms of contraception. It is considered prudent before prescription of the OCP or the insertion of an IUCD. Sometimes the pelvic examination may be left to the second visit to help build confidence. Pelvic examination is necessary for women wishing to use the diaphragm to judge the appropriate size of the device.

PERINEUM/VULVA – Look for signs of infection, specifically STDs, particularly if an IUCD is to be fitted.

VAGINA – Vaginal inspection should exclude any congenital malformations preventing the use of vaginal contraception or an IUCD.

CERVIX – Exclude cervical pathology and pelvic sepsis.

BIMANUAL EXAMINATION – Uterine enlargement may alter the options chosen especially for the OCP, which may increase the size of fibroids, and for the IUCD, whose efficacy may be reduced by a large endometrial cavity.

Relevant Initial Investigations

For most individuals/couples there is no indication for investigation, but medical tests are sometimes necessary to screen for occult medical conditions which may influence choice.

Haematology

Hb – Heavy menstrual loss may lead to anaemia and should be screened for if surgery is contemplated.

Biochemistry

URINE PREGNANCY TEST – This is advised by some before insertion of an IUCD.

Microbiology

CHLAMYDIAL SEROLOGY – Women with high titres are at greater risk of getting recurrent pelvic infection and this may influence the choice of IUCD.

BACTERIOLOGY – Vaginal and endocervical swabs should be taken if there is any suspicion of PID before insertion of an IUCD. Some units now do this routinely.

Diagnostic Imaging

PELVIC ULTRASOUND – Any suspicion of uterine or ovarian pathology should be investigated with pelvic ultrasound. This may help with insertion of the IUCD by indicating size and axis of uterus. In the future, women may have a scan immediately after insertion, to check positioning. With lost IUCD strings, scanning can help to identify the location of the IUCD.

Cytology

CERVICAL – An opportunity for cervical cytology screening.

COMMON METHODS OF CONTRACEPTION

I. Intrauterine Contraceptive Device (IUCD)

Background

DEFINITION – The IUCD is a manufactured foreign body made from plastic and coated with copper or progestogen. The device is placed in the uterine cavity, preventing sperm transport, fertilisation and implantation. Non-medicated devices are no longer available. Some groups see these devices as abortifacients.

MODE OF ACTION – The IUCD sets up a **foreign body reaction** in the endometrium, leading to leucocyte infiltration, rendering the endometrium hostile to implantation. Sperm transport may also be affected.

METHODS – Non-medicated devices such as the Lippes loop have now been withdrawn from the market. Copper-containing devices were developed in the 1960s. The copper increases the inflammatory reaction and efficacy, allowing a smaller device to be used which in turn decreases side-effects such as bleeding, pain and expulsion.

Effective hormone-releasing devices have been developed in the last ten years. They have a similar action to oral progestogen preparations, causing atrophy of the endometrium and thickening of the cervical mucus. The levonorgestrel device releases 20 mcg/day from the hormone reservoir lasting up to 5 years. The amount of progestogen in the circulation is small compared with depot progestogen contraception.

ADVANTAGES – Single act of motivation. Relatively cheap. Does not interfere with sexual act. Rapidly reversible (with aid of doctor). Success rates vary depending on the type of IUCD. Modern copper-containing devices (multiload 375, copper T380) have a pregnancy rate of less than 1 per hundred women after 1st year of use, making it one of the most effective methods of contraception. The levonorgestrel-containing device has an even higher success rate and the advantage of reduced menstrual loss.

DISADVANTAGES – Requires skilled practitioner. **Bleeding and pain** are the two commonest reported symptoms, in copper-containing devices, causing 10% to be removed by the end of 1 year. The copper-containing devices are associated with an increase of menstrual loss of up to 50%, whereas hormone-releasing devices actually reduce

blood loss by up to 50%, but there is more likely to be erratic bleeding in the first 3 months. Cramping pain experienced in the first few weeks usually settles. Extreme pain on insertion may cause a profound vasovagal reaction.

Spontaneous expulsion occurs in around 5% by the end of 1 year, but the majority occur in the first 3 months, and the woman should be advised to check for the threads regularly. Careful choice of size and correct placement will help reduce this. **Ectopic pregnancy** is more common if a woman does conceive (5% risk vs 1% in pregnancy without IUCD), but overall the chance is lower because the chance of conception is much reduced. If a woman has an **intrauterine pregnancy**, the chance of (infected) miscarriage is higher and the chance of preterm prelabour rupture of membranes is increased. It is advisable to remove the IUCD as soon as pregnancy has been confirmed, if the strings are visible.

Pelvic inflammatory disease is more common with copper devices (but not hormone systems) but only in younger women, and the increased chance is more modest than originally suspected. Careful selection is essential. Lost threads are not uncommon and usually found in the cervix but they should be retrieved to exclude perforation or expulsion. If the threads cannot be located, ultrasound should be used to check position, but it is advisable to retrieve and replace the IUCD (Figure 24.1).

Uterine perforation is rare, occurring in 1 per thousand insertions and may be prevented by carefully assessing the uterine size and orientation, allowing accurate insertion. Retrieval can be difficult, requiring radiology to confirm position and laparoscopy to remove it.

IDEAL USE – Parous women who wish effective method but for whom OCP is undesirable or contraindicated.

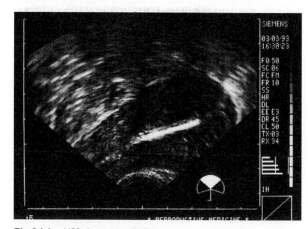

Fig 24.1   *USS showing an IUCD.*

SCREENING/PREVENTION – Take measures to avoid pelvic infection. Ask woman to report pregnancy early so that ectopic pregnancy can be diagnosed early, and so that the device can be removed if it is an intrauterine pregnancy. Teach woman to feel for strings so that expulsion can be detected early.

OVERVIEW – The IUCD is extremely popular with some women, but careful selection is essential. The progestogen-releasing IUCD which has fewer contra-indications may well become the most commonly used reversible contraceptive in the next ten years.

Follow-up

SHORT TERM – After insertion, the woman should be seen at 4 weeks to check the threads can still be felt.

LONG TERM – Yearly follow-up should be encouraged to check the threads and assess any problems that may have arisen. These clinics provide an ideal opportunity for general health and pelvic screening to take place. The devices need changing every 3 to 7 years depending on type.

2. Oral Hormonal Contraception

Background

DEFINITION – The use of sex-steroid hormones to suppress ovulation and/or alter endometrium and cervical mucus.

METHODS – Combined oestrogen and progestogen preparation (COPP) and low-dose progestogen-only preparation (PoP).

- **COPP** – **Ethinyloestradiol** is by far the most commonly used synthetic oestrogen in the COPP. Various **progestogens** have been used. Norethisterone, a derivative of testosterone, and levonorgestrel have detrimental effects on blood lipids, decreasing levels of HDLs and increasing the levels of LDL. The newer progestogens, gestodene and desogestrel, are more lipid friendly but have been linked with a higher risk of venous thromboembolism. A typical cycle is for the pills to be taken for 21/28 days, allowing 7 pill-free days for a withdrawal bleed. If pill is missed (over 12 h) at the beginning or the end of the cycle there is more chance of contraception failure, and extra contraception (barrier) should be used for the next 7 days with continuation of the COPP. Similar precautions should be taken when changing pill or prescribed antibiotics.

  Various regimens are available including **monophasic** formulations with the same dose of oestrogen and progestogen each day. **Biphasic** and **triphasic** preparations alter the daily dose of progestogen across the cycle to prevent erratic bleeding. These have been met with limited enthusiasm.

- **PoP** – The **progestogen-only pill** contains a low dose of a progestogen which is taken every day. About 50% of women will continue to ovulate regularly, and its principal actions are thought to be alteration of the cervical mucus and atrophy of the endometrium. If the pill is missed by more than 3 h the protective effect may be lost and covering protection should be used.

ADVANTAGES –

- **COPP** – **Failure rate** less than 1 per hundred woman years. Good control of menstrual cycle. **Protective against PID** – acts by thickening cervical mucus. Often **improves acne and mild hirsutism** (use Dianette – combination of ethinyloestradiol and an anti-androgen). Protective against **endometrial and ovarian cancers**.
- **PoP** – Fewer serious complications.

DISADVANTAGES –

- **COPP** – **Premeditation**: requires forethought by the woman. **Weight gain** is probably one of the commonest complaints, but studies show the average weight gain is zero! Breast tenderness and nausea are common initially but these generally subside.

  Psychological effects may occur, with some women describing a loss of libido and episodes of depression. These are probably progestogenic effects.

  Metabolic effects have been seen, with glucose tolerance being reduced; thus may require alteration in insulin therapy for diabetics.

  Cardiovascular effects are seen and can be fatal. The risk of venous thromboembolism is increased three-fold for users of the COPP and even more in smokers, women with a previous history of thrombosis, and in those with obesity. The chance of arterial thrombosis is increased, but fatal stokes and myocardial infarctions are still very rare, occurring in less than 1 per 10 000 users. Cerebral haemorrhage is twice as likely but again is very rare and is also related to smoking and hypertension.

  Hepatic disease is not common, but there is an increased incidence in women developing obstructive jaundice secondary to gallstones, and rare hepatic tumours are slightly more common on the COPP.

  Breast cancer – despite intensive study the relationship between COPP and breast tumours is still poorly defined. If there is any effect it is likely to be modest. **Drug interactions** occur as discussed above.

- **PoP** – Although this formulation carries far fewer medical risks, it must be taken regularly at the same time each day. Abnormal menstrual bleeding is seen frequently in PoP users but this is well tolerated by many women. Failure rate is higher at 2–3 per hundred woman years.

IDEAL USES –

• **COPP** – Good all round contraceptive for women of all ages.
• **POP** – Good for women breast feeding and for more elderly women; efficacy of POP at 40 years is the same as for the COPP at 20 years.

SCREENING/PREVENTION – In order to avoid serious adverse effects, careful screening should take place and contraindications for the COPP observed (Box 24.1). It should be remembered that the PoP contains a low-dose progestogen and does not present the same risks as the COPP. Tell women to report symptoms of venous thrombosis early. Women undergoing surgery should have heparin prophylaxis.

Box 24.1 Contraindications to COPP

Absolute contraindications to COPP
   Past or current cardiovascular disease
      thrombosis
      cerebral haemorrhage
      infarction
      hypertension
      valve disease
      coagulopathies
   Hepatic disease
      viral hepatitis
      adenoma
      cholestasis
   Pregnancy
   Undiagnosed genital tract bleeding
   Oestrogen sensitive neoplasms

Relative contraindications
   Risk for cardiovascular disease
      smoking
      obesity
      over 35 years of age
   Migraine
   Family history of breast cancer
   Renal disease
   CIN
   On medication likely to interact with th COPP
      antibiotics
      anticonvulsants
   Past history of oestrogen-dependent neoplasm
   Sickle cell disease — homozygous
   Breast feeding

OVERVIEW – **COPP** is an excellent form of reversible contraception. Despite much adverse media attention, it remains very popular. Compliance is important, and it is advised that the pill be taken at the same time every day. **PoP** is safer but has a much higher failure rate. Compliance is even more critical.

Information for the Patient
The woman should be warned of the effects of antibiotics and gastrointestinal upset and advised to report adverse symptoms early.

Follow-up
SHORT TERM – It is advised to see the woman 4 weeks after starting the pill to check that she is complying with the instructions and that there are no problems. Blood pressure should be checked then and again yearly. There is no indication for yearly pelvic examination if there are no symptoms.

3. Depot Progestogen Preparations

Background
DEFINITION – The insertion of a slow-release hormonal reservoir.

METHODS – High-dose progestogen acts by supressing ovulation and by altering the endometrium and cervical mucus. The **depot injection** (medroxyprogesterone acetate, Depo Provera) is stored in a crystalline suspension and given as an intramuscular injection. It needs repeating after 3 months. **Subdermal implants** using levonorgestrel have been manufactured with silastic rods which last for 5 years.

ADVANTAGES – Very safe; may be used in women with history of venous thrombosis. Cheap. Do not have to think of contraception daily or at time of sex.

DISADVANTAGES – **Irreversibility** – once a depot injection is given, it cannot be reversed. **Erratic bleeding**, which may be heavy, is probably the commonest complaint. This is usually temporary, although occasionally the implants need to be removed. **Weight gain** may be severe in a small proportion of women, possibly due to fluid retention.

   Amenorrhoea is common and, though usually not seen as a problem by most women, it makes others concerned about the possibility of pregnancy. **Oestrogen deficiency** – ovulation is suppressed and oestradiol levels are low. The effects of this on bone mass are not yet well known. **Skin reaction** – the silastic rods may cause disfiguring fibrosis. **Removal of silastic rods** may be difficult.

CONTRAINDICATIONS – Unexplained abnormal bleeding; depression.

IDEAL USES – For women who want very reliable contraception but who cannot reliably take the OCP or for whom oestrogen is contraindicated. As a short-term contraception after delivery prior to sterilisation. For sexually active, mentally incompetent women.

SCREENING/PREVENTION – Nil relevant.

OVERVIEW – All depot preparations should be inserted at the time of termination/miscarriage or within the first 5 days of the menstrual cycle. The **depot injection** is easily inserted and does not need repeating for 3 months. The **subdermal implants** comprise 6 small sticks that are inserted on the inside of the upper arm. They can be difficult to locate and remove but are licensed for 5 years.

Information for the Patient

PROGNOSIS – Very low failure rates (0.2 per hundred woman years) makes depot progesterone an attractive option, especially for women who have difficulty complying with other methods. The levonorgestrel IUCD may revolutionise future contraception because of the associated reduction in menstrual loss and protection over infection and ectopic pregnancy.

Follow-up

SHORT TERM – A 6 week appointment to assess satisfaction and routine long-term follow-up.

4. Barrier Methods

Background

DEFINITION – Devices designed to prevent live sperm from entering the cervical canal. Best used in conjunction with spermicidal cream (e.g. nonoxynol).

METHOD – They come in a variety of shapes and sizes. They are either worn on the penis or inserted into the vagina. The diaphragm, vault cap, cervical cap, female condom and vaginal sponge are all inserted into the vagina prior to intercourse.

The **diaphragm** and **cervical cap** should be fitted after careful examination of the vagina by a trained nurse or doctor (Figure 24.2). Once the correct size has been fitted in the clinic, the woman is instructed to fit it herself. Spermicidal cream should be applied to the device, which is inserted prior to intercourse. The device should be left in place for 8 h after intercourse for the spermicidal cream to work. If further intercourse is planned, a spermicidal cream or pessary should be inserted.

Condoms/sheaths are placed over the penis just before penetration. Again they should be applied before intercourse is started, remember 'a kettle spits before it boils'.

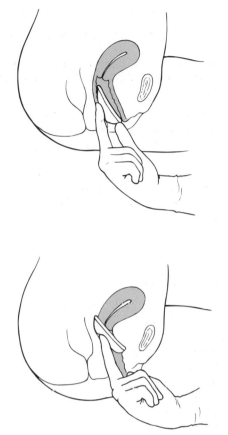

Fig 24.2 *Insertion of a diaphragm.*

ADVANTAGES – Sheaths are widely available in public areas and are useful for unexpected encounters. They are also important for couples practising safe sex. Major side effects are extremely rare.

DISADVANTAGES – **Failure rates** are higher, ranging from 3 to 12 per 100 woman years, mainly on account of the varying motivation and compliance. They tend to interfere with the spontaneity of sex and reduce sensitivity. **Vaginal irritation** may be caused by allergy to the device or the spermicidal cream.

IDEAL USE – Spacing of family, safe sex, extra cover if OCP tablet missed and for 'one-night stands'.

CONTRAINDICATIONS – Mentally incompetent or latex allergy.

SCREENING/PREVENTION – May help reduce risk of STDs, including HIV and hepatitis B, and also of cervical cancer. Hypoallergenic non-spermicidal-containing condoms have been developed which reduce vaginal irritation.

OVERVIEW – Main advantage for young people is their accessibility and value in safe sex. However, efficacy is low unless compliance is very good.

Information for the Patient

PROGNOSIS – Methodical use of the barrier methods can make them nearly as effective as hormonal contraception.

Follow-up

SHORT TERM – A 6 week check to ensure that the diaphragm is being fitted correctly.

LONG TERM – Diaphragms should be checked annually in clinic for damage and correctness of size.

5. Non-medical Contraception

Background

DEFINITION – Prevention of contraception using knowledge of the menstrual cycle to avoid intercourse during fertile phase or by withdrawal prior to ejaculation. These methods stem from the days when other forms were not available and are used today when religious and cultural beliefs ban the use of contraception.

METHODS – Ovulation takes place 14 days before the onset of menstruation in women with **regular** cycles. Avoidance of intercourse 4–5 days either side of predicted day of ovulation is known as the **rhythm method**. Detection of fertile mucus and mucus change is **Billing's method**. Withdrawal of penis before ejaculation is called **coitus interruptus. Home urine hormone monitoring** can be used to test for fertile days. **Regular breast feeding** inhibits ovulation, and in undeveloped countries this is still an important method of contraception. In the United Kingdom, breast feeding tends to be stopped earlier, and the failure rate is therefore higher.

ADVANTAGES – No major physical side effects. All that may be available for devout Catholics. Inexpensive.

DISADVANTAGES – **Failure rates** are as high as 20 per 100 woman years, mainly because of the varying motivation and compliance.

IDEAL USE – Spacing of family in women with religious beliefs or those who wish to avoid medical complications.

CONTRAINDICATIONS – Mentally incompetent.

OVERVIEW – The success of the **rhythm method** depends on the regularity of the cycle and motivation of the couple, but it can be extremely effective in a stable relationship. Education is an essential component of these methods.

6. Emergency (Postcoital) Contraception

Background

DEFINITION – Contraception given after intercourse to prevent fertilisation or implantation.

METHODS – Used after failed contraception (burst condom or missed OCP), unprotected intercourse or rape. The morning-after pill (ethinyloestradiol 100 mcg and levonorgestrel 300 mcg) and the IUCD have been used.

MAIN COMPLICATIONS – Nausea and vomiting are common with the morning-after OCP. The OCP may also cause cycle disruption. IUCD insertion may exacerbate any infection and should be used with caution after rape. Method failure is not associated with fetal malformation, but there is some evidence to suggest that the incidence of ectopic pregnancy is higher.

PRECAUTIONS – Do pregnancy test to rule out possibility of early conception.

Treatment Options

The morning-after pill must be given within 72 h of intercourse. Extra tablets are given in case the first set is vomited back up. Insertion of an IUCD can be performed up to 5 days after intercourse.

Information for the Patient

PROGNOSIS – The morning-after pill has over 95% success rate, whereas the IUCD is nearly 100% effective.

Follow-up

SHORT TERM – After the morning-after pill a withdrawal bleed should occur within a week and the next periods may be delayed. A 4 week appointment should be made to check menstruation has occurred and there is no pregnancy. The IUCD should be removed after the next period.

LONG-TERM – Appointment with the GP or family planning clinic to get advice about long-term contraception.

GOLDEN POINTS

1. Listen to the woman's/couple's needs and wishes. Dissatisfaction will lead to poor compliance.

2. Consider safe sex issues for young adults and give information on emergency contraception.

3. Pay careful attention to medical indications and contraindications.

4. Give clear information about practical issues and operate open-door policy if problems arise.

5. Remember that menopause does not immediately indicate end of fertility and that HRT is not a form of contraception.

25 Request for sterilisation

CLINICAL SIGNIFICANCE

Sterilisation is permanent contraception. For women it involves an intermediate-category operation, but it is popular because it requires a single episode of motivation. It is highly effective, and serious complications are rare. Perhaps the greatest problem is regret, which is more common in younger women, women with small families, and those who are sterilised shortly after pregnancy.

For women over 30 years, female sterilisation is one of the most popular methods of contraception because of its efficacy, simplicity, relatively low cost and lack of need for maintenance. Worldwide, hundreds of thousands of women are sterilised each year, and the vast majority are pleased with their decision.

METHODS OF STERILISATION

MAIN CATEGORY	TECHNIQUES
1. *Female*	Laparoscopic tubal clip application
	Open tubal ligation
	Bilateral salpingectomy
	Laparoscopic tubal diathermy
	Laparoscopic tubal ring application
	Hysterectomy (if associated medical problems)
	(Hysteroscopic cornual diathermy)
2. *Male*	Vasectomy

This chapter is largely concerned with female sterilisation.

As with reversible forms of contraception the views about sterilisation vary widely and are influenced by religious and cultural beliefs.

Sterilisation is a joint decision for many couples, but a woman does not need the permission of her partner to have the procedure performed.

There is a view that vasectomy is simpler, cheaper and associated with fewer complications than female sterilisation, and some doctors try to persuade women not to have the operation themselves. The decision to undergo sterilisation is not simply an assessment of the medical issues, however. Some women cannot influence their husbands to undergo vasectomy, some might not trust their husbands, others may have husbands whose work is under pressure, and some women may have more than one partner. Ultimately, therefore, the decision should be left to the woman to make, and undue pressure should not be applied.

CLINICAL ASSESSMENT

Organisation of Care

Sterilisation involves counselling and surgery. Tradition-ally, gynaecologists have taken part in both roles, but there is an argument for the GP to undertake the counselling and for the gynaecologist simply to act as a technician.

Views about sterilisation vary amongst clinicians. Some believe that if there is no contraindication to surgery then the decision is solely for the woman to make. Others maintain that the final decision should be that of the gynaecologist. Many women come to the clinic anxious that they have to prove their case for sterilisation. For those with a liberal philosophy, it may help to state at the start of the consultation that the choice will be hers and you are simply there to advise her.

It is important that the woman (and her partner) have a good understanding of the nature of sterilisation. Leaflets will help to reiterate that which is discussed. The issues that must be discussed are shown in Table 25.1.

Relevant History

Presenting Complaint

MAIN ISSUE - **Reason for request** - it is helpful to hear the woman's story and occasionally to explore what she has to say in some detail. She may have misconceptions about her current form of contraception or about the safety of further pregnancy.

Table 25.1   Issues to be discussed about sterilisation

Information to be discussed	Potential effect on woman
Permanent form of contraception[a]	Regret
Failure rate	5/1000 chance of conception
Unable to see Fallopian tubes	Mini-laparotomy
Trauma during laparoscopy	Major laparotomy
Tubal damage	Ectopic more common if do conceive[b]

[a]Sterilisation can be reversed, but the operation is generally not funded by the NHS.
[b]But overall the ectopic rate is lower because the conception rate is greatly reduced.

ASSOCIATED ISSUES – **Menstrual problems** may make hysterectomy an attractive proposal.

EFFECT ON PATIENT – Concerns about becoming pregnant can lead to problems with intercourse and even psychosexual problems. These are not necessarily relieved by sterilisation.

Gynaecological History

GYNAECOLOGICAL DISEASE – A history of pelvic inflammatory disease, ectopic pregnancy or endometriosis may make surgery difficult. This should be explained.

MENSTRUAL HISTORY – A full menstrual history should be taken and any irregularities investigated. If there are severe problems, hysterectomy may be an appropriate option to consider. Sterilisation does not make periods lighter or heavier, though cessation of the OCP may make periods increase to their former level.

CERVICAL CYTOLOGY – If the woman is due to have a cervical smear it should be offered.

CONTRACEPTION – The current method should be recorded. It is particularly important to note the presence of an IUCD, as this can be removed at the time of surgery. The woman should be encouraged to maintain contraceptive cover until the day of surgery. There is no indication to stop OCP before surgery; the chance of postoperative thrombosis is outweighed by the chance of unwanted pregnancy. An opportunity should be given to discuss all available methods, particularly novel forms which may not be known to the woman, e.g. progestogen-containing IUCD.

FERTILITY REQUIREMENTS – Future fertility requirements are important. It is essential for the woman to be sure she has completed her family.

Obstetric History

DELIVERY – Multiple caesarean sections may make visibility of the tubes difficult, but this is unusual compared with other pelvic surgery. f the woman has had a recent delivery or termination, it may be wise to consider leaving a period of a few months before undertaking the operation.

Medical History

MEDICAL CONDITIONS – Severe cardiac or respiratory diseases may be contraindications to surgery.

SURGERY – Previous laparotomy may make laparoscopy more difficult. This should be explained to the woman.

PSYCHOLOGICAL DISORDERS – Psychosexual problems will not be resolved by sterilisation.

Social History

AGE – A woman's age is an important factor in regret, and a very young woman with a small family must be counselled extremely carefully; it may be wise to give a few months for her to reflect on her wish for sterilisation.

DEPENDANTS – May affect whether day-care is suitable or not.

Relevant Clinical Examination

General Examination

BODY-MASS INDEX – Obesity may make anaesthesia unsafe and laparoscopy more difficult.

Abdomen

PALPATION – Provides an opportunity to screen for abdominal or pelvic tumours. Surgical scars may make laparoscopic surgery more difficult and dangerous.

Pelvic

Pelvic examination is not necessary if there are no symptoms, but some gynaecologists prefer to do a check to make sure there are no current problems.

CERVIX – Exclude cervical pathology.

BIMANUAL EXAMINATION – Uterine enlargement or ovarian tumours make laparoscopy more dangerous. Fixation may make access to the Fallopian tubes more difficult to identify.

Initial clinical investigations

Other than any preoperative checks, investigations are generally not needed.

MEDICAL IMAGING – If an IUCD has been inserted in the

past, but the strings cannot be seen, radiological imaging should be undertaken to identify its position.

METHODS OF STERILISATION

Background

DEFINITION – **Female sterilisation** is the permanent obstruction, destruction or removal of the Fallopian tubes, preventing fertilisation. **Male sterilisation** (vasectomy) is the ligation and transection of the vas deferens, preventing the passage of sperm.

METHODS – The Fallopian tubes can be obstructed by using **clips** (Filshie/Hulka-Clemens) or **rings** (Fallope), or be ablated using **diathermy**. See Figure 25.1.

MAIN COMPLICATIONS – Sterilisation can lead to minor problems such as wound infection, bruising and pain. The most serious complications relate to laparoscopy and include trauma to bowel, bladder and major vessels. **Chronic pain** occurs in up to 1% of women following diathermy sterilisation. **Menstrual disturbance** is commonly seen but this is either a subjective symptom or simply because many women will previously have been using hormonal contraception which has regulated their menstrual flow. **Vasectomy** is a much simpler procedure, but scrotal haematoma and/or infection occur in about 5% of men, and 1% are left with severe chronic testicular pain.

SCREENING/PREVENTION – **Female sterilisation** – the woman should be advised to maintain contraceptive cover until the operation day. Unless the woman is menstruating, any IUCD should be left in situ until the start of the next menstrual cycle to avoid implantation of a conceptus. Any OCP cycle should be completed. A **pregnancy test** should be taken before the procedure. All discussions should be carefully documented in the notes for **medico-legal** purposes. The pelvic organs should be inspected to look for occult disease during the laparoscopy. **Vasectomy** – all men produce seminal samples at about 3 months. Contraceptive cover is maintained until three consecutive samples show no sperm.

OVERVIEW – Female clip sterilisation is a highly effective form of contraception. It is very easy to perform with serious complications being rare. Its efficacy is similar to that of other techniques, and, if there is a need for reversal, the success of microsurgery is very high. Tubal ligation requires open surgery and is more difficult to reverse. Diathermy was associated with a small risk of bowel trauma and chronic pelvic pain, and it is also harder to reverse.

Vasectomy is a comparatively simpler procedure and it can be performed under local anaesthesia. It is of similar efficacy, but there is a 1% incidence of chronic testicular pain, and unprotected intercourse must be avoided until three seminal analyses have confirmed azoospermia. Vasectomy is technically easier to reverse, but fertility rates are low because of the production of antisperm antibodies.

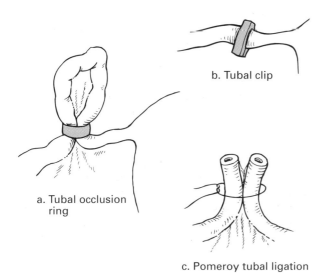

a. Tubal occlusion ring

b. Tubal clip

c. Pomeroy tubal ligation

Fig 25.1 *Types of tubal occlusion.*

GOLDEN POINTS

1. Female sterilisation is highly effective, and satisfaction rates are high.

2. Counselling is essential to help avoid regret and medico-legal problems.

3. Vasectomy may seem an easier option from a medical perspective, but the woman's wishes should be paramount.

4. Hysterectomy should be considered if there are other gynaecological problems in conjunction.

5. Advise woman to continue with contraception until day of surgery.

26 Request for termination of pregnancy

CLINICAL SIGNIFICANCE

In 1967 an act of Parliament was passed allowing termination of pregnancy to be undertaken for certain medical indications. Overnight the number of women dying of severe pelvic infections secondary to criminal interference fell dramatically.

At the same time, the advent of contraception and the social change of the 1960s led to a large increase in unplanned pregnancy, especially amongst teenage women. The demand for termination has increased year-on-year since, and currently about 150 000 terminations are performed each year in England and Wales.

Many women have terminations each year without problem, but the procedure carries risks of uterine trauma, pelvic infection and emotional problems. It is essential therefore that the women are counselled carefully and that the procedure is performed carefully by expert gynaecologists. Support should be available freely afterwards.

LEGAL CRITERIA

The 1967 Abortion Act provided five reasons that allowed women to request a termination.

- '… continuation of the pregnancy would involve risk to the life of the pregnant woman greater than if the pregnancy were terminated'
- '… termination necessary to prevent grave permanent injury to the physical or mental health of the pregnant woman'
- '… the pregnancy has not exceeded 24 weeks gestation and the continuation of the pregnancy would involve risk of injury to the mental and physical health of the woman greater than if the pregnancy were terminated'
- '… the pregnancy has not exceeded 24 weeks gestation and the continuation of the pregnancy would involve risk of injury to the mental and physical health of any existing child(ren) of the pregnant woman greater than if the pregnancy were terminated'
- '… that if the child were born it would suffer from such physical or mental abnormalities as to be seriously handicapped'.

For a termination of pregnancy to be carried out, two registered medical practitioners must sign a legal form. In practice many units appear to operate a policy of termination on request, and most seem to be performed for women who feel the pregnancy has arisen at the wrong time.

This chapter is largely concerned with request for termination for social indications.

CLINICAL ASSESSMENT

The woman may present to her GP, the family planning clinic or specialist termination clinic. Termination of pregnancy creates an ethical dilemma for a number of doctors who will not consent on moral grounds, but they are obliged to refer the woman to someone who will deal with things.

Termination of pregnancy is a difficult decision, and women deserve advice from expert counsellors and not simply from general gynaecologists. Ideally, the women should be seen in a dedicated clinic with specialist counsellors and doctors.

Guidelines have been set out by the Royal College of Obstetricians and Gynaecologists stating that any woman should be able to have her first consultation within 5 days of initial presentation. It is also recommended that if the woman's request is in keeping with the Abortion Act, the termination should be available within 7 days of that appointment.

Relevant History

Presenting Complaint

MAIN SYMPTOM – **Amenorrhoea** is usually the first indication of pregnancy. The last menstrual period is recorded to estimate the gestational age, but ideally an ultrasound scan should be performed to date the pregnancy accurately.

OTHER IMPORTANT ISSUES – Request for termination may be for a wide variety of reasons, and it is sometimes important to explore these in detail. Factors include social reasons such as unplanned pregnancy, young age, old age, abandonment by partner, and financial problems. Medical indications include severe maternal diseases such as cyanotic heart disease and cancer, and severe psychological disorders. Fetal problems include inherited disease such as cystic fibrosis, sporadic malformations such as spina bifida, Down's syndrome, and high-order multiple pregnancy. Rape is a very rare but very important issue that requires special attention and follow-up. A full evaluation should be made of the woman and her reasons for requesting a termination.

EFFECT ON PATIENT – The woman should be allowed to make the decision appropriate to her but it should be remembered that the emotional reaction to termination can be very mixed. Even women who have been raped may have very conflicting emotions. It is important to recognise these dilemmas and allow women to talk of them freely. Support is an important part of counselling for termination of pregnancy, both before and after the procedure.

Gynaecological History

CONTRACEPTION – A full contraceptive history of the methods used and problems encountered should be recorded. If conception has occurred with an IUCD in place its site must be determined before any surgical procedure. *The most important issue is to jointly plan future contraception*.

CERVICAL CYTOLOGY – This is an opportunity to offer cervical cytology.

GYNAECOLOGICAL DISEASE – Some of these women may have a history of pelvic inflammatory disease or other sexually transmitted diseases. Such women are at increased risk of post-termination infection.

FERTILITY REQUIREMENTS – Women who have completed their family may wish to have sterilisation performed at the same time. This is fraught with problems of regret but should be considered in very exceptional cases.

Obstetric History

Record the number of pregnancies and any complications, particularly a previous caesarean section which may affect late termination.

Medical History

PSYCHOLOGICAL DISORDERS – Careful counselling is imperative, as the decision to terminate a pregnancy could lead to psychological problems. **Psychiatric** disease on its own may be an indication for termination.

Social History

AGE – The risks of surgical termination (**cervical trauma** and **uterine perforation**) are greater in women under 18 years of age and over 10 weeks gestation. Teenage women may require special counselling together with support from their parents. The issue of child sex abuse needs to be considered in girls under 16 years of age and they should be seen by appropriately trained professionals if possible.

FAMILY AND OCCUPATION – Other aspects of the woman's social history do not necessarily alter the management, but asking questions gives the woman an opportunity to raise other difficult issues in her life which might be dealt with at a later stage.

Relevant Clinical Examination

Abdomen

CONTOUR/PALPATION – The uterus may be visible, and the fundal height should be determined if a scan is not routinely performed. A large uterus may indicate wrong menstrual dates, twins or an ovarian mass.

Pelvic

The main reason for performing a vaginal examination is to screen for infection.

PERINEUM/VULVA – Screen for sexually transmitted disease such as viral warts or the ulcers associated with herpes.

VAGINA – Offensive discharges from infection may be noted.

BIMANUAL EXAMINATION – This is best replaced by an ultrasound scan.

Relevant Initial Investigations

Haematology

Hb – Anaemia may present in pregnancy and should be detected prior to termination as there is a risk of haemorrhage.

BLOOD GROUP – ABO grouping and rhesus status should be checked, with blood grouped and saved for surgical terminations. Rhesus negative women should be given anti-D prophylaxis after the termination.

Endocrine Tests

β-hCG – A urine test should be performed to confirm the diagnosis of pregnancy. These are very accurate and can diagnose pregnancy before a missed period.

Microbiology

BACTERIAL CULTURE – There is an increased risk of pelvic infection after termination, and pathogenic organisms should be screened for or prophylactic antibiotics given. Vaginal swabs should be taken to screen for infection (bacterial vaginosis, trichomonas and gonorrhoea) and endocervical swabs sent for chlamydial ELISA.

Diagnostic Imaging

PELVIC ULTRASOUND – Provides confirmation of the site of the pregnancy and the number of sacs. Occasionally an ectopic pregnancy will be suspected.

Cytology

CERVICAL – Cervical cytology testing should be offered if the woman has never had a smear or one is due.

Histopathology

TROPHOBLAST – Many units send a small sample of trophoblast to confirm removal of the pregnancy and to rule out the small possibility of trophoblastic tumours.

FETUS – If there is suspicion of fetal abnormality, the fetus should be sent for examination for confirmation.

DETAILS OF METHODS OF TERMINATION

First Trimester Suction Termination

Background

INDICATIONS – Request for termination of a pregnancy before it has reached 12–14 weeks gestation.

METHODS – **Surgical** – suction evacuation of uterus. This method is the most common, with 70% of all terminations in the first trimester being performed surgically. The women tend to be admitted for day care and given a general anaesthetic, although local anaesthesia carries a lower risk of complications. The cervix is then mechanically dilated to accommodate the suction cannula (10 mm for a 10 week pregnancy and 12 mm for a 12 week pregnancy, etc.). Using suction is faster with less blood loss than medical termination. The endometrial cavity should be checked for retained products using gentle curettage. Cervical preparation is advisable in very young women (under 18 years) or pregnancies over 10 weeks gestation. A prostaglandin (misoprostol) pessary is inserted vaginally prior to cervical dilatation to reduce the risk of trauma.

Medical – induction of termination using mifepristone (antiprogesterone) and misoprostol (prostaglandin analogue). Medical termination of pregnancy is advised before 6 weeks gestation, and may be chosen by the woman between 7 and 9 weeks gestation. On its own, mifepristone may induce expulsion of the fetus in 60% of cases, but this increases to over 95% when combined with misoprostol or gemeprost, which induce cervical dilatation and uterine contractions but have side effects such as nausea, vomiting and, occasionally, severe diarrhoea. A typical regimen would be 200 mg of mifepristone given orally on day 1 of the termination. The woman stays on the ward for 2 h to ensure the tablet is not vomited back. She is then allowed home to return on day 3 when a prostaglandin pessary (misoprostol or gemeprost) is inserted vaginally. The fetus is usually expelled 4 to 6 h afterwards. These women should be on fluid only in case a surgical evacuation is required because of failure of the technique or retained products of conception. An ultrasound scan will help to confirm complete expulsion.

MAIN COMPLICATIONS – Termination of pregnancy is very safe and, overall, is said to carry fewer risks than a pregnancy going to term. **Failure** to terminate the pregnancy is commoner with surgical evacuation under 6 weeks gestation, when it is easy to miss the sac and fetus. For this reason medical termination is preferred under 6 weeks. **Pelvic infection** is significantly increased after termination but more so after surgical procedures. **Haemorrhage** is experienced with both methods, but with medical termination it is more likely to be heavy and prolonged.

SCREENING/PREVENTION – Sexual education and the widespread use of effective contraceptive methods will help reduce unwanted and untimely pregnancies. Screening for vaginal/pelvic infection is advised, with prophylactic antibiotic being given as routine or if organisms are grown (a single dose of metronidazole 1 g rectally and 7 days of oral doxycycline 100 mg b.d.).

OVERVIEW – **Non-directive counselling** should be available together with support for the woman. Details of methods and complications should be explained in detail but sympathetically. Medical termination is offered to women under 6 weeks pregnant. Beyond 6 weeks, the woman should make an informed choice between the medical and surgical options. These women should have a plan for **contraception** to start immediately after the termination. Infection is the most important complication, and screening and antibiotic prophylaxis are essential.

Follow-up

SHORT TERM – A 2 week appointment should be offered to make sure the bleeding has stopped and that there is no evidence of risk of a continuing pregnancy. Contraception intentions can be checked. Post-termination counselling should be made available.

LONG TERM – Contraception should have been arranged prior to the termination, but women should be encouraged to attend family planning on a regular basis to make sure they are happy with their chosen method.

Midtrimester Termination of Pregnancy

Background

INDICATIONS – Request for cessation of a pregnancy beyond 14 weeks gestation but before the end of the 24th week of pregnancy. The indications for later termination mimic those of the first trimester, but social indications are less common, and there is a larger proportion of cases of fetal problems.

METHODS – **Surgical** – Dilatation of cervix and evacuation (D+E) by fragmentation and removal of fetus under ultrasound guidance. Preparation of the cervix with prostaglandin and laminaria tents is essential for this method. D+E is not suitable if the fetus needs to be examined but is used by some units for women wishing late termination for social reasons. Laparotomy and opening of uterus (hysterotomy) is rarely used now but may still be indicated for women with several previous caesarean deliveries.

Medical – induction of uterine contractions and vaginal delivery of fetus. Methods used include vaginal prostaglandin analogues (misoprostol), trans-cervical passage of Foley catheter and intra-amniotic prostaglandin.

MAIN COMPLICATIONS – Haemorrhage, infection and pain are seen. With dilatation and evacuation there is a risk of uterine perforation. With medical induction there is a risk of uterine rupture. Misplaced intra-amniotic injections of prostaglandin may cause maternal cardiovascular collapse.

SCREENING/PREVENTION – For infection (see above). The mechanism for referral for social termination of pregnancy should be streamlined to reduce the need for late termination.

OVERVIEW – Late termination is more difficult for women both physically and emotionally. The method used will depend on the needs of the woman and the expertise of the gynaecologist.

Follow-up

SHORT TERM – A 2 week appointment is advisable to check there have been no problems afterwards and that a plan for contraception is in place.

LONG TERM – An indication of fetal abnormality should be followed up to explain the results of any investigations on the fetus. The woman should be advised to book early for her next pregnancy.

Third Trimester Termination

Background

INDICATION – Cessation of pregnancy after the end of the 24th week of pregnancy for severe fetal abnormality and severe (life-threatening) maternal disease. Some clinicians believe that the fetal indication is restricted to those with lethal abnormalities.

METHODS – Injection of fetal heart under ultrasound guidance to induce asystole (fetocide) and then induction of contractions (see above) and vaginal delivery. The indications for stopping a pregnancy after 24 weeks are few. Severe maternal disease may require ending the pregnancy, but it is more commonly for severe fetal abnormality.

COMPLICATIONS – Those of labour. Failure to induce contractions may make hysterotomy necessary. This is very rare with the combination of mifepristone and misoprostol.

SCREENING/PREVENTION – Antenatal screening in the second trimester may avoid the late diagnosis of fetal abnormality.

GOLDEN POINTS

1. Offer a streamlined dedicated service with facilities for counselling and support.

2. Perform ultrasonography on all women to establish dating and number of fetuses.

3. Screen for infection and give antibiotic prophylaxis if appropriate.

4. Cervical preparation is necessary for women under 18 years old or over 10 weeks gestation.

5. Give anti-Rh(D) gammaglobulin for rhesus negative women.

6. Give advice on contraception.

Clinical Problems in Obstetrics

27 Nausea and vomiting in pregnancy

CLINICAL SIGNIFICANCE

Nausea and vomiting in pregnancy affect up to 70% of women. They constitute the commonest complaint during the first 5 months of pregnancy, leading to nearly 9 million hours of paid unemployment per year. When mild, the complaint is an irritation, but in its severest form leads to electrolyte disturbance and dehydration. It may be an indication of systemic disease and should therefore not be dismissed too easily.

DIFFERENTIAL DIAGNOSIS

MAIN CATEGORY	DIAGNOSIS
1. *Physiological*	Mild nausea and vomiting
	Hyperemesis gravidarum
	Large uterus (big baby or hydramnios)
2. *Infection*	Urinary tract infection
3. *Multiple pregnancy*	
4. *Hydatidiform mole*	
5. *Metabolic*	Diabetes
6. *Mechanical*	Large for dates
	Reflux oesophagitis
7. *Non-obstetric causes*	Ovarian cysts
	Appendicitis
	Obstructed bowel/liver disease
	Raised intracranial pressure

Physiological vomiting is the commonest, occurring in up to 70% of pregnancies. This may be a normal response to pregnancy. Occasionally it becomes severe, causing electrolyte disturbance, when it is known as hyperemesis gravidarum. This is seen more commonly with molar and multiple pregnancy.

CLINICAL ASSESSMENT

Rapid Emergency Assessment

Initial assessment of the physical state should be carried out. Resuscitation should involve gaining intravenous access and starting fluid replacement. These women often present in a dehydrated state, and intravenous fluid (crystalloid) replacement is required initially.

Relevant History

Presenting Complaint

MAIN SYMPTOM – **Nausea** on its own is a recognised symptom of early pregnancy but may lead to **vomiting**. In its mildest form women just bring back solids occasionally, and this is referred to as morning sickness.

As the severity increases, they describe vomiting all solids and fluid, sometimes not being able to tolerate anything orally. **Last menstrual period** will indicate the possibility of pregnancy, and the gestation can be calculated. Nausea and vomiting in the first and second trimester is almost physiological, whereas in the third trimester it may be due to more sinister causes.

COMMONLY ASSOCIATED SYMPTOMS – Associated **diarrhoea** or **abdominal pain** may be caused by gastroenteritis or other non-pregnancy related causes (appendicitis, torted cyst, inflammatory bowel disease). Urinary frequency or loin pain are signs of urinary tract infections which commonly cause nausea and vomiting. If **pruritus** is present then liver disease may be a problem. Other **symptoms of pregnancy** such as weight gain, breast enlargement, and tiredness are other signs of early pregnancy. **Vaginal bleeding** in early pregnancy may indicate a threatened miscarriage or even a molar pregnancy. Associated headaches are common, but, if associated with visual disturbance, raised intracranial pressure must be considered.

EFFECT ON PATIENT – This can be an extremely distressing problem during an already emotional period.

Obstetric History

DELIVERY - More commonly seen in women during their first pregnancy. There may be a history of multiple pregnancies.

OBSTETRIC COMPLICATIONS - If the woman suffered from hyperemesis in her first pregnancy, it is more likely to occur in the next one. Molar pregnancies may recur, along with pregnancy-associated liver disease.

Medical History

MEDICAL CONDITIONS - Diabetics are prone to nausea and, if they develop vomiting, require close attention and often require an insulin sliding scale to avoid ketoacidosis.

PSYCHOLOGICAL DISORDERS - High anxiety levels and depressive states are associated with increased nausea.

Drug History

MEDICATIONS - They may have been started on a course of antibiotics which can lead to nausea.

SMOKING AND ALCOHOL - Heavy smoking may induce nausea and also increases the risk to the pregnancy.

Social History

AGE - Nausea and vomiting (NAV) is commoner in younger and older women.

DEPENDANTS - If admission is required, child care may have to be arranged.

LIFESTYLE - There is an increased incidence of hyperemesis gravidarum in single mothers or those with poor home support.

Relevant Clinical Examination

General Features

GENERAL DEMEANOUR - There may be signs of dehydration or anaemia. Jaundice may occur in severe cases. Signs of pregnancy, such as pigmentation, may be present on the face (chloasma), nipples or abdomen (linea nigra, striae gravidarum). Check blood pressure in later pregnancy for hypertension.

BODY-MASS INDEX - Prolonged vomiting can lead to dramatic weight loss.

Abdomen

OLD SCARS - Scars from previous surgery or pregnancies should be observed.

PALPATION - The fundus may be larger than expected and may contain a multiple pregnancy. In the third trimester the fetal parts should be palpated and position defined along with assessment of growth and liquor volume. The site of tenderness may indicate possible causes: Suprapubic pain may indicate a urinary tract infection, and loin pain may mean it has spread to pyelonephritis. Pruritus and jaundice with hepatic tenderness may

indicate liver disease. Guarding and rebound should be assessed to look for peritonitis.

BOWEL SOUNDS - Auscultation should take place for bowel sounds and the fetal heart.

Pelvic

VAGINA/CERVIX - Inspection may reveal a darkening and thickening of the vaginal walls and cervix - an early indicator of pregnancy. If there has been any bleeding, the cervix should be examined for an ectropion or any signs of miscarriage.

BIMANUAL EXAMINATION - Bimanual examination will help to date early pregnancies and allows the adnexa to be palpated for cysts or tenderness.

Relevant Clinical Investigations

Haematology

Hb - Anaemia may present because of anorexia.

WCC - The white cell count will be raised if infection is present.

PLATELET COUNT - Only if hepatic disease is suspected.

Biochemistry

SERUM U+Es - To assess renal function and check for electrolyte disturbance with dehydration.

SERUM LFTs - Exclude liver disease, especially if jaundiced or there is a chance of pre-eclampsia.

RANDOM BLOOD SUGAR - In diabetics.

Endocrine Tests

β-hCG - Very high levels are seen in molar pregnancies.

Microbiology

URINE - A urine dipstick will reveal ketones if the women is dehydrated, leucocytes and blood with urinary tract infection. Proteinuria in later pregnancy is possibly a result of liver disease, and pre-eclampsia should be considered.

BACTERIAL CULTURE - Urine should be sent for culture and sensitivity if infection is suspected. Urinary infections are more common in pregnancy. Diarrhoea should also be sent for culture if present.

Diagnostic Imaging

ULTRASOUND - Allows the pregnancy to be confirmed, excluding multiple pregnancy and molar pregnancies.

DETAILS OF INDIVIDUAL CONDITIONS

I. Physiological

Background

DEFINITION - Nausea and vomiting in pregnancy when it is mild (nausea only) or moderate (nausea and vomiting).

AETIOLOGY – This is felt to be a natural reaction of the body to pregnancy, complicating up to 70%. There is an association with a reduced incidence of miscarriage in these women. It starts after the first missed period and frequently is one of the first signs of early pregnancy. The peak incidence is at the 10th week, slowly reducing after 16 weeks. In the first trimester it is felt to be due to the rapid rise in β-hCG levels, but in later pregnancy the rapidly enlarging uterus and the associated relaxation of the pyloric sphincter play an important part. It has been shown that threatened miscarriage associated with nausea and vomiting has a better prognosis than when not, and this tends to support the theory that not vomiting is abnormal in pregnancy. There is also a psychological element involved with the process.

MAKING THE DIAGNOSIS – The diagnosis will be made from the history, with mild vomiting and an associated pregnancy. Investigations are used to exclude other causes.

MAIN COMPLICATIONS – **Nausea** is the biggest complication, with **occasional vomiting**. At worst it is an inconvenience to the woman.

Treatment Options

REASSURANCE – This is a normal sign of pregnancy and seldom associated with disease. They should be reassured that it will settle.

CHANGE OF LIFESTYLE/DIET – General dietary advice is usually all that is required. The woman should eat small meals and try to avoid fatty foods. Eating dry toast can be helpful during bad periods. It is important to keep fluid intake high.

DRUG THERAPY – Metoclopramide can be useful, although oral antiemetics can be difficult to take. Rectal prochlorperazine is well tolerated and provides effective relief. Antacids may be useful in later pregnancy to combat oesophageal reflux.

OVERVIEW – Reassurance and dietary advice are the mainstay of treatment; if the woman's condition is worse the diagnosis should be hyperemesis gravidarum.

Follow-up

SHORT TERM – Routine antenatal care providing the vomiting resolves.

LONG TERM – This may reoccur in subsequent pregnancies.

2. Hyperemesis Gravidarum

Background

DEFINITION – This is the severest form of nausea and vomiting of pregnancy, which leads to dehydration, electrolyte disturbance or weight loss. It is rare, complicating up to 1% of pregnancies.

AETIOLOGY – Human chorionic gonadotrophin has been implicated, as women with multiple pregnancies and hydatidiform mole have greater than normal levels. Other theories implicate adrenal and thyroid disease. There is an association with social factors, with women in unfamiliar surroundings having an increased risk. It has been shown to have a protective effect against postnatal depression.

MAKING THE DIAGNOSIS – A history of severe nausea and vomiting with associated dehydration and weight loss. The urinary electrolytes may be deranged, and significant pathology will be excluded. Multiple and molar pregnancies will be diagnosed by ultrasound scan.

MAIN COMPLICATIONS – Severe vomiting leading to electrolyte disturbance, proteinuria and anorexia.

SCREENING – Antenatal screening will reveal multiple and molar pregnancies.

Treatment Options

CHANGE OF LIFESTYLE/DIET – The same dietary advice should be provided, but it is seldom successful during acute episodes.

DRUG THERAPY – Admission with intravenous access. Fluid replacement should be designed to correct the electrolyte disturbance and should include glucose if there are ketones on urinary dip testing. Diabetics will require a sliding scale. Rectal prochlorperazine is generally as successful as intravenous antiemetics.

SURGERY – In the severest situation, termination has been offered with normal pregnancies, but this is extremely rare.

Follow-up

SHORT TERM – Regular antenatal appointment should be made to check progress with maternal weight gain and fetal growth.

3. Liver disease

Background

DEFINITION – Disorders of liver function, leading to nausea and vomiting in pregnancy.

AETIOLOGY – There are specific disorders associated with pregnancy which can present with nausea and vomiting. The commonest is pre-eclampsia, which usually does not present until the third trimester and is dealt with in Chapter 31. **Acute fatty liver of pregnancy** – cause is unknown but presents in the third trimester. Biopsy shows microvesicular fat infiltration. It is commoner in primigravid women and twin pregnancies. It is diagnosed by excluding viral infection, with the bilirubin being less than 100 and the aspartate transaminase (AST) mildly raised.

MAKING THE DIAGNOSIS – With **acute fatty liver of pregnancy** there may be pruritus and jaundice with a raised AST, and associated raised TNR. Diagnosis is by excluding infective causes (hepatitus). **Cholestasis of pregnancy** presents with pruritus, nausea and signs of obstructive jaundice, usually after 30 weeks gestation.

MAIN COMPLICATIONS – Nausea and vomiting with liver involvement, leading to jaundice, pruritus and deranged liver function.

Treatment Options

REASSURANCE – **Acute fatty liver of pregnancy** is very rare, with an incidence of only 1 in 14 000 pregnancies **Cholestasis of pregnancy** occurs in less than 0.1% of pregnancies and is the second commonest cause of jaundice in pregnancy, with viral hepatitis being the first. It resolves spontaneously after delivery, which is usually carried out at 38 weeks.

SURGERY – **Acute fatty liver of pregnancy** – the only cure is delivery in a specialised unit with support for the liver failure and neonatal support if required.

Follow-up

SHORT TERM – Careful monitoring should take place if liver function has been deranged to make sure a full recovery takes place.

LONG TERM – High risk in further pregnancy.

4. Hydatidiform mole

See Chapter 6.

5. Pre-eclampsia

See Chapter 31.

GOLDEN POINTS

1. Confirm pregnancy.

2. Exclude multiple and molar pregnancies.

3. Check renal and liver function.

4. Give dietary advice early.

5. Admit early if severe vomiting occurs before electrolyte disturbance occurs.

6. In later pregnancy it can be more sinister, and pre-eclampsia should be excluded.

28 Abnormal fetal screening test results

CLINICAL SIGNIFICANCE

Since the 1970s the perinatal mortality has halved, and at least part of this reduction has been ascribed to the increased detection of fetal abnormalities at a gestation when termination may be offered. Even so, approximately 1% of pregnancies are complicated by a major anomaly.

Screening aims to provide information such that individual choices can be made about treatment options. During pregnancy there are few treatment options except secondary prevention by selective termination of pregnancy in affected cases. Because of these limited options, adequate counselling is vital prior to any testing, particularly with respect to the accuracy of the tests and potential outcomes.

Any screening test should be accurate, acceptable, cost effective and be able to identify an early stage of the disorder when treatment will improve the outcome to a greater extent than later treatment – screening tests must do more good than harm. Particularly, screening tests with a high false positive rate can cause a great deal of angst, may prompt unnecessary invasive investigation and possibly even termination of a normal fetus. Similarly, a low-risk result does not mean no risk; note the sensitivity (detection rate) of the tests.

Some tests, usually those with minimal associated miscarriage rates, are offered to the whole obstetric population, whereas more invasive testing is reserved for 'high-risk' groups.

DIFFERENTIAL DIAGNOSIS

MAIN CATEGORY	DIAGNOSIS
Chromosomal disorders	
1. *Serological tests*	AFP Down's risk
2. *Ultrasound scan*	Nuchal translucency Other ultrasound markers
3. *Invasive testing*	Amniocentesis Chorionic villus sampling (CVS) Cordocentesis
Structural anomalies	
1. *Ultrasound*	Craniospinal Renal tract Gastrointestinal tract Skeletal Cardiac

FETAL SCREENING TESTS

A plethora of screening tests are employed for both maternal and fetal abnormality, and the number of tests available rises exponentially each year. However, many of these tests are only used in specialist centres for relatively uncommon conditions and will not be encountered by most medical students. Therefore in this chapter we will concentrate only on those tests, for fetal abnormality, commonly used in routine clinical practice which all students should meet. For details of other screening tests for occult maternal problems, please refer to the introductory chapter on routine antenatal care.

It is important to remember that these tests are not mutually exclusive; tests are often used in combination, e.g. the identification of markers for chromosomal abnormality at routine scan may prompt further invasive testing using amniocentesis.

CLINICAL ASSESSMENT

Making the Diagnosis

A history and examination can usefully identify women at increased risk of fetal abnormality so that screening and diagnostic tests can be concentrated in high-risk groups.

Relevant History

Age

The risk of fetal chromosomal abnormalities, particularly trisomies, increases with maternal age and exponentially after 35 years. For example the risk of Down's syndrome rises from 1:2000 at 20 years to 1:350 at 35 years and 1:40 at 44 years. Although the risk of Down's syndrome increases with age, fewer older women get pregnant, and therefore over 50% of Down's syndrome babies are born to women less than 35 years old.

Maternal age is such a significant risk factor that many of the tests used to screen for chromosomal abnormality modify the age-related risk to produce an individual risk (see nuchal translucency and serum screening, below).

Obstetric History

A history of previous fetal anomaly increases the risk of future problems. For example, a previous history of Down's increases the risk in future pregnancy by a factor of 4.

Similarly, a woman whose previous baby was born with a structural defect increases the risk of future anomalies. The risk of cardiac abnormalies is doubled after a previous episode, and the mother should be offered a fetal echocardiogram in future pregnancies.

The risk of neural tube defects rises after 1 child to 1:25, and 1:10 after two or more affected children. This recurrence risk can be substantially reduced by folate supplementation, taken from 1 month preconception to about 8 weeks of pregnancy.

Medical History

There may be a history, or family history, of a potentially heritable condition: autosomal disorders including Huntington's chorea and autosomal recessive conditions, e.g. cystic fibrosis, sickle cell anaemia and thalassaemia. Many of these disorders can potentially be diagnosed antentally using molecular probes. However, most of the tests require an initial aminocentesis or CVS, and the associated increased miscarriage risk may not be acceptable to the parents.

Social History

Neural tube defects are more common in lower social groups. This may be related to poor nutrition and a lack of folate in particular.

Relevant Clinical Examination

Abdomen

There are a number of clinically detectable complications of pregnancy that are associated with fetal and/or chromosomal abnormality and should prompt further investigation.

PREGNANCY – Inconsistent uterine size: small for dates fetus, oligohydramnios and polyhydramnios are all associated with anomalies. See relevant chapters. Breech presentation is also, more rarely, associated with fetal anomalies. However, most anomalies are detected during routine screening tests.

Booking Tests

See Chapter 3.

SCREENING TESTS FOR GENETIC DISORDERS

Prenatal screening is now routine for some disorders and optional for others where a patient is deemed to be at increased risk.

1. Serological tests:
   - AFP
   - Down's risk
2. Ultrasound scan:
   - diagnosis
   - nuchal translucency
3. Invasive testing:
   - amniocentesis
   - chorionic villus sampling
   - cordocentesis.

The serological tests are screening tests, which identify a high-risk population who may require further testing to make a diagnosis, whereas the others are diagnostic tests.

AFP

Screening for neural tube defects (NTD) aims to detect the leakage of alphafetoprotein, a protein manufactured in the fetal yolk sac and fetal liver, across an open defect in the skin, i.e. a neural tube defect. The leakage produces a high AFP concentration in the amniotic fluid and a correspondingly high maternal serum level.

NB: any disorder that involves potential leakage of fetal serum into the maternal system, however indirect, can produce a high level of AFP. Therefore, anterior abdominal wall defects, some skin defects, fetomaternal haemorrhage and intrauterine death can all produce a high AFP without a NTD.

Natural History of NTDs

There is a marked geographical variation in incidence – rising towards the west. The overall incidence is 3–10/1000. NTDs vary in their severity: anencephaly is uniformly fatal, whilst isolated spinal lesions can produce a range of problems from paraplegia to normal.

Optimum Gestation

A blood test is usually performed at 16–18 weeks. The normal levels of AFP alter with gestation, and therefore accurate dating is necessary. The results are expressed as multiples of the median (MoM), and 2.5 MoM is commonly deemed a positive result.

Accuracy

The cut off of 2.5 MoM will identify approximately 80% (sensitivity = detection rate) of NTDs. Only 3% of the normal population will produce a value of this magnitude. Therefore 20% of NTDs will be missed using this test, whilst 3% of pregnancies will be falsely identified as high risk.

Maternal/Fetal Risks

A routine blood test.

Secondary Investigations

A positive result identifies the pregnancy as high risk for NTD; further investigation is required to make a diagnosis. Amniocentesis looking for high AFP concentrations in the amniotic fluid has now been largely superseded by ultrasound scanning. They are safe and accurate with high sensitivities and low false-positive rates.

Conclusion

AFP screening is now rarely used primarily to screen for NTDs, as ultrasound scans are more accurate. However, it is now used as part of the serum screening for Down's syndrome, and incidentally discovered raised levels should still prompt a thorough search for possible causes.

Down's Syndrome

Down's syndrome is the most common cause of mental handicap in the UK. Trisomy 21 has an overall incidence of 1:700 in a general obstetric population. There is again a wide spectrum of outcomes with Down's syndrome, and there are no specific antenatal tests available to predict the severity of possible handicap. Methods of screening are shown in Table 28.1.

Table 28.1	Methods of screening for Down's syndrome	
	Serum screening	Nuchal translucency
Test gestation	14–16 weeks	9–13 weeks
Sensitivity (detection rate)	60%	80%
Advantages	Simple blood test.	Early diagnosis may permit 1st trimester TOP
Disadvantages	Low sensitivity and later diagnosis.	Very operator dependent

Serum Screening

By combining a number of serum markers for Down's syndrome: low AFP, low unconjugated oestriol (uE_3) and raised levels of human chorionic gonadotrophin (hCG) with a known risk factor – maternal age – an overall numerical risk can be produced for any given pregnancy. A risk of > 1:300 is deemed to be high enough to warrant counselling for further investigation.

OPTIMUM GESTATION – A blood test is usually performed at 16 weeks; accurate dating is again necessary. The results are expressed as a risk which commonly ranges from 1:10 to 1:5000.

ACCURACY – The accuracy of this test is very dependent on maternal age: the sensitivity ranges from over 70% in mothers aged 37 or over, to less than 30% in women aged 20 years. 5% of normal pregnancies will fall into the 'high-risk' group.

MATERNAL/FETAL RISKS – A routine blood test.

SECONDARY INVESTIGATIONS – A positive result identifies the pregnancy as high risk for Down's syndrome. Invasive testing, commonly amniocentesis or chorionic villus sampling, is required to confirm the diagnosis. However, both are associated with increased miscarriage rates.

CONCLUSION – Serum screening has been introduced to replace screening on maternal age alone, and it undoubtedly identifies more Down's syndrome fetuses. However, because it has a relatively high false-positive rate, many normal pregnancies are falsely identified as high risk, causing a great deal of anxiety. The majority (75%) of these women opt for invasive testing, which increases both the anxiety and the miscarriage rate of potentially normal fetuses. The test should therefore be an opt-in test, after counselling, rather than opt-out as it commonly is.

Nuchal Translucency

NUCHAL FOLD THICKNESS – The nuchal fat pad (nuchal translucency) at the back of the neck can be enlarged in fetuses, in the first trimester, with Down's syndrome. Therefore measuring the nuchal fat pad by transvaginal scanning in the first trimester can be used for Down's risk assessment (Figure 28.1). It can be combined with maternal age to produce a numerical relative risk (see Table 28.2).

It has been suggested that using this screening test will detect a greater number of affected fetuses (80%) than serum screening, with the same false-positive rate. Nuchal translucency screening (followed by CVS) also allows first trimester diagnosis of Down's syndrome thus allowing suction TOP. The test is gaining popularity, but not all units routinely use it yet.

Both serum screening and nuchal translucency will also incidentally detect some other trisomies (Patau's and Edward's syndrome).

Invasive Procedures

Invasive procedures sample fetal cells, directly or indirectly, to identify characteristic fetal cellular defects,

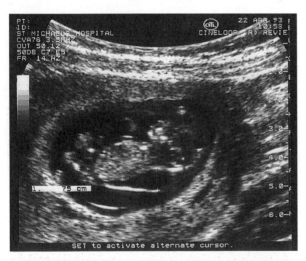

Fig 28.1 *USS of nuchal translucency. With kind permission of Mr Sanjay Vyas, Bristol.*

Table 28.2 Nuchal translucency material risk	
Nuchal fold thickness	× maternal age-related risk
2 mm	0.5
3 mm	1
4 mm	3

e.g. chromosomal abnormalities. Ultrasound is used to allow accurate direction of the instruments during all invasive procedures. Advantages and disadvantages of the procedures are given in Table 28.3.

Rhesus-negative women should be given anti-Rh(D) to prevent the potential rhesus isoimmunisation common to all invasive procedures.

Fetoscopy is the introduction of a relatively large-bore endoscope into the amniotic cavity. It has a 10% miscarriage rate and has been largely superseded by the improvements in ultrasound.

Ultrasound Screening for Structural Anomalies

Ultrasound scanning is used, in this context, primarily to identify morphological abnormalities (Figure 28.2). However, there are ultrasound markers for chromosomal abnormalities that can be used as a method of screening e.g. nuchal fold translucency – see above.

OPTIMUM GESTATION – The Royal College of Obstetricians has recently recommended that routine ultrasound scans should be undertaken between 18 and 20 weeks.

ACCURACY – The accuracy of ultrasound scanning is very operator dependent, however; in most major centres detection rates of 90–100% can be expected for major anomalies. The false positive rates are low, in the order of 1%.

MATERIAL/FETAL RISKS – Ultrasound is considered extremely safe.

Abnormalities

1. **Craniospinal** – Over 50% of fetal abnormalities are craniospinal, including **neural tube defects, hydrocephalus, microcephaly, choroid plexus cysts** (markers of chromosomal abnormalities) and **cerebellar abnormalities**.

2. **Renal tract** – Fluid-filled structures are easily visualised by ultrasound: **polycystic kidneys**, dilated ureters associated with an **obstructive uropathy** and a dilated bladder, commonly secondary to posterior urethral valves. **Renal agenesis** is often diagnosed indirectly: severe oligohydramnios and no bladder.

3. **Gastrointestinal** – Bowel obstruction and anterior wall defects are the most commonly diagnosed abnormalities. Bowel obstruction produces dilatation proximal to the obstruction, e.g. the double bubble of **duodenal atresia** is the stomach and dilated first part of the duodenum (Figure 28.3). NB: bowel obstruction above the ileum causes polyhydramnios. An **omphalocoele** is a midline defect, within the cord, through which a peritoneal sac and a variable amount of abdominal contents protrude. They are

Table 28.3   Advantages and disadvantages of invasive procedures

	Amniocentesis	Chorionic villus sampling (placental biopsy)	Cordocentesis (fetal blood sampling)
Procedure	The needle is introduced abdominally into a pool of liquor away from the fetus 10 ml of fluid is withdrawn	CVS obtains fetal tissue from the chorion at the edge of the placenta. The sample can be obtained using either a transcervical or a transabdominal route	Fetal blood is obtained from the umbilical vein where the umbilical cord inserts into the placenta 1–2 ml of blood is withdrawn
Gestation	15 weeks onward	10 weeks onward	20 weeks onward
Procedure-related miscarriage rate (related to operator experience)	0.5–1%	1–2%	1–2%
Other complications	Related to oligohydramnios, i.e. talipes and respiratory problems	Fetal limb anomalies with early CVS < 9/40. Ruptured membranes and infection	Fetal exsanguination, cord haematoma and chorioamnionitis
Time for result	3 weeks	48 h to 1 week	48 h to 1 week
Advantages	• Least procedure-related loss	• Early gestation allows STOP • Genetic material allows use of gene probes • Rapid results	• As CVS except gestation • Direct haematological assessment of fetus, i.e. Hb

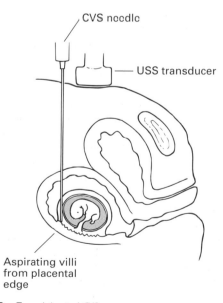

Fig 28.2   *Transabdominal CVS.*

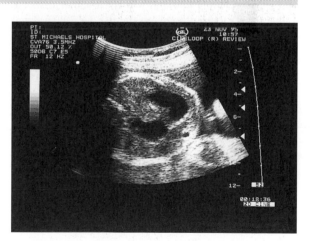

Fig 28.3   *Double bubble of duodenal atresia in cross-section of abdomen.*

commonly associated with chromosomal abnormalities. **Gastroschisis** is an anterior wall defect lateral to the cord, and the prognosis is generally good.

4. **Skeletal** – **Dwarfism** can be identified by measuring the fetal long bones. Facial abnormalities, including **cleft palates**, can be visualised.

5. **Cardiac** – Cardiac anomalies are often difficult to visualise using the standard four-chamber view, though large **septal defects** and abnormal ventricles, e.g. **hypoplastic left ventricle**, can be identified.

Treatment Options

An abnormal screening test result always provokes a great deal of anxiety, and its management requires sensitivity and understanding.

Newsbreaking

Arrange a quiet room and time to reach any partners or relatives that the pregnant woman feels necessary. There should be sufficient, uninterrupted time available for a full discussion. The exact nature of the result should be discussed, and, ideally, written information could be provided, as it is often difficult to comprehend and take in all the information presented immediately after bad news. This would include the following.

Risks – A positive screening test is not diagnostic, though many couples given a positive Down's risk assume it is diagnostic. For example, for a risk of 1 in 300, couples commonly only see the 1 rather than the 300. It may be helpful to invert the risk, i.e. 299/300 will be absolutely normal.

Potential outcomes – A paediatrician should be involved to provide an overview of paediatric outcomes where necessary.

Further investigation – The potential for further investigation and risks should be discussed. Invasive testing, in particular for karyotype, is often recommended even where the initial abnormality is structural only.

Therapeutic options – There may be antenatal or postnatal therapeutic interventions available. Discuss termination of pregnancy and what exactly it entails – commonly the induction can take a long time and it is a 'mini-labour'.

• **Further counselling** – Offer further counselling and time to make a decision.

Follow-up

SHORT TERM

• Conservative
  – Follow-up visits with ultrasound scans if required

  – Delivery in a tertiary unit where appropriate
  – Postnatal paediatric follow-up
• TOP – Prostaglandin induction of labour.

A postmortem should be offered after TOP, as this may yield information relevant to the management of future pregnancies. A follow-up appointment is vital to discuss both the index pregnancy and also to make any plans for future pregnancies.

LONG TERM

• Pre-pregnancy
  – counselling if required.
  – folate supplementation to reduce the recurrence risks for NTDs.
• Early USS for reassurance
• Referral to tertiary unit if required.

SELF-HELP GROUPS – Bereavement counselling can also be offered as well as contact with support groups such as SATFA (Support after Termination for Fetal Abnormality).

GOLDEN POINTS

1. Major fetal abnormality occurs in about 1% of pregnancies.

2. Couples must be fully informed about the tests and, where an abnormality is discovered, about the prognosis and therapeutic options before they can make an appropriate choice.

3. Serum screening and nuchal translucency are the most commonly used screening tests for Down's syndrome.

4. Most screening tests produce a risk assessment, and further invasive testing is often required to make a diagnosis.

5. There is an excess, procedure-related risk of miscarriage after invasive tests.

6. Ultrasound scans can be used both for screening and diagnosis of structural anomalies.

7. Termination of pregnancy is not the only therapeutic option, and couples must be allowed sufficient time and information to make their own decision.

29 Abdominal pain in the second half of pregnancy

CLINICAL SIGNIFICANCE

Abdominal pain is a common antenatal complaint; indeed most women will experience pain at least once during the pregnancy. In general the pain is benign in nature and can be managed conservatively, but there are dangerous causes including premature labour and abruption. The diagnosis of 'ligamentous' pain, in particular, requires exclusion of more sinister causes.

Pain in pregnancy can be directly related to the pregnancy or incidental to it. Any cause of pain outside of pregnancy can also present in pregnancy, and therefore it is important to keep an open mind and not always assume pain is pregnancy related; consider potential medical and surgical causes of pain. The list of differential diagnoses below is therefore not exhaustive.

One of the most important differential diagnoses is premature labour, premature labour is the single most important cause of neonatal mortality and morbidity. It accounts for only 5–10% of deliveries but 85% of neonatal deaths!

DIFFERENTIAL DIAGNOSIS

MAIN CATEGORY	DIAGNOSIS
Pregnancy related	
1. *Uterus*	Premature labour/ miscarriage
	'Red degeneration' of a fibroid
	Uterine rupture
	'Ligamentous pain'
2. *Liquor*	Polyhydramnios
3. *Placenta*	Placental abruption
4. *Other*	Right upper quadrant pain secondary to PET
Indirectly related to pregnancy	
1. *Renal*	Urinary tract infection
	Pyelonephritis
2. *Musculoskeletal*	General aches and pains secondary to ligamentous relaxation
3. *GI tract*	Oesophagitis
	Haemorrhoids
	Constipation
Incidental	
1. *Gynaecological*	Ovarian cyst accident
2. *Surgical*	Appendicitis
	Cholecystitis
3. *Medical*	Sickle cell crisis

CLINICAL ASSESSMENT

Once again, the spectrum of presentation is enormous, ranging from mild abdominal pain, mentioned in passing in the antenatal clinic, to a severely distressed woman in premature labour. Consequently the urgency of the assessment varies, though the latter situation is much less common.

Rapid Emergency Assessment

It is important to exclude premature labour.

Making the Diagnosis

Relevant features include site and severity of the pain, associated vaginal loss, history of fetal movement, urinary and bowel symptoms.

Relevant History

Presenting Complaint

MAIN COMPLAINT – Pain – the site and nature of the pain are obviously important.

UTERUS – distension secondary to polyhydramnios is characteristically diffuse over the uterus, whereas the pain of premature labour is characteristically intermittent. Central period-like pain can herald a miscarriage. Red degeneration of fibroids (haemorrhagic necrosis) is painful, and the pain is often localised over the fibroid.

LOW ABDOMINAL PAIN AND ASSOCIATED BACK PAIN — Common in pregnancy, and most commonly they are related to the progesterone-induced relaxation of the ligaments and muscles that support the skeleton. Other more serious causes of pain should be excluded prior to making a diagnosis of ligament pain. Stretching of the round ligaments in the second trimester can cause pain anywhere along their course from the fundus to the groin.

VAGINAL LOSS – **vaginal bleeding** in association with abdominal pain should prompt exclusion of placental abruption (see Chapter 30). A history of ruptured membranes is important, as this would alter future management (see Chapter 37).

URINARY – **renal colic**, **UTIs** and **pyelonephritis** are associated with loin pain and low abdominal pain. Also note a history of **dysuria** and frequency, which may suggest a UTI with the caveat that most women describe increased frequency in pregnancy.

GI – **constipation** is more common in pregnancy, again probably because of progesterone's smooth-muscle relaxant effect. Similarly, there is an increase in oesophageal reflux symptoms (**heartburn**) because the upper oesophageal sphincter is less competent in the high-progesterone environment.

OTHER – **Upper abdominal pain**, particularly over the right upper quadrant, is usually hepatic in origin, and, although gallstones and hepatitis can complicate pregnancy, it is important to exclude **HELLP syndrome**. **Appendicitis** can present as right lower quadrant pain in pregnancy but it also can present with pain much higher up than McBurney's point because the caecum can be pushed upwards towards the liver by the gravid uterus.

Obstetric History

INDEX PREGNANCY – A previous history of ruptured membranes predisposes to ascending infection and chorioamnionitis. Multiple pregnancy and polyhydramnios both predispose to premature labour. In severe PET/ HELLP, hepatic distension stretches the hepatic capsule, causing pain, and is associated with high maternal and fetal mortality.

OBSTETRIC HISTORY – The recurrence risk of premature labour is increased in future pregnancies. Indeed, the risk of premature labour is low in women whose previous pregnancies have gone to term; therefore it is important to establish the gestation of previous deliveries.

Gynaecological History

Fibroids may have been identified outside pregnancy in association with menorrhagia. Ovarian cysts can reoccur in pregnancy, and tort/rupture as outside pregnancy.

Medical History

Sickle cell crises are more common in pregnancy. Diabetes mellitus is associated with premature labour, partly through it association with polyhydramnios.

Drug History

DRUGS – Crack cocaine can increase the risk of an abruption.

Relevant Clinical Examination

It is important to exclude potential dangerous complications first.

General Features

GENERAL – Exclude signs of shock and premature labour. However, most commonly, the signs are quite diffuse. It is also important to remember that more than one condition can coexist, and indeed one may precipitate another. For example: pyelonephritis can precipitate premature labour, ruptured membranes and preterm labour, etc., so do not confine yourself to one diagnosis unnecessarily.

Abdomen

PREGNANCY – The uterus is classically hard and tender – 'woody' – after a severe abruption, as retroplacental blood irritates the myometrium. Palpable tightenings are found in premature labour. Tightenings should be confirmed by abdominal palpation and their frequency recorded as a baseline. A tense abdomen with a larger than expected symphyseal–fundal height may be related to polyhydramnios or multiple pregnancy, both of which predispose to premature labour. Presentation should also be determined, as a lower segment caesarean section (LSCS) can be considered in preterm breech presentations. Where the abdomen is tender to palpation and there is a history of spontaneous rupture of membranes (SRM), amnionitis should be excluded. Fibroids can be palpable as discrete tender 'lumps' on the uterus.

GENERAL – Peritonism is obviously an important finding and usually warrants laparotomy. Loin pain and tenderness is a feature of pyelonephritis. There may be other symptoms of sickle cell anaemia, such as bone pain, in a sickle cell crisis. A maternal pyrexia suggests a primary infection and can precipitate premature labour.

Pelvis

VAGINAL EXAMINATION – **Speculum** – a speculum examination should be performed to confirm a history of ruptured membranes or if there is a history of antepartum haemorrhage (APH), to identify the source of the bleeding. **Vaginal examination** – The effacement and dilatation of the cervix should be determined as a baseline. Vaginal examination should also be avoided after a history of ruptured membranes, to reduce the risk of ascending infection.

Relevant Investigations

Haematology

A FBC should be undertaken as part of the baseline investigation. Low haemoglobin can be a feature of sickle cell anaemia. A raised white count is a feature of underlying infection, e.g. UTI, chorio-amnionitis, etc. Likewise a raised white count is a feature of appendicitis. A low platelet count is a feature of HELLP (Haemolysis, Elevated Liver enzymes, Low Platelets) syndrome. A Kleihauer test should be performed where an abruption is suspected in a rhesus-negative woman.

Biochemistry

Liver function tests should be performed to exclude HELLP syndrome in women with right upper quadrant pain. C-reactive protein is a non-specific marker of inflammation/infection and therefore may be useful where infection is suspected, especially chorio-amnionitis.

Microbiology

An MSU should be sent for microscopy and culture where a UTI is suspected. Group B streptococcal colonisation of the vagina predisposes to premature labour and can lead to a severe neonatal pneumonia, therefore an HVS is useful for the paediatricians in the event of a preterm labour.

Diagnostic Imaging

USS – Ultrasound scans are useful to exclude potential causes of preterm labour such as polyhydramnios.

CTG – The fetus is at increased risk of compromise after an abruption and with premature labour. Therefore the fetal heart should be auscultated as part of the initial assessment, followed by more sophisticated CTG monitoring where appropriate.

DETAILS OF INDIVIDUAL CONDITIONS

1. Premature Labour

Background

DEFINITION – Premature labour is strictly defined as labour (progressive cervical dilatation and effacement) prior to 37 weeks gestation. However, there is obviously an enormous difference in potential outcomes between those infants born at 24 weeks and 36 weeks. Therefore, because of differences in outcomes and management, it is possibly more appropriate to use 34 weeks gestation as a watershed.

AETIOLOGY – Preterm labour is associated with a number of maternal and fetal conditions, but in up to 40% of cases there is no obvious precipitating cause.

Maternal:
- Medical disorders, e.g. diabetes mellitus.
- Maternal pyrexia can precipitate preterm labour.
- Urinary tract infections, particularly pyelonephritis, are frequently implicated.
- Abnormal vaginal flora have been implicated in the pathogenesis of premature labour, at least in association. They appear to produce proteolytic enzymes, which attack the membranes, leading to premature rupture and thence labour.

Fetal: Multiple pregnancy is the single most frequent cause of preterm labour, secondary to uterine overdistension.

Liquor:
- Polyhydramnios also predisposes to premature labour, again secondary to uterine overdistension.
- Premature rupture of the membranes often precedes preterm labour. This may in itself start labour through local prostaglandin release or follow an ascending infection leading to chorio-amnionitis.

Placenta: Extravasated retro-placental blood following a placental abruption irritates the myometrium and can cause uterine contractions.

MAIN COMPLICATIONS – **Fetal** – premature labour is the single biggest cause of perinatal mortality in the UK. The 8% of babies that deliver before 34 weeks gestation account for 75% of all perinatal mortality (85% if congenital abnormalities are excluded). Within this group there is an enormous variation in outcome: at 34 weeks gestation the outcomes are generally good, but at the other end of the spectrum the outcomes can be dire. At 24 weeks gestation the perinatal mortality improves by 1% per day!

The main risks are linked to respiratory distress syndrome (RDS). Premature infants lack surfactant and therefore their lungs function less well. This leads to hypoxia and thence other complications like intra-ventricular haemorrhage (IVH). Therefore anything that reduces RDS will improve survival. The administration of steroids reduces the incidence of RDS by up to 50%.

Treatment Options

There should be a multidisciplinary approach to preterm labour, including the neonatologists, because the management varies with gestational age, neonatal facilities, cause of labour, maternal and fetal condition. As a rule of thumb, labour should be inhibited before 34 weeks gestation to allow administration of steroids and, if necessary, transfer to appropriate neonatal facilities as long as maternal or fetal welfare is not prejudiced. There is no apparent benefit of treatment > 48 h.

CONSERVATIVE AND REASSURANCE – Approximately 50% of 'premature labours' will cease spontaneously. Appropriate treatment of causes, for example adequate treatment of a UTI, may also be sufficient to arrest the labour without additional tocolysis.

All women presenting with preterm labour should be given steroids to enhance fetal lung maturity. This will ensure those babies that do deliver have received steroids, and it will not harm those who remain in utero. Caution should be used with concurrent maternal diabetes, as the steroids will increase the blood glucose and there will be a transient increase in insulin requirement. This should be anticipated.

MEDICAL – Tocolysis is unlikely to be successful where the cervix is > 3 cm dilated and should only be used with caution after SRM or an APH, as they may lead to an amnionitis or abruption, respectively.

β-sympathomimetics – intravenous ritodrine is commonly used to inhibit labour through its agonist effect on β2 receptors on the uterus (smooth-muscle relaxation). However, their agonist effects at other sites – tachycardia, tremor, hypotension, hypokalaemia, hyperglycaemia (important in diabetics) and nausea – can limit the use of these drugs.

Calcium channel blockers – again, these work through a direct effect on smooth-muscle relaxation. Nifedipine is administered orally and is less invasive with fewer side effects than ritodrine. The side effects are headache and, classically, facial flushing.

Other smooth muscle relaxants, e.g. glycerol trinitrate patches, have been tried. In the USA, NSAIDs, particularly indomethacin, are used. Their tocolytic effect is mediated through the reduction in prostaglandins. However, their use can lead to premature closure of the fetal ductus arteriosus and oligohydramnios.

SURGICAL – Caesarean should be performed for usual obstetric indications.

Information for Patients

PROGNOSIS – The fetal prognosis is largely dependent on gestation. Neonatal advice is invaluable, and the parents should ideally be counselled by the neonatologists about both prognosis and likely neonatal course on special care baby unit (SCBU). A visit to SCBU should be arranged where possible.

Follow-up

SHORT TERM – Premature labours are associated with increased postnatal morbidity, particularly infection and depression. Close obstetric follow-up should continue in the postnatal period.

LONG TERM – There is an increased risk of preterm labour in subsequent pregnancies, and therefore women should be offered preconception counselling and an early booking visit in the future to discuss potential treatments and outcomes.

2. Other

Background

The management of the other causes of abdominal pain in the second half of pregnancy is largely problem specific and ideally conservative.

UTI/PYELONEPHRITIS – Pyelonephritis complicates 1% of pregnancies, and asymptomatic bacteriuria complicates 5% of pregnancies. Treatment of pyelonephritis is

---

GOLDEN POINTS

1. Abdominal pain is a common complication of pregnancy, and it is important to exclude potential dangerous causes, particularly premature labour.

2. Premature labour complicates 5–10% of pregnancies but accounts for 85% of perinatal mortality.

3. Steroids should be administered to all women at risk of preterm labour < 34 weeks gestation.

4. Exclude and treat potentially treatable causes of preterm labour.

5. Reserve tocolysis for women < 34 weeks gestation, < 3 cm dilated and for a maximum of 48 h to allow maximum benefit of the steroids and transfer to a unit with appropriate SCBU facilities.

6. Discuss likely outcomes with neonatologists.

7. Other causes can usually be managed conservatively.

aggressive: intravenous antibiotics, intravenous hydration and paracetemol to reduce maternal pyrexia. Penicillin-based antibiotics are generally safe in pregnancy.

APPENDICITIS – The management of appendicitis in pregnancy is similar to that outside pregnancy, i.e. appendicectomy, except it may be sensible to administer steroids prior to the operation in anticipation of the occasional preterm labour.

FIBROIDS – **Red degeneration** – The treatment is conservative: simple analgesia. Occasionally, hospital admission is required and topical application of ice packs.

30 Vaginal bleeding in the second half of pregnancy

CLINICAL SIGNIFICANCE

Antepartum haemorrhage (APH) after 20 weeks gestation is a common (3% of pregnancies) and potentially life-threatening complication of pregnancy for both mother and baby. Placenta praevia and placental abruption should be considered in all women presenting with APH, as they are both serious and demand specific management. Approximately half of the women who present after an APH are subsequently discovered to have either a placental abruption or praevia. No firm diagnosis is made in the other half.

DIFFERENTIAL DIAGNOSIS

MAIN CATEGORY	DIAGNOSIS
1. *Placental causes*	Placenta praevia
	Placental abruption
	Marginal bleed
2. *Fetal causes*	Vasa praevia
3. *Uterine/cervical causes*	Cervical ectropion
	Cervical carcinoma
	Cervical polyp
	Uterine rupture
4. *Miscellaneous*	Vulval varices
	Trauma

CLINICAL ASSESSMENT

There is an enormous range in the severity of pain and bleeding: from the shocked woman with a massive placental abruption to the much more common painless vaginal loss, often less than a period. The majority of women who present are not acutely unwell, and emergency resuscitation is rarely necessary. However, there should be a low threshold for aggressive resuscitation where there is evidence of 'shock'.

Rapid Emergency Assessment

There should be a rapid assessment of maternal haemodynamic condition followed by appropriate **resuscitation** with early recourse to blood transfusion:

- oxygen
- large-bore intravenous access – two venflons
- cross-match and intravenous fluids
- theatre for EUA.

Make an assessment of the maternal abdomen and fetal heart. Vaginal examination is absolutely contraindicated until a placenta praevia can be excluded.

The haemorrhage of an abruption can be concealed inside the uterus, and therefore the degree of shock may be out of keeping with the revealed loss. Aggressive fluid replacement is essential.

Making the Diagnosis

The initial assessment includes diagnosis; major placental abruption and placenta praevia in particular should be excluded. Relevant features include degree of haemorrhage, abdominal pain and precipitating events. The diagnosis of a marginal bleed requires the exclusion of more sinister causes.

Relevant History

Presenting Complaint

MAIN COMPLAINT – **Bleeding** – An estimate of the volume should be noted. This can be difficult as a 'little blood goes a long way' and a small amount can look enormous to an anxious couple. Comparison with a normal period can be a useful baseline, i.e. is it heavier or lighter? Both placenta praevia and placental abruption can present with heavy bleeding, whereas the less serious causes are characteristically lighter. However, light bleeding does not exclude either an abruption or a praevia. **Repeated episodes** of bleeding are a feature of **placenta praevia**, and therefore it is important to document any previous episodes.

Pain – Painful bleeding is most suggestive of an **abruption** as it separates from the uterine side wall. However, be careful: there may be two separate pathologies, i.e. preterm labour and a placenta praevia. **Low back pain** can be present with **abruption** of a posterior placenta. **Painless bleeding** is a feature of **placenta praevia**, though this is rather non-specific in that most of the other differentials are painless too.

PRECIPITATING CAUSES – **Vaginal examination** can provoke heavy bleeding with an undiagnosed placenta **praevia** and this may be the first presentation of a significant praevia. An **abruption** can be precipitated by the sudden deceleration of a **car crash** where the pregnant woman is a passenger. **Post-coital bleeding** commonly indicates a **cervical pathology** and may, most commonly, be due to a cervical ectropion or a cervical polyp, though, rarely, carcinoma of the cervix can present in pregnancy and should be excluded – ask about recent cervical smear results. Vaginal bleeding can be caused by trauma; elicit any relevant incidents.

Obstetric History

INDEX PREGNANCY – Fetal maturity/**gestation** is very important, particularly where delivery would be contemplated after resuscitation, i.e. the fetus is of sufficient maturity or steroids should be administered for prematurity.

An early scan may have identified a low-lying placenta. However, this finding is rather non-specific, as 90% of the women with a low placenta at 20 weeks have a normally sited placenta at 36 weeks. The placenta itself does not move 'amoeba-like' up the uterine wall; the placenta is stationary and the lower segment grows away from it.

Sudden decompression of the uterus can precipitate a placental abruption, i.e. artificial rupture of membranes (ARM) for a patient with polyhydramnios or trauma. External cephalic version can also precipitate an abruption, therefore, any history of intervention or injury should be noted.

OBSTETRIC HISTORY – There is an increased risk of both placenta praevia and a placental abruption after a previous episode. **Placenta praevia** is more common after uterine surgery, and therefore a history of **previous LSCS** is important. The risk of placenta accreta is also increased after previous LSCS. Placenta accreta is a potentially serious complication where the placenta grows through the normal endometrium and invades the myometrium. There may be a slightly thinner endometrium over the previous scar, predisposing to accreta.

Gynaecological History

A **recent normal smear** virtually **excludes cervical carcinoma** and should be documented. However, pre-pregnancy smear abnormalities should prompt further investigation after an APH.

Medical History

There is an increased risk of abruption with hypertension, including pre-pregnancy essential hypertension as well as pre-eclampsia. The risks of abruption are increased with antiphospholipid antibody syndrome, other manifestations of which include recurrent miscarriage and venous thrombosis.

Drug History

DRUGS – Crack cocaine can increase the risk of an abruption. Aspirin was thought to increase the risk of an abruption, but this has been disputed in the recent CLASP trial.

CIGARETTES – There is an increased risk of both abruption and praevia with smoking, although the mechanism is unclear.

Social History

High parity and poor nutrition are associated with abruption, though again the exact mechanisms are unclear.

Relevant Clinical Examination

Remember that vaginal examination is absolutely contra-indicated until placenta praevia has been excluded.

General Features

GENERAL – Remember that most women who present will be haemodynamically stable. However, be aware of these more sinister findings. Exclude signs of **shock** – pallor, sweating, hypotension and tachycardia. The degree of shock may be completely out of keeping with the observed haemorrhage, as the blood can pool behind the placenta or be forced into the myometrium in a severe abruption. This is a **concealed haemorrhage**. Remember also that hypotension is rare, and hypertension may be a more likely finding as a risk factor for placental abruption. Recurrent bleeding may cause anaemia; check the conjunctiva.

Abdomen

GENERAL – On abdominal palpation try to identify pointers towards either placenta praevia or an abruption first. Check for abdominal scars, including a previous LSCS scar.

PREGNANCY – The **uterus** is classically **hard and tender** after a severe **abruption** as retro-placental blood irritates the myometrium. The uterus often appears normal with a placental praevia although there may be low uterine muscle tone. Recurrent placental haemorrhages from a low-lying placenta may reduce placental function and predispose to fetal intrauterine growth retardation (IUGR). Therefore the symphyseal–fundal height may be smaller than expected. **Malpresentation** is more common with placenta **praevia** as the low-lying placenta displaces the presenting part. The **presenting**

part may therefore also be **higher** than expected. APH of all causes is more common with multiple pregnancy; this can be confirmed by the palpation of multiple fetal parts. To monitor **fetal condition** the fetal heart should be auscultated as part of the initial assessment, followed by more sophisticated CTG monitoring where appropriate. A severe **abruption** can cause intra-uterine death, and therefore the **fetal heart** will be **absent**. Less severe abruptions may cause fetal distress which can be determined with the CTG.

Pelvis

VAGINAL EXAMINATION – **Speculum** – a speculum examination should be performed to visualise the cervix and to exclude cervical pathology. Ideally, this should only be performed after an ultrasound scan has excluded a placenta praevia. **Vaginal examination** – only after an ultrasound scan has excluded a low-lying placenta should a vaginal examination be performed. An abruption can precipitate a labour, and then the cervical dilatation should be noted as part of the assessment. Where the ultrasound findings are equivocal, then a vaginal examination can be performed in the operating theatre with everyone ready for a LSCS if there is a heavy bleed – examination without anaesthetic (EWA). Vaginal examination can then determine whether or not there is any placenta below the presenting part.

Relevant Investigations

Haematology

Blood should be taken immediately as part of the initial assessment and resuscitation. A FBC should be taken to provide a baseline haemoglobin. Blood should be cross-matched for all women who present with either a heavy loss or have the potential for further loss, e.g. a placenta praevia confirmed on USS.

Abruptions can allow the passage of fetal cells into the maternal system resulting in rhesus sensitisation in rhesus-negative women. A small abruption can be difficult to diagnose; therefore a Kleihauer test should be performed and/or anti-Rh(D) administered prophylactically to all rhesus-negative women presenting with an APH. A Kleihauer should not be used to diagnose a placental abruption; it is not sensitive or specific.

Diagnostic Imaging

USS – USS is the gold standard to visualise a **low-lying placenta**. Abdominal USS is used routinely, although transvaginal scanning can be used in difficult cases, e.g. posterior placenta where the fetal head can obscure the lowest edge. Transvaginal scanning is safe. Retro-placental haemorrhage is only rarely seen on USS, and therefore USS is less useful for the diagnosis of an abruption.

MRI – Recently, MRI scans have been used as a method of placental localisation as they are very accurate and seem safe in pregnancy. However, their use is confined to centres with easy access to MRI scanning – a very few!

DETAILS OF INDIVIDUAL CONDITIONS

1. Placenta Praevia

Background

DEFINITION – The placenta is partly or wholly implanted in the lower segment of the uterus. It is usually divided into four grades:

I   Placenta encroaches into the lower segment.
II   Placenta extends to the edge of the internal os.
III Placenta partially covers the internal os.
IV   Placenta completely covers the internal os.

Placenta praevia (Figure 30.1) classically presents with recurrent, painless bleeding which can vary from spotting to a life-threatening haemorrhage. The bleeding is

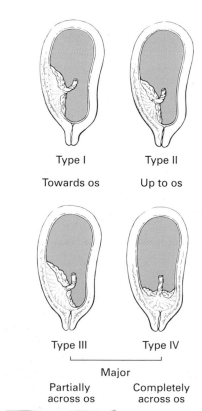

Type I
Towards os

Type II
Up to os

Type III

Type IV

Major

Partially
across os

Completely
across os

Fig 30.1   *Types of placenta praevia.*

maternal unless there are **vasa praevia**, when the bleeding originates from one of the placental vessels across the cervix with a velamentous (side-on) insertion of the cord.

There is an increased risk of **post partum haemorrhage** (PPH) with a placenta praevia. This is because the lower segment of the uterus does not contract very efficiently, thus the maternal blood vessels supplying the placenta are not closed and there is an increased loss.

Placenta accreta is the attachment of the placenta directly to the myometrium. This is more likely in the lower segment and to areas of uterine scarring where the endometrium is thinner. The placenta is more difficult to remove, leading to PPH, and occasionally a caesarean hysterectomy is required where it is impossible to remove the entire placenta.

AETIOLOGY –
Maternal:
- age and multiparity
- cigarette smoking
- previous uterine surgery, including LSCS.

Fetal:
- multiple pregnancy due to the increased placental area.

MAKING THE DIAGNOSIS – See Table 30.1.

MAIN COMPLICATIONS –

Maternal: The main complications are life-threatening haemorrhage, caesarean section, placenta accreta and PPH.

Fetal: There can be a significant fetal morbidity and mortality secondary to acute blood loss. Before the introduction of conservative management of placenta praevia, the fetal loss rate was over 80%, primarily because of prematurity. With modern care, a perinatal mortality rate of 50–60 per 1000 is achievable

(background rate for UK: 8–9 per 1000).

Treatment Options

The aim of treatment is supportive until fetal maturity allows delivery by LSCS, ideally > 37 weeks gestation or the blood loss compromises maternal/fetal health.

CONSERVATIVE AND REASSURANCE – **Admission** to hospital is often recommended in symptomatic placenta praevia. This is to allow early recourse to delivery if there is a life-threatening haemorrhage. However, some obstetricians allow selected women home, and, whilst they may require readmission, there is no difference in outcome except women prefer it.

Where early delivery is anticipated, **steroids** should be administered to enhance fetal lung maturity. **Four units of blood** should be cross-matched and be constantly available until delivery.

MEDICAL – There is almost no indication for vaginal delivery because the risks are enormous: haemorrhage, dystocia and premature placental separation. One exception maybe a dead or abnormal fetus with a low grade praevia – grade I.

SURGICAL – Delivery by **LSCS** for grade II placenta praevia upwards should be by the most senior obstetrician available. Where accurate ultrasound facilities are available for the diagnosis of placenta praevia, examination prior to LSCS is unnecessary. The caesarean section should be undertaken under a **GA** as there can be better haemodynamic control in the event of major haemorrhage.

At least 4 units of blood should be available at the time of LSCS, as there is a high risk of significant haemorrhage. The possibility of placenta accreta is increased after previous LSCS, and the woman should be counselled about possible hysterectomy if the blood loss is otherwise uncontrollable.

Information for Patients

PROGNOSIS – With care the prognosis is generally good. The messages from previous Confidential Enquiries into Maternal Death in the UK have largely been heeded – senior obstetricians should conduct delivery. The fetal prognosis is largely dependent on gestation.

Follow-up

SHORT TERM – Routine management requires **hospital admission** until delivery, although there is a significant psychological morbidity associated with prolonged hospital admission. Therefore a pragmatic policy of discharge sometimes prevails in selected patients.

LONG TERM – There is an increased recurrence risk after previous placenta praevia, and therefore an appointment for prenatal counselling may be appropriate.

Table 30.1	Diagnosing placenta praevia
Making the diagnosis	Placenta praevia
History	Recurrent, painless bleeds
Examination	Soft, non-tender uterus
	Abnormal fetal lie/ presentation, as the placenta prevents engagement of the fetal presenting part
Investigation	Identification of low-lying placenta on scan
	X-match 4 units

2. *Placental Abruption*

Background

DEFINITION – The placental attachment to the uterine wall is disrupted by haemorrhage, i.e. there is premature separation of the placenta. The placental separation is associated with retro-placental bleeding which tracks down between the membranes and the uterus to be revealed as an APH. The **separation** is usually much **more extensive** than a placenta praevia, causing more disruption to the fetal blood supply. This results in a much higher number of **intrauterine deaths** and a higher incidence of fetal distress requiring early delivery. The increased perinatal mortality associated with abruption is partly due to prematurity.

PPH is increased by the associated release of thromboplastins into the maternal circulation, resulting in a **disseminated intravascular coagulation (DIC)**. Where a significant amount of blood has infiltrated the myometrium the uterus cannot contract – a **Couvelaire uterus** – and this also increases the risk of **PPH**. The major blood loss can result in **hypovolaemia** with subsequent **acute renal failure** and oliguria.

AETIOLOGY –
Maternal:
- hypertension (50% of cases)
- sudden decompression of an overdistended uterus, i.e. SRM, after polyhydramnios or after delivery of the 1st twin
- age and multiparity
- cigarette smoking, cocaine use
- antiphospholipid antibody syndrome
- folate deficiency.
Fetal: multiple pregnancy.
Liquor: polyhydramnios.

MAKING THE DIAGNOSIS – See Table 30.2.

MAIN COMPLICATIONS

Maternal: Placental abruption is a potentially life-threatening complication with significant morbidity, notably haemorrhage, shock, DIC, and renal failure caused by hypotension.

Fetal: The perinatal mortality of confirmed placental abruption is high – 300 per 1000 – and more than half the perinatal losses are due to death before the mother arrives at hospital. Most of the other morbidity is related to prematurity, whilst the increased disruption to the placental architecture increases the risk of fetal anaemia compared with placenta praevia.

Treatment Options

Treatment depends on the severity of the abruption and the fetal condition.

Table 30.2 Diagnosing placental abruption	
Making the diagnosis	Placental abruption
History	Painful bleeds
Examination	Hard, tender uterus
Investigation	Confirm fetal wellbeing on CTG DIC

CONSERVATIVE – Small abruptions are often self-limiting; therefore, where the bleeding ceases and the fetal condition is satisfactory, the woman may be allowed home after a period of observation. Delivery may be more appropriate at term.

MEDICAL – More severe abruptions require a more intensive approach – maternal resuscitation and analgesia are priorities. Blood should be taken for cross-match and to exclude a clotting abnormality. Four units of blood should be cross-matched and be constantly available until delivery. Urine output should be monitored for the oliguria of acute tubular necrosis, and haemodialysis used where appropriate. **DIC** should be managed in conjunction with the haemotologists. The precipitant, the fetus, must be delivered followed by **fresh frozen plasma** and platelet transfusion. Where early delivery is anticipated, **steroids** should be administered to enhance fetal lung maturity.

SURGICAL – When the fetus is alive and of sufficient maturity to deliver, vaginal delivery is encouraged and labour should be induced or augmented. LSCS is required for obstetric indications, e.g. transverse lie, and for fetal distress or when clinical shock from haemorrhage is otherwise uncontrollable.

Where the fetus is dead the risks of LSCS are not warranted, and vaginal delivery should be planned. If the abruption is severe enough to cause fetal death then the complication rates are increased and the maternal risk is considerable. Increased vigilance for potential complications is required.

Information for Patients

PROGNOSIS – If the fetus is viable on admission to hospital the prognosis is generally good. However, where the fetus is dead, not only is the fetal prognosis zero, the maternal risks are also increased. There is an increased risk of placental abruption in future pregnancies.

Follow-up

SHORT TERM – Follow-up is required for those women discharged home after a suspected mild abruption, and they should be treated as high risk with frequent antenatal clinic visits. A 'debriefing' visit may be required after a complicated postnatal period, usually scheduled for 6 weeks.

LONG TERM – Prenatal counselling may be required, as there is an increased risk of abruption after a previous abruption.

3. Other Causes

The management of the other causes of APH is problem specific, though it is largely conservative.

Marginal Haemorrhage

Marginal haemorrhage is a diagnosis of exclusion. There are minimal maternal or fetal risks, and no specific treatment is required. Anti-Rh (D) should be administered. The woman should be counselled to return for monitoring should there be any further APHs.

Cervical Pathology

Ectropions are more common in the pregnancy, because of the high oestrogen levels. They usually present as postcoital bleeding and they can be visualised with a speculum. No treatment is required save expectant management. Cervical polyps can be removed if they are symptomatic.

Cervical carcinoma presents in 1 in 5000 pregnancies, usually as postcoital bleeding or vaginal discharge. The diagnosis is confirmed by cervical biopsy If the disease is diagnosed before fetal viability a termination of pregnancy is often recommended to allow treatment. However, in the third trimester, treatment can be delayed to allow lung maturation followed by delivery by LSCS, as a large cervical lesion can cause excessive bleeding. Treatment is otherwise as for non-pregnant patients:

primary surgery or radiotherapy for early stage disease (stage Ib or less) and radiotherapy for more advanced lesions.

GOLDEN POINTS

1. Bleeding in the second half of pregnancy is a common and potentially life-threatening complication.

2. Over half of the women who present with APH will subsequently be diagnosed as either placental abruption or praevia.

3. Aggressive resuscitation is essential where there are any signs of shock.

4. Vaginal examination is contraindicated unless praevia has been excluded.

5. Consider anti-Rh(D) prophylaxis and steroids where appropriate.

6. Placenta praevia should be managed expectantly in hospital until delivery by LSCS at term.

7. The management of placental abruption depends upon gestation and fetal condition, but labour should be induced or augmented unless there are specific contraindications.

8. Other causes can usually be managed conservatively.

31 Raised blood pressure in pregnancy

CLINICAL SIGNIFICANCE

Hypertension is one of the commonest complications of pregnancy, affecting 10–15% of all pregnancies. There is an enormous spectrum of disease from mild hypertension which is associated with minimal risk to both mother and baby to life-threatening pre-eclampsia.

Hypertension in pregnancy may be pre-existing (chronic) or pregnancy induced. Although the two disorders are quite separate, both in aetiology and effect, there can be an overlap, as chronic hypertension can predispose to pre-eclampsia.

There are at least two forms of pregnancy-induced hypertension: pre-eclampsia, which increases the maternal and fetal risk but which completely resolves post delivery, and a transient, non-proteinuric hypertension which does not increase the maternal and fetal risks but may predispose to hypertension later in life.

DIFFERENTIAL DIAGNOSIS

MAIN CATEGORY	DIAGNOSIS
1. *Chronic hypertension*	Essential Renal disease Diabetes Coarctation of the aorta Drug abuse: cocaine Hormone-secreting tumours: Cushing syndrome, phaeochromocytoma
2. *Pregnancy induced*	Pre-eclampsia Transient, non-proteinuric hypertension

CLINICAL ASSESSMENT

Pre-eclampsia (PET) is a difficult diagnostic problem and requires an appreciation of the maternal manifestations of the syndrome. Antenatal visits are a screening system for PET where the blood pressure and degree of proteinuria are routinely measured.

Women who present with symptoms of PET or are identified as at risk on routine antenatal testing can be referred to hospital for further investigation. There is often a day assessment unit (DAU) where women can be investigated as outpatients. Those women with severe disease can be admitted for close monitoring, whereas those with less severe problems can be monitored as outpatients with appropriate follow-up.

Rapid Emergency Assessment

Pre-eclampsia can present as a potentially terminal crisis. There are a number of sinister symptoms which should prompt rapid action:

- **Frontal headache** or visual symptoms, i.e. glitter or 'seeing stars', may indicate **severe hypertension** or impending eclampsia.
- **Oliguria** may herald **renal failure**.
- **Right sided upper abdominal pain** should prompt investigation for **hepatic swelling**.
- Fitting in late pregnancy, without any previous history, is **eclampsia** until proved otherwise.
- Hyper-reflexia is a sinister finding that may be associated with cerebral oedema.

Intravenous access must be established followed by appropriate resuscitation. Caution should be exercised with the administration of i.v. fluids. Careful monitoring of the maternal and fetal condition is required.

Relevant History

Presenting Complaint

MAIN COMPLAINT – **Hypertension** is most commonly detected during antenatal visits, by the GP or the midwife.

A rise of more than 20 mmHg in the **diastolic** blood pressure from booking, or a blood pressure of greater than **140/90**, is significant and warrants further investigation.

COMMONLY ASSOCIATED SYMPTOMS – Both chronic hypertension and early pre-eclampsia can be symptomless. There are symptoms of more advanced or more severe disease that warrant further investigation. These are detailed above in the rapid assessment section.

Many patients will complain of swelling. This may manifest as simple ankle oedema or more difficult problems, i.e. the symptoms of carpal tunnel syndrome. Remember that ankle oedema is not a specific sign of pre-eclampsia – 80% of normal pregnancies will have some degree of oedema.

Gynaecological History

CONTRACEPTION – Previous hypertension on the oral contraceptive pill is important, as this can indicate a susceptibility to pregnancy-induced hypertension. This is an oestrogen effect.

Obstetric History

DELIVERIES – Pre-eclampsia is primarily a condition of primigravid women, though the recurrence risk of severe pre-eclampsia is approximately 15%. Therefore a previous history of PET is an important feature to elicit, as well as the gestational age at delivery, the mode of delivery and any complications. A history of previous miscarriage is associated with a reduced incidence of PET.

Medical History

MEDICAL CONDITIONS – Some medical conditions and pre-existing hypertension should be documented. Pregnancy can affect and be affected by many of the causes.

Renal disease is not usually affected by pregnancy; the outcome of the pregnancy is determined by the degree of renal impairment and the blood pressure: creatinine > 200 µmol/L or BP > 140/90 in the non-pregnant state can compromise the pregnancy.

A history of hypertension secondary to coarctation of the aorta requires careful monitoring in pregnancy. It can predispose to aortic dissection and heart failure during pregnancy as well as hypertension.

Endocrine tumours are rare but important causes of chronic hypertension. Both Cushing syndrome and phaeochromocytoma are associated with a high maternal and fetal morbidity. Specific treatment can reduce these risks, though pregnancy is inadvisable until the condition is stable.

Diabetes mellitus also predisposes to PET: up to 15% of diabetic pregnancies.

Drug History

MEDICATIONS – Chronic hypertension is controlled using a wide variety of antihypertensives, some of which are contraindicated as they have adverse effects on pregnancy. In particular, ACE inhibitors should be stopped, as they are associated with severe, early IUGR, oligohydramnios and fetal death. There are many other drugs which are contraindicated in pregnancy, and standard recommendations apply.

SMOKING – The incidence of PET is slightly reduced in women who smoke, but the problems associated with smoking far outweigh any benefits. All pregnant women should be encouraged to stop smoking.

DRUGS – Cocaine use has been associated with hypertension, an increased risk of PET and fetal death.

Social History

AGE – Chronic hypertension is more common in older women, whilst pre-eclampsia is more common in women at the extremes of reproductive age: < 20 or > 35 years.

Relevant Clinical Examination

General Features

GENERAL – Oedema is a feature of PET, particularly pretibial, though this may be anywhere, including facial.

NEUROLOGICAL – Chronic or severe hypertension can produce papilloedema, and the fundi should be examined. Tendon reflexes may be brisk immediately prior to eclampsia as the degree of cerebral irritation increases. Brisk reflexes are not specific, though the demonstration of clonus should raise the index of suspicion.

BODY-MASS INDEX – Hypertension is more common in obese women. A broad sphygmomanometer cuff should be used in obese women to avoid an artificially high BP reading.

CVS

Coarctation of the aorta is rare, and can be excluded by a normal CVS examination and palpation of normal femoral pulses.

The blood pressure should be measured, and there is now accumulating evidence that the 5th Korotkov sound should be used to measure the diastolic blood pressure, as it is more consistent. The measurement should be repeated if the blood pressure is > 140/90.

Abdomen

PREGNANCY – Both chronic hypertension and PET are associated with IUGR and oligohydramnios; therefore the symphyseal–fundal height may be less than expected. An enlarged uterus in the first trimester with a recent onset of hypertension should alert the clinician to the possibility of hydatidiform mole.

TENDERNESS – The liver may also become oedematous, enlarge and stretch the hepatic capsule, producing pain and tenderness over the liver.

Pelvis

VAGINAL EXAMINATION – Where there is severe PET and delivery is contemplated, the state of the cervix should be determined. Induction of labour is more likely to be successful where the cervix is 'favourable'.

Relevant Investigations

There is no specific diagnostic test for PET, but there are a number of biochemical features.

Haematology

A full blood count and clotting screen should be completed as part of the further investigation. **Haemoconcentration** can be present, as the 'leaky' damaged endothelium cannot prevent the osmotic movement of water out of the intravascular space into the interstitium (oedema). **Thrombocytopaenia** and **clotting disorders** can occur, provoked by the damaged endothelium.

Biochemistry

Proteinuria is one of the hallmarks of PET: > 0.3 g protein in 24 h. Where there is doubt about the dipstick measurement of proteinuria, a 24 h urine collection will produce a quantitative result. A 24 h urine with raised catecholamines can confirm a phaechromocytoma. **Hyperuricaemia** is a feature of PET and is related to the perinatal mortality, and therefore it can be used as an indirect measure of the severity of the PET.

Microbiology

Proteinuria can be secondary to an incidental UTI, and this should be excluded where there is a high clinical suspicion.

Diagnostic Imaging

Fetal growth retardation is more common in pregnancies complicated either by chronic hypertension or PET. USS is used both to diagnose fetal growth retardation and also to monitor in-utero fetal condition, i.e. biophysical profile.

DETAILS OF INDIVIDUAL CONDITIONS

1. Pre-eclampsia

Background

DEFINITION – Pre-eclampsia is an endothelial disorder, primarily of primigravid women, in the last half of pregnancy, which is characterised by proteinuria and hypertension. It affects virtually all maternal organ systems and the fetus indirectly by affecting the placenta.

Pre-eclampsia affects 10% of the primigravid obstetric population, but it is the commonest cause of maternal death in the UK and a significant cause of fetal morbidity and mortality. There is no specific diagnostic test for pre-eclampsia, and treatment requires delivery. The management of a pregnancy complicated by PET entails fetal/ maternal surveillance and pre-emptive delivery.

There is a sequence of events leading to the development of pre-eclampsia: abnormal implantation leads to underperfusion of the placenta which produces an agent that damages the endothelium (toxaemia). The damaged endothelium loses its anticoagulant properties and activates the coagulation cascade. The damaged endothelium is also more sensitive to circulating pressors producing vasospasm, hypertension and a reduced end-organ perfusion. The damaged endothelium is also more permeable, resulting in a shift of intravascular fluid to the interstitium – oedema – and a leak of protein through the glomerulus – proteinuria.

AETIOLOGY –
Maternal factors:
- primigravidae or new partner
- extremes of reproductive age
- racial origin
- history of PET in previous pregnancy
- family history of PET.

Medical:
- chronic hypertension
- diabetes mellitus
- antiphospholipid syndrome.

Fetal:
- multiple pregnancy
- molar pregnancy.

MAIN COMPLICATIONS –
Fetal: The fetal syndrome comprises nutritional and respiratory deprivation secondary to poor placental function:
• intrauterine growth retardation
• oligohydramnios
• consequences of prematurity – where maternal disease necessitates preterm delivery.
• perinatal death.

Maternal: Almost all maternal organ systems can be affected; the pathophysiology of individual conditions is secondary to endothelial damage and/or hypertension. Think of each system from the head downwards, as an aide-memoire:

- Cerebral
  - haemorrhage
- Eyes
  - retinal detachment
  - cortical blindness
- Chest
  - pulmonary oedema
- Liver
  - hepatic capsule distension secondary to hepatic oedema
  - HELLP
- Kidney
  - acute cortical necrosis
  - acute tubular necrosis
- Clotting
  - thrombocytopaenia and disseminated intravascular coagulopathy
- Placenta
  - abruptio placentae
- Maternal death
  - The most common causes of death, in a recent report, were cerebral haemorrhage, pulmonary oedema and adult respiratory distress syndrome. Unfortunately, in 80% of the deaths the medical care was deemed substandard.

PREVENTION – There are no effective clinical interventions apart from abstinence or multiparity. Fish oil rich in long-chain, omega-3 unsaturated fatty acids may have some protective effect. Aspirin may have a small protective effect in women who have previously had severe PET necessitating delivery prior to 32 weeks gestation.

Treatment Options

CONSERVATIVE AND REASSURANCE – The mainstay of PET management is delivery. Hospital admission and observation is required where the disease deteriorates remote from term and conservative treatment is employed to prolong the pregnancy. Bed rest is now known not to be helpful. In severe disease the amount of time that can be gained is limited – about 15 extra days before a pre-eclamptic crisis becomes imminent.

Where delivery is anticipated before 34 weeks gestation, steroids should be administered to accelerate fetal lung maturity.

MEDICAL – **Delivery** – PET is a complex multisystem disorder which requires delivery to fully effect a cure. Induction of labour (IoL) is employed for disease > 36 weeks gestation; before this, IoL is more likely to fail. Prostaglandin preparations are the agents of choice where the cervix is unfavourable.

Delivery is usually by LSCS where there is severe PET preterm or there are other obstetric indications for LSCS, e.g. breech presentation. Careful fetal monitoring is mandatory in labour, and an epidural anaesthetic is often recommended to reduce the hypertension.

Antihypertensives – Treatment of PET with antihypertensives does not reduce the progression or development of PET as a multisystem disorder; rather it can reduce the hypertensive morbidity to a minimum, i.e. CVA secondary to severe hypertension. Antihypertensives are used in two different ways: acutely to control the severe hypertension of PET during or immediately prior to delivery, and as long-term treatment to be used for non-proteinuric hypertension.

Labetolol and hydralazine intravenously are used for immediate treatment of severe hypertension. Once the hypertension is stabilised or the hypertension less severe, then oral medication can be used. Methyldopa is commonly used antenatally because of the large body of experience associated with its use in pregnancy. Nifedipine and oral labetolol are also used, though β-blockers are associated with an increased rate of IUGR.

Anticonvulsants – magnesium sulphate is now the treatment of choice for prevention of recurrent eclamptic fits after an initial seizure. It should be continued for up to 48 h postpartum, as up to 25% of fits occur in the postnatal period. Magnesium sulphate has overtaken phenytoin as the agent of choice after eclampsia. It is more effective and it may have a cerebroprotective effect in preterm infants. Magnesium sulphate can also be used for initial seizure prophylaxis. The use of nifedipine and magnesium sulphate together is contraindicated, as there is a potential risk of extreme hypotension. Magnesium sulphate is excreted primarily by the kidneys, and the dose must be reduced if the urine output is low, to reduce the risks of toxicity. This can manifest as a spectrum of clinically apparent neuromuscular disorders ranging from absent reflexes to respiratory depression.

Adjuvant therapy – potential complications include oliguria and renal failure, HELLP and pulmonary oedema which may be iatrogenic, secondary to overaggressive fluid management. The renal and hepatic complications require treatment in specialist centres.

OVERVIEW – PET represents a spectrum of disease from mild to potentially life threatening for both mother and fetus. Mild pre-eclampsia remote from term (< 36/40) can be managed conservatively with close fetal and maternal monitoring for disease progression. PET at term or severe PET merits delivery followed by appropriate monitoring for potential complications.

Information for Patients

PROGNOSIS – The prognosis for mothers with pregnancies

complicated by PET is generally good. There is a recurrence rate of 10–15% in future pregnancies, though the disease is likely to be less severe and occur at a later gestation.

SELF-HELP GROUPS – Severe PET can cause both high morbidity and mortality. Self-help groups may provide a useful means of support, e.g. APEC (Action on Pre-eclampsia).

Follow-up

SHORT TERM – The disease process spontaneously resolves in the majority of women within 48 h of delivery, and monitoring can be discontinued. Severe PET, in particular with HELLP, may take longer to resolve, and monitoring should be continued.

LONG TERM – Most women will be normotensive at discharge from hospital, they will not need specific follow-up and they may use the oral contraceptive pill without increased risk. However, those women who are still hypertensive at the 6 week check will require further investigation to exclude an underlying cause, particularly renal, so that appropriate long-term management can be instituted.

2. Chronic Hypertension

Background

DEFINITION – Chronic hypertension is usually defined as a persistent elevation of the blood pressure > 140/90 mmHg. Severe hypertension is defined as a systolic > 160 mmHg and/or a diastolic blood pressure ≥ 100 mmHg.

AETIOLOGY – Chronic hypertension complicates approximately 1% of pregnancies, and essential hypertension is responsible for 90% of those. Essential hypertension is more common in older mothers. Secondary causes of chronic hypertension are listed at the beginning of the chapter.

MAIN COMPLICATIONS – Mild hypertension is not associated with any increase in maternal or fetal morbidity. However, the risk is increased where PET is superimposed or there are severe underlying disorders. Maternal risks include placental abruption (5× increase in risk) and PET (4× increase in risk). Poor placental function can result in fetal IUGR.

PREVENTION – Weight loss may help in those women whose hypertension is related to obesity. Good control of underlying disorders is essential.

Treatment Options

CONSERVATIVE – Ideally, the cause of the hypertension will have been elucidated or investigated at a prenatal clinic so that treatment of any underlying problems can be instigated. The principles of management are surveillance for potential complications and appropriate treatment of the hypertension. Monitoring consists of regular hospital clinic visits and serial fetal growth scans.

MEDICAL – The use of antihypertensive medication does not reduce the incidence of superimposed PET or abruption. Often, the physiological decrease in blood pressure in the middle trimester of pregnancy will allow discontinuation of previous antihypertensive medication, at least temporarily. A blood pressure consistently > 140/95 may merit oral treatment to reduce the hypertensive morbidity.

The antihypertensives used are similar to those used in mild pregnancy-induced hypertension or PET. Some antihypertensives are contraindicated in pregnancy: ACE inhibitors produce severe early IUGR and oligohydramnios, for example, and should be discontinued.

SURGICAL – Delivery should again be considered where the hypertension is severe or the fetus is compromised by superimposed complications.

Information for Patients

PROGNOSIS – The prognosis for pregnancy outcome is determined by the severity of any underlying disorders. The prognosis is generally good for women

---

GOLDEN POINTS

1. PET and mild chronic hypertension are completely different disorders.

2. PET is a multisystem disorder with increased perinatal and maternal mortality, whilst mild hypertension is only associated with an increase if there is a severe underlying pathology or PET develops.

3. PET cannot be reliably predicted or prevented, and there is no standard diagnostic test.

4. Antenatal management consists of maternal and fetal surveillance.

5. The only cure for PET is delivery!

6. Antihypertensive medication reduces the hypertensive morbidity only. It does not reduce the development of PET or its progression.

7. Magnesium sulphate has become the anticonvulsant of choice after an eclamptic seizure.

with essential hypertension, unlike those women with underlying problems. For example, severe renal disease can compromise the pregnancy, and also the condition itself may be exacerbated by pregnancy, resulting in a progression of the disease. A multidisciplinary approach with combined medical/obstetric care is essential.

Follow-up

SHORT TERM – After delivery, oral antihypertensive medication needs to be continued. Most antihypertensives are not contraindicated in breast-feeding mothers.

LONG TERM – Long-term follow-up is rarely necessary with essential hypertension. Those women with underlying disorders will require routine medical follow-up.

32 Diabetes in pregnancy

CLINICAL SIGNIFICANCE

There are two different types of diabetes in pregnancy: pre-existing insulin-dependent diabetes mellitus (IDDM or type 1) and gestational diabetes which is characteristically non-insulin-dependent (NIDDM or type 2). There is an excess perinatal morbidity and mortality for babies of diabetic (pre-existing IDDM) mothers, though the risks of gestational diabetes are less clear.

Pre-existing IDDM is both affected by, and affects, pregnancy. For example: maternal proliferative retinopathy characteristically deteriorates in pregnancy; there is an increase in the rate of fetal congenital abnormalities; and there is an increase in other complications of pregnancy, i.e. polyhydramnios and PET. Mothers with IDDM should be managed by a multidisciplinary team with a specialist interest in diabetes. Under this umbrella, many women can be treated almost as normal with tight diabetic control.

Identification of women with gestational diabetes can help improve their obstetric care, but it may be most useful in identifying a subpopulation of women who are at risk of NIDDM in later life and therefore may benefit from long-term measures to reduce that risk after pregnancy, i.e. diet, etc.

Occasionally the margins between these apparently disparate groups are blurred, as up to 1% of women with gestational diabetes may require insulin and occult IDDM may be unmasked by pregnancy, but for practical purposes the groups are quite different.

DIFFERENTIAL DIAGNOSIS

1. *Pre-existing diabetes mellitus*
2. *Gestational diabetes*

CLINICAL ASSESSMENT

Clinical assessment for women with pre-existing IDDM should include a thorough medical examination of the diabetic mother to exclude any diabetic complications, i.e. examination of the fundi for retinopathy and hypertension associated with nephropathy as well as the pre-pregnancy insulin requirements. Tight control of blood sugar levels at the time of conception is important, as poor control around the time of conception increases the risk of fetal anomaly.

Relevant History

Presenting Complaint

Screening for gestational diabetes is an inexact science. There are a plethora of different tests using different glucose loads and different threshold serum levels to define overt and gestational diabetes, and even where a positive result is obtained the tests are not reproducible at least 50% of the time. Despite this, screening remains popular. Some units screen their whole obstetric population between 20 and 28 weeks, whereas some screen only where there is an indication – see below.

Table 32.1 DDM and NIDDM in relation to pregnancy

	IDDM	NIDDM
Definition – random	Blood glucose > 11	Blood glucose 8–11
75 g glucose		> 9
Maternal risks	Innumerable	Risk of NIDDM in later life
Perinatal risks	10 x background	Minimal excess risks
Treatment	Strict control of blood glucose – insulin	Diet

Obstetric History – Index Pregnancy

ANTENATAL – Maternal weight > 100 kg or > 20% above ideal body weight predisposes to diabetes and warrants a GTT. Persistent glycosuria (> 2 occasions) on urine dipstick testing also merits further investigation. Poly-hydramnios and/or fetal macrosomia are both related to diabetes, and a GTT should be undertaken as part of the routine investigation of these conditions.

Obstetric History

A previous history of stillbirth, unexplained neonatal death, congenital anomaly or large baby (> 4.5 kg) also merits a GTT.

Drug History

Steroids are diabetogenic and can precipitate gestational diabetes or hyperglycaemia or even ketoacidosis in women with IDDM. Care should therefore be taken when administering steroids, e.g. in preterm labour to promote fetal maturity.

Social History

The epidemiology of gestational diabetes parallels other social ills. Like obesity it is more common in class IV and V than in women from class I.

Relevant Clinical Examination

General Features

GENERAL – Excepting obesity there are few specific features of gestational diabetes. However, complications of established IDDM should be excluded, i.e. retinopathy, vascular disease, etc. Pre-eclampsia is more common in IDDM mothers, and therefore the blood pressure should be monitored regularly.

Abdomen

PREGNANCY – Measurement of the symphyseal–fundal height is essential, as it can be smaller where the pregnancy is complicated by IUGR, or, more commonly, larger than would be anticipated in the presence of polyhydramnios and/or macrosomia.

TENDERNESS – Uterine overdistension caused by poly-hydramnios can give rise to a tender uterus – see Chapter 33.

Relevant Investigations

Haematology

Glycosylated haemoglobin can be used as a measure of long-term diabetic control. HbA1 levels of > 12% are associated with increased rates of fetal anomaly. They should be measured 4 weekly.

Biochemistry

Biochemical monitoring of the blood glucose is one of the mainstays of the management of diabetes in pregnancy. The blood glucose should be maintained between 4 and 7 mmol/L for maximum benefit. Fructosamine is a measure of long-term glucose control and can be used in an analogous manner to glycosylated haemoglobin.

In gestational diabetes, women whose pre-prandial blood glucose is persistently > 6 mmol/L may be offered insulin.

Urinalysis is of no benefit for monitoring diabetic control in pregnancy. Renal function should be assessed as part of the booking or baseline investigations. Significantly impaired renal function, i.e. creatinine > 200, is associated with increased perinatal mortality and morbidity, particularly IUGR and stillbirth.

Microbiology

Diabetes is associated with an increase in the incidence of bacteriuria which, untreated, predisposes to ascending infection. Therefore regular MSUs should be performed antenatally to exclude asymptomatic infection.

Diagnostic Imaging

Ultrasound scanning is now an essential part of the management of pregnancies complicated by diabetes: to assess gestational age, to identify fetal anomalies, to measure fetal growth, liquor volume and assess fetal wellbeing.

DETAILS OF INDIVIDUAL CONDITIONS

1. Insulin-dependent Diabetes Mellitus

Background

IDDM complicates approximately 4/1000 pregnancies and is the most common pre-existing medical condition to complicate pregnancy in the UK.

Main Complications

IDDM is a high-risk state for both the woman and her fetus in pregnancy. The fetal and neonatal loss rate is increased nine-fold and the major congenital malformation rate is increased six-fold. There is also an increased maternal morbidity and mortality. Tight diabetic control can minimise these potential complications. Differential characteristics of IDDM and NIDDM in relation to pregnancy are given in Table 32.1.

MATERNAL – Diabetes can both affect and be affected by pregnancy.

Diabetic complications – diabetic retinopathy classically deteriorates during pregnancy, though early and aggressive laser treatment can reduce the rate of deterioration back to non-pregnancy rates. Nephropathy and small-vessel disease can, rarely, worsen in pregnancy. Similarly, ischaemic heart disease can also deteriorate. Autonomic neuropathy can be associated with intractable vomiting in pregnancy.

Obstetric complications – the list of potential obstetric complications is daunting. Pre-eclampsia complicates 14% of pregnancies, a 3–4-fold increase compared with non-diabetic women. Polyhydramnios complicates 25% of diabetic pregnancies, predominantly because of the osmotic diuretic effect of fetal hyperglycaemia. Polyhydramnios contributes to the higher rates of preterm labour (17%) and rupture of membranes. Maternal infection rates are also increased, particularly UTIs.

FETAL – There are potential fetal complications in each trimester. The rate of miscarriage is increased in diabetic pregnancies. There is also a six-fold increase in the number of congenital anomalies, and the incidence of anomalies is related to the diabetic control immediately

pre-pregnancy, i.e. the better the control the lower the risk of anomalies. There are some anomalies that are particularly associated with diabetes, e.g. caudal regression syndrome, but there is also a general increase in the incidence of cardiac and neurological abnormalities.

Macrosomia is a common complication of diabetic pregnancies (Figure 32.1). High maternal blood glucose levels cross the placenta, leading to a fetal hyperglycaemia. The fetal pancreas responds appropriately, producing insulin, which promotes growth. Macrosomic babies are at increased risk of obstructed labour and, in particular, shoulder dystocia. Shoulder dystocia occurs at lower birth weights in diabetic pregnancies than in non-diabetic ones, and this may be because they have proportionally larger shoulders. Therefore size and wellbeing should be monitored regularly.

The perinatal mortality is increased to approximately 70/1000, and, although this is a significant improvement

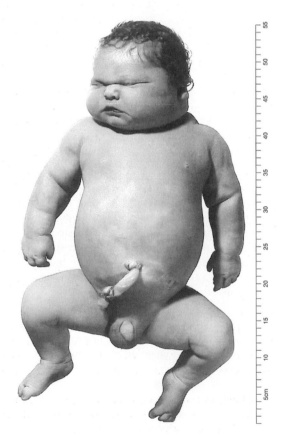

Fig 32.1 *Macrosomic baby of a diabetic mother. Reproduced, with the author's permission, from N.A. Beischer, E.V. Mackay, P.B. Colditz, Obstetrics and the Newborn, 3rd edn, 1997, W.B. Saunders.*

over historical controls, there is obviously still a long way to go to reduce this to 'normal' levels.

NEONATAL – Babies of diabetic mothers are at risk of severe hypoglycaemia after birth because of their high levels of circulating insulin – see above. Therefore, monitoring of blood glucose and early feeding are mandatory with resort to tube feeding where required.

Babies of diabetic mothers are also relatively polycythaemic and therefore at increased risk of neonatal jaundice. There are also potential metabolic complications: hypocalcaemia and hypomagnesaemia.

There is also an increase in the incidence of respiratory distress syndrome (RDS) in babies of diabetic mothers, and this is thought to be due to a change in surfactant secondary to fetal hyperglycaemia. RDS can complicate deliveries at significantly later gestations than in non-diabetic pregnancies, sometimes > 37/40.

Treatment Options

PREVENTION – Prevention of potential complications is the key to the care of diabetic pregnancies, in particular tight diabetic control. Preventative measures, including good diabetic control, should be encouraged at all stages of pregnancy: pre-pregnancy, antenatal, during labour/delivery and also postnatally.

PRE-PREGNANCY – Good prenatal care can reduce both the perinatal morbidity and mortality rate in the infants of diabetic mothers, and all diabetic women of childbearing age should be counselled, with these advantages in mind, about contraception so that pregnancy can be as planned as possible. Women should be assessed for pre-existing diabetic complications and treated prior to pregnancy.

Control of diabetes should be optimised, as good control in early pregnancy can reduce the incidence of major anomalies from 12% to under 2%. This may require a change in insulin regime, and partners should be taught how to recognise and treat hypoglycaemia. Folate supplements should also be prescribed prenatally to reduce the excess risk of neural tube defects in infants of diabetic mothers.

ANTENATAL CARE – Appropriate surveillance followed by pre-emptive delivery or delivery at term is, as usual, the key to antenatal care. Antenatal care should ideally be undertaken in a dedicated clinic, by a multidisciplinary team: obstetrician, midwife, physician and a diabetic nurse.

Diabetic antenatal care - good diabetic control particularly reduces perinatal mortality and morbidity, i.e. incidence of stillbirth, RDS, polycythaemia, etc. Therefore all women should perform regular glucose monitoring; usually 4 times a day, before meals. Women should aim to maintain their glucose levels between 4 and 7 mmol/L. Long-term control can be assessed using glycosylated haemoglobin, aiming to achieve non-diabetic levels. Multiple injections of short-acting human insulin are preferable to other regimes, but some women may require longer-acting insulins. The insulin requirement rises in pregnancy as the diabetogenic hormones increase, and therefore an increase in insulin dosage will often be required. Both hypoglycaemia and ketoacidosis are more common in pregnancy and can cause fetal death. Rapid recognition and accurate treatment are essential. Surveillance for other potential maternal diabetic complications is important. Therefore, fundi and renal function should be assessed at least each trimester.

Obstetric antenatal care – fetal anomalies are more common in diabetic pregnancies, and therefore screening is important. Refer to Chapters 3 and 28. PET is more common in diabetic pregnancies, and therefore blood pressure and urine should be checked regularly.

Fetal macrosomia, polyhydramnios and IUGR are all important complications of diabetic pregnancies, and, although they can be detected clinically by measuring the symphyseal– fundal height, most women are scanned 4 weekly until 36 weeks and 2 weekly thereafter. Fetal monitoring is important to reduce the incidence of sudden fetal death and usually includes CTGs and/or ultrasound biophysical profiles. The frequency of monitoring depends on risk assessment. Routine fetal monitoring often includes twice-weekly monitoring after 36 weeks until term. In the presence of complications, i.e. maternal vascular disease, macrosomia or polyhydramnios, monitoring should be more frequent, as fetal compromise is also more common.

LABOUR AND DELIVERY – **Timing of delivery** – ideally, all women should be allowed to proceed to full term and aim for a vaginal delivery. Prolonging pregnancy beyond term is not recommended and indeed may increase the stillbirth rate. Earlier delivery may be required in the presence of complications, as the risk of fetal compromise is increased.

Labour – it is difficult to ensure a normal intake of food in labour, and therefore to avoid a diabetic ketoacidosis and maintain normal blood glucose it is necessary to administer intravenous dextrose and insulin using a sliding-scale regime. Labour should be managed as normal, with routine continuous fetal heart monitoring. One of the most significant potential complications of diabetic labour is shoulder dystocia. Infants of diabetic mothers are at particular risk of shoulder dystocia, and shoulder dystocia might be anticipated after a slow labour. Therefore, an experienced team of midwives and obstetricians should manage the labour. Immediately after delivery the insulin requirement falls almost to pre-pregnancy levels, and as soon as the woman is eating normally again after delivery she can be restarted on her pre-pregnancy subcutaneous insulin regime.

POSTNATAL –

Neonatal: Neonatal hypoglycaemia is a very dangerous complication of the immediate postnatal period, which can lead to severe cerebral damage. Therefore feeding must be established early, with frequent blood glucose monitoring.

Maternal: Pre-pregnancy insulin should be restarted. Breast feeding reduces the insulin requirement and therefore the dose may need to be similarly reduced for breast feeding mothers.

Contraception should be discussed in hospital.

OVERVIEW – The management of a diabetic pregnancy demands tight blood glucose control from before conception to after delivery, together with appropriate surveillance and monitoring of both the mother and baby by a multidisciplinary team.

Information for Patients

PROGNOSIS – The prognosis for diabetic pregnancies has improved markedly over recent years, though the perinatal mortality and morbidity is still higher than the background rate. Both maternal and fetal complications can be reduced to a minimum by tight glucose control. The prognosis is worst for mothers with poor control and/or diabetic complications.

Follow-up

SHORT TERM – The short-term follow-up depends on the pregnancy. Many diabetic mothers may be offered the standard antenatal schedule of visits, though the frequency should be increased where complications arise.

LONG TERM – All diabetic women should be seen 6 weeks after delivery and before any planned pregnancies.

Gestational Diabetes

Background

DEFINITION – Gestational diabetes is defined as carbohydrate intolerance of variable severity with onset during pregnancy. The exact diagnostic criteria for gestational diabetes are those identified in Table 32.1.

AETIOLOGY – The exact aetiology is uncertain. Women who develop gestational diabetes are also at risk of developing NIDDM later in life. This suggests that there is a predisposition to glucose intolerance, which is revealed at times of increased stress: an inherent insulin resistance is exacerbated by the increase in anti-insulin hormones, i.e. human placental lactogen. Obesity and polycystic ovarian syndrome are related to insulin resistance and to both gestational and late-onset diabetes.

MAIN COMPLICATIONS – The risks of gestational diabetes are unclear. Whilst there is a slightly increased perinatal mortality associated with an abnormal glucose tolerance test, this is equally well predicted by the indication for the test as by the result: i.e. obesity, previous large baby or stillbirth. Therefore, there is little evidence to support the widespread screening of all pregnant women for abnormal glucose tolerance.

Maternal: Perhaps the most significant risk is the development of NIDDM later in life with all its associated potential complications. Unlike pre-existing IDDM, there is no increase in PET.

Fetal: The predominant fetal risk is macrosomia and its sequelae, e.g. shoulder dystocia. However, it is important to note that fetal size correlates with maternal weight. Therefore, obesity itself may predispose to both fetal macrosomia and an abnormal glucose tolerance.

Treatment Options

Treatment is as conservative as possible, and insulin is rarely required. However, there is no evidence that any treatment reduces the excess perinatal mortality.

DIET – Women who are overweight or who have an abnormal glucose tolerance test should be encouraged to eat a low-fat, low-refined-sugar and high-fibre diet and increase their exercise (as should everyone). In the majority of cases this will be sufficient.

INSULIN – A very small proportion of women whose pre-prandial blood glucose is consistently > 6 mmol/L may require insulin. Insulin has been demonstrated to reduce the incidence of macrosomia, though there is no associated decrease in CS rates or perinatal mortality.

Information for Patients

PROGNOSIS – The prognosis for pregnancy is generally excellent; however, the increased risk of future NIDDM is significant – 60% within the next 20 years. Obesity increases that risk, and therefore weight loss should be encouraged, though this is a general public health measure and not specific to the postpartum period.

Follow-up

SHORT TERM – Women with an abnormal glucose tolerance test should ideally be followed in a specialist multidisciplinary antenatal clinic, though there is no requirement for the additional scans, fetal monitoring, etc., obligatory for the pregnancies of women with pre-existing IDDM. Pregnancies may also be permitted to continue beyond term.

GOLDEN POINTS

1. There is an enormous difference between pre-existing IDDM in pregnancy and gestational diabetes.

2. Tight blood glucose control before, during and after pregnancy will reduce the excess perinatal mortality and morbidity to a minimum in women with IDDM.

3. Women should be cared for by a multidisciplinary team in a dedicated clinic.

4. The fetus should be monitored regularly throughout pregnancy for fetal compromise, using ultrasound scans and CTGs.

5. The mother should be monitored for potential complications, and even where the pregnancy is otherwise uncomplicated it should not progress past term.

6. Gestational diabetes is an entirely different entity where the main risk is fetal macrosomia and future development of NIDDM.

7. Screening for abnormal glucose tolerance is a variable feast and should not be offered routinely to low-risk women.

8. Insulin is very rarely required for gestational diabetes.

3

33 Large for dates

CLINICAL SIGNIFICANCE

Inconsistent uterine size is a relatively common antenatal finding. Although the majority of pregnancies are deemed to be normal after investigation it is important to exclude potentially dangerous complications of pregnancy.

Where the uterus is larger than anticipated for the gestation it is important to exclude macrosomia and polyhydramnios because of the associated increase in perinatal mortality. However, the most common causes are incorrect dates and clinical error.

The main risks are those associated with uterine overdistension, i.e. preterm labour or rupture of membranes, abnormal lie and PPH are common to all the major causes of large for dates and contribute to the excess perinatal morbidity/mortality of the condition.

DIFFERENTIAL DIAGNOSIS

MAIN CATEGORY	DIAGNOSIS
Fetus	
1. *Large fetus*	Racial differences
	Medical causes
	- Diabetes mellitus
	- Gestational diabetes
2. *Multiple pregnancy*	
Liquor	
Polyhydramnios	Fetal anomalies
	- Swallowing difficulties
	- Gut atresias
	Hydrops fetalis
	- Rhesus iso-immunisation
	- Congenital cardiac defects
	- Idiopathic
	Medical causes
	- Diabetes mellitus
	- Gestational diabetes
	Monozygotic twins
	- Twin–twin transfusion
Uterus	
Fibroids	
Miscellaneous	
Incorrect dates	Unsure
Obesity	Post-pill conception

CLINICAL ASSESSMENT

Clinical assessment of the gravid uterus can be inaccurate: there is a wide 'normal range', and measurement of the fundal height is often not reproducible. However, a suspicion of large for dates should prompt further investigation if only to exclude potential abnormalities.

After 20 weeks the symphyseal fundal height should be the same number of centimetres as weeks gestation ± 3 cm.

Rapid Emergency Assessment

A diagnosis of large-for-dates uterus rarely requires emergency assessment unless there are signs of premature labour.

Making the Diagnosis

Unlike the small-for-dates uterus, where there are few specific symptoms, a woman with a larger than expected uterus will often complain of symptoms directly related to the uterine enlargement: abdominal pain secondary to distension, difficulty sleeping and dyspnoea. The symptoms are exaggerated by rapid changes in uterine size, i.e. acute polyhydramnios.

However, the main complaint may be as simple as the endless comments about her size from her immediate peer group. Do not dismiss these comments without some further investigation, even if it is only palpation and measurement of the fundal height; you may otherwise miss something!

Relevant History

Presenting Complaint

DATES – As with the small-for-dates uterus it is first essential to verify, and correct if necessary, the gestational age. Dating from menstrual data can be wrong in up to 40% of cases, and therefore the dates should be checked against the first available scan. If there has been an ultrasound scan in the first trimester then use that, but more commonly the first routine scan is the 19–20 weeks anomaly scan.

PAIN – Pain is the commonest presenting complaint. This can vary from a diffuse abdominal pain, or a feeling of her skin being stretched, to 'contraction-like' pains. Although women with early polyhydramnios may complain of pain from 24 weeks gestation, the pain of large for dates is more common in the third trimester. Acute polyhydramnios is characteristically painful, probably because of the sudden distension of the uterus. Fibroids can be painful in pregnancy, particularly in the second trimester. See Chapter 29.

'Feels large for dates' – the patient may be asymptomatic but thought to be large.

MINOR SYMPTOMS OF PREGNANCY – Many of the minor symptoms of pregnancy are exaggerated by a large-for-dates uterus, particularly those that are related to the size of the uterus, i.e. pressure-dependent ankle oedema, varicose veins and haemorrhoids, where increased pressure is put on pelvic venous return and the effects are seen downstream. Oesophageal reflux is also more common.

The mother may also complain of dyspnoea. This is because the increased size of the uterus exaggerates the normal flaring of the lower margin of the rib cage and reduces the movement of the diaphragm, which gives rise to short shallow breaths and consequently a feeling of breathlessness.

Obstetric History

INDEX PREGNANCY – An early scan may have identified a fetal anomaly predisposing to polyhydramnios (see above) or identified a multiple pregnancy or indeed incidentally identified fibroids. Equally, the woman may have been noted as being rhesus negative on routine booking blood tests, and this should raise the index of suspicion for rhesus disease in the presence of polyhydramnios. It is important to note the gestation where there is a possibility of preterm labour.

OBSTETRIC HISTORY – A previous large baby predisposes to further large babies, and it is important to note a previous baby with weight > 4.5 kg. Note a previous history of gestational diabetes or an abnormal glucose tolerance test in pregnancy. Rhesus disease classically complicates multigravid women, as the commonest time for rhesus isoimmunisation is at delivery of the first child. However, it is not exclusive to multips. Rhesus isoimmunisation classically recurs in future pregnancies, and it is therefore important to note previous episodes. There are some rare genetic diseases that are potentially recurrent and predispose to polyhydramnios i.e. myotonic dystrophy. Ensure that previous children are normal and that there are no diseases that run in the family.

Gynaecological History

Fibroids may be symptomatic outside pregnancy, classically causing menorrhagia (see Chapter 7).

Medical History

Both gestational NIDDM and pre-existing IDDM are associated both with polyhydramnios and fetal macrosomia (see Chapter 32).

Drug History

For once there is little association with drugs or smoking.

Social History

Low socioeconomic status correlates with abnormal glucose tolerance, possibly due to poor-quality nutrition and the increased incidence of obesity.

Relevant Clinical Examination

General Features

GENERAL – Large mothers have large babies. Maternal weight directly correlates with fetal weight, and obesity is associated with abnormal glucose tolerance; therefore an assessment of maternal size is important. General examination should confirm the presence of lower-limb oedema, varicose veins, etc., where present.

Abdomen

GENERAL – On abdominal palpation, try to identify whether the uterine contents are 'all baby' or 'all water.'

PREGNANCY – A large-for-dates uterus would be > 3 cm above the expected size. The measurement of abdominal girth is not used in routine clinical practice.

Polyhydramnios distends the uterus and produces a tight feeling uterus. Fetal parts are not readily palpable, because of the increased amount of liquor separating the examining hand from the fetus. Similarly, the fetal heart may also be difficult to hear. Polyhydramnios also predisposes to abnormal presentation and lie, as there is a greater intrauterine volume than normal.

Fetal macrosomia palpates differently: the fetal parts are easily palpable and there is rarely an abnormal lie, as there is little room for manoeuvre. The fetal head may not be engaged if it is very large. Remember that polyhydramnios and fetal macrosomia can coexist, so the picture may not always be completely clear.

Multiple pregnancy is usually diagnosed on routine booking scan, though the palpation of more than two fetal poles should prompt further investigation.

Occasionally, it is possible to palpate individual fibroids, particularly if they are large and sited anteriorly or at the fundus. They can be tender. The presence of a cervical fibroid may also prevent engagement of the fetal head.

Pelvis

VAGINAL EXAMINATION – There is no need to routinely perform a vaginal examination, except perhaps where there is a suspicion of preterm labour or that a cervical fibroid may obstruct labour.

Relevant Investigations

Haematology

It is important to assess rhesus status. If the mother is rhesus (antigen) negative and rhesus isoimmunisation is suspected then her own anti-D antibody levels can be measured. Obviously the higher the maternal antibody level, the more likely the baby is to be affected, because the antibodies can easily cross the placenta and produce haemolysis of the fetal red cells. Maternal anti-D > 15 i.u. is abnormal and warrants further investigation.

Biochemistry

The problems of screening for abnormal glucose tolerance are described in Chapter 32. However, a large-for-dates uterus merits a glucose tolerance test.

Cytology

Chromosomal abnormalities are associated with gut atresias and many fetal cardiac abnormalities. In the presence of these and other abnormalities, a cordocentesis, or amniocentesis, is often undertaken to obtain fetal blood for cytology.

Microbiology

Similarly, fetal blood obtained at cordocentesis can be examined serologically for intrauterine viral infection, e.g. parvovirus infection leading to fetal anaemia and subsequent polyhydramnios.

Diagnostic Imaging

USS – Ultrasound scanning is essential for the diagnosis, investigation and management of the large-for-dates uterus. Ultrasound is used to:

- identify fetal number and chorionicity, i.e. monozygotic or dizygotic twins
- identify and quantify polyhydramnios/macrosomia
- identify any underlying aetiologies
- monitor fetus/liquor volume.

LIQUOR VOLUME – There are a number of different methods used to measure liquor volume. Most commonly the deepest pool is measured and should normally be between 2 and 8 cm.

FETAL SIZE – Fetal macrosomia is a measurement of size. The abdominal circumference (ac) is classically used, and an ac > 90th centile is deemed macrosomic. Fetal fat can also be visualised in macrosomic infants, particularly around the abdomen and head. Fetal growth per se is less important than in small-for-dates babies.

ANOMALIES – Major structural anomalies are more common, especially in association with polyhydramnios. See below for details.

CTG

Similarly, CTGs are also used to monitor fetal wellbeing. See also Chapter 32.

DETAILS OF INDIVIDUAL CONDITIONS

1. Polyhydramnios

Background

Polyhydramnios is associated with risks of uterine overdistension, and these risks are compounded by the related increase in major structural fetal abnormalities.

DEFINITION – Polyhydramnios is defined as a pool depth at ultrasound of > 8 cm.

AETIOLOGY – Amniotic fluid is produced by the cells that line the amniotic cavity. There is a normal circulation of the amniotic fluid where the fetus swallows liquor, absorbs it in the gut and excretes it as urine. Therefore conditions where excess fluid is produced, characteristically by a large placenta, or conditions where fetal swallowing or gut absorption is impaired, will cause polyhydramnios.

Hydrops fetalis is basically fetal heart failure, precipitated by a number of different causes. Adult heart failure is characterised by excess interstitial fluid, and likewise so is hydrops fetalis, with generalised oedema of the skin, ascites and polyhydramnios. See Box 33.1.

MAIN COMPLICATIONS –

Maternal: The main maternal complications are related to uterine overdistension:

- antenatal: premature rupture of membranes, premature labour, unstable lie

Box 33.1 Aetiology of polyhydramnios

Maternal

Increased placental area	– Multiple pregnancy
	– Diabetes mellitus

Fetal

Anomalies that impair swallowing	
	– Anencephaly
	– Spina bifida
	– Myotonic dystrophy
Reduction in the area of the gut available to absorb fluid	– Gut atresias
	– Oesophageal
	– Duodenal
	– Jejunal
Hydrops fetalis	– The most common causes are related to 'high output' heart failure particularly anaemia. Rhesus iso-immunisation and some intrauterine viral infections, particularly parvovirus, can cause fetal anaemia
	– Other causes include structural heart defects, some associated with chromosomal abnormalities, and there are of course idiopathic causes

Neonatal

Tracheo-oesophageal fistula	– TOF predisposes to polyhydramnios and should be excluded prior to feeding in babies born with associated polyhydramnios

– intrapartum: cord prolapse
– postpartum: postpartum haemorrhage (see Chapter 43).

Fetal: The main fetal complications are related to premature delivery and fetal asphyxia secondary to complications including cord prolapse. Other complications relate to the fetal anomalies which initially precipitated the polyhydramnios, i.e. chromosomal abnormalities, cardiac defects and gut atresias.

Treatment Options

Once a diagnosis has been made, it is important to exclude any treatable causes, e.g. fetal anaemia, and rule out any intrinsic fetal conditions. Paediatricians should be alerted to attend the delivery to examine the baby immediately.

CONSERVATIVE AND REASSURANCE – Mild polyhydramnios can be managed conservatively, particularly where the pregnancy is > 34 weeks and the potential dangers of preterm labour are reduced.

MEDICAL – Simple analgesia, e.g. paracetemol, can also be prescribed. NSAIDs, especially indomethacin, have been used both to directly reduce polyhydramnios by reducing fetal urine output and also to inhibit preterm labour. However, there are theoretical risks of premature closure of the ductus arteriosus associated with treatment, and it is not used routinely in the UK.

SURGICAL – In more severe cases (< 35 weeks), serial amniocentesis is used to directly reduce the liquor volume, although half the women will go into labour. After 35 weeks gestation, induction of labour should be considered.

Fetal anaemia, secondary to rhesus isoimmunisation or parvovirus infection, can be treated by direct blood transfusion into the umbilical vein at cordocentesis. This often needs repeating at intervals. Treatment of the anaemia will reduce the hydrops.

Information for Patients

PROGNOSIS – The fetal prognosis for pregnancies complicated by polyhydramnios is largely dependent on gestation and any underlying causal defects. Overall, the prognosis is good, particularly for fetal anaemia treated by transfusion. Maternal prognosis can be improved by anticipating potential problems and invoking preventative measures, e.g. prophylactic oxytocics for the third stage of labour.

Follow-up

SHORT TERM – The follow-up regime for women with pregnancies complicated by polyhydramnios depends on the precipitating cause. Uncomplicated polyhydramnios can be managed on an outpatient basis, and even fetal transfusions are managed on that basis. However, severe symptomatic polyhydramnios should be managed in hospital and particularly where there is a risk of preterm labour.

LONG TERM – Prenatal counselling may be required after poor perinatal outcomes and potentially recurrent causes of polyhydramnios, e.g. rhesus isoimmunisation.

2. Multiple Pregnancy

See Chapter 35.

3. Large Fetus/Macrosomia

Background

DEFINITION – There is no universally accepted definition for macrosomia, although an estimated fetal weight > 90th centile and/or a birth weight > 4.5 kg are both used. There is less concern about the rate of growth in these infants than in their small-for-dates peers, as intra-uterine compromise is not such a feature; indeed rather the reverse.

AETIOLOGY – There is a wide racial difference in birth weights and Afro-Caribbeans characteristically have the largest babies. Maternal size is also a significant factor; heavy mothers have heavy babies. Therefore there are a number of constitutional factors that can contribute to a normal, large baby.

However, macrosomia is a much more sinister finding in the infants of diabetic mothers (see Chapter 32). A high maternal blood glucose crosses the placenta and stimulates the fetal pancreas. The resultant hyper-insulinaemia stimulates growth and therefore macrosomia. However, this hyperinsulinaemia has a number of potentially dangerous consequences both in and ex utero (see Chapter 32).

MAIN COMPLICATIONS –

Maternal: The main maternal complication of fetal macrosomia is obstructed labour (see Chapter 40).

Fetal: In diabetic pregnancies a macrosomic fetus, particularly with associated polyhydramnios, can be a sign of poor diabetic control, and the fetus is at risk of metabolic compromise; therefore it is important to regularly monitor the fetus as described in Chapter 32. Where the mother is not diabetic the risks of fetal compromise are significantly less.

One potential complication common to all large babies is shoulder dystocia. This is a very dangerous complication of delivery where the shoulders impact against the inside of the maternal bony pelvis after delivery of the head. Simply pulling on the head will not expedite delivery, there are a series of manoeuvres that must be performed, including pushing down on the anterior shoulder by suprapubic pressure, rotating the shoulders into an oblique position and finally delivering the posterior arm and using this to 'corkscrew' the baby out.

Overzealous pulling on the head in shoulder dystocia can injure the brachial nerve plexus and result in nerve palsies, particularly Erb's palsy. There is also a risk of fetal bony fractures, particularly the humerus and clavicle. Where attempts to deliver the baby are unsuccessful the baby can die on the perineum, an obviously devastating occurrence.

Treatment Options

Once a diagnosis has been made, it is important to exclude an occult abnormal glucose tolerance, and therefore a GTT should be performed. The treatment options are limited; there is no treatment that will 'shrink' the baby. In women with gestational diabetes, diet control does not seem to prevent macrosomia, and although putting these women on insulin will reduce the incidence of macrosomia, the incidence of obstructed labour and shoulder dystocia remains unchanged!

The main treatment options are, as usual in obstetrics, surveillance followed by pre-emptive delivery. Induction of labour may seem a likely option but there is an increased risk of an emergency caesarean section and instrumental delivery. In the USA there is an increasing trend towards performing a caesarean section for mothers whose babies have an estimated weight > 4 kg, but this will mean that many babies will be delivered by caesarean section unnecessarily with the consequent increased maternal and fetal risks of CS. In the UK, women are encouraged to deliver in a consultant unit with experienced obstetricians and midwives in attendance. A slow labour should alert the obstetric team to the possibility of shoulder dystocia.

Information for Patients

PROGNOSIS – The prognosis for macrosomic fetuses is generally good, especially where the mother is not diabetic.

SELF-HELP GROUPS – Self-help groups are available for women with diabetes, and there is also an Erb's Palsy self-help group.

Follow-up

SHORT TERM – Diabetic mothers should be managed as per the regime outlined in the chapter on diabetes in pregnancy. In non-diabetic mothers, the risks of fetal compromise are much less, and therefore the monitoring can be less intensive – kick charts and scans for growth.

LONG TERM – There is an increased recurrence risk after one baby > 4.5 kg, and therefore it is important to exclude an occult gestational diabetes and be aware of the risks of shoulder dystocia.

4. Other Causes

The management of the other causes of large for dates is problem specific though it is largely conservative.

Fibroids

Fibroids rarely cause problems in pregnancy. Occasionally they can cause pain if they infarct during pregnancy – haemorrhagic infarction ⇒ red degeneration. They may also obstruct labour if big enough and at the cervix, but this is extremely uncommon.

GOLDEN POINTS

1. Check the dates carefully before making a diagnosis of large for dates.

2. The main risks of the large-for-dates uterus are related to overdistension – premature labour and PPH.

3. It is important to exclude or identify polyhydramnios and/or fetal macrosomia, as these are associated with an increased perinatal mortality.

4. Polyhydramnios is mainly related to maternal diabetes, rhesus disease and fetal disorders that obstruct the GI tract.

5. Polyhydramnios can be treated conservatively or by serial amniocenteses until the fetus is sufficiently advanced to merit delivery.

6. Shoulder dystocia and obstructed labour are two potential complications common to all large babies. Concurrent maternal diabetes can compound these.

7. Other causes can usually be managed conservatively.

34 Small for dates

CLINICAL SIGNIFICANCE

Inconsistent uterine size is a relatively common antenatal finding. Although the majority of pregnancies are deemed to be normal after investigation, it is important to exclude potentially dangerous complications of pregnancy.

Where the uterus is smaller than anticipated for the gestation it is important to exclude intrauterine growth retardation and oligohydramnios because of their associated increase in perinatal mortality. However, the most common causes are incorrect dates and clinical error.

One of the most important, and difficult, concepts to understand in the small-for-dates (SFD) fetus is the distinction between fetal size and fetal growth: babies below the 10th centile, or >2 standard deviations below the expected mean for the gestation, are defined as small though not necessarily growth retarded. IUGR is a reduction of growth velocity and therefore the diagnosis can only be made after estimating size on at least two occasions. The estimated fetal weight will not follow the projected growth pattern, i.e. the baby is not fulfilling it's growth potential (see Figure 34.1).

Small babies are usually genetically small; there is an intrinsic cause (low growth potential), e.g. babies of Asian mothers, mothers of small stature, or babies compromised by a very early insult such as viral infection or congenital defects. In contrast, the main aetiology of growth retardation is extrinsic: inadequate nutrition often secondary to poor placental function.

DIFFERENTIAL DIAGNOSIS

MAIN CATEGORY	DIAGNOSIS
Fetal causes	
Small fetus	Constitutional
	Racial differences
	Chromosomal abnormality
	− Trisomies 13, 18, 21
	Fetal infection
	− Cytomegalovirus
	Intrauterine growth
	− Medical complications
	− PET
	Retardation (IUGR)
	− Socio-economic
	− Placental insufficiency
	Intrauterine death
Liquor	
Oligohydramnios	Fetal anomalies
	− Renal agenesis
	− Urethral obstruction
	Placental insufficiency
	Premature rupture of
	membranes
Miscellaneous	
Incorrect dates	Unsure
	Post-pill conception

CLINICAL ASSESSMENT

Clinical assessment of the gravid uterus is notoriously inaccurate. There is an enormous 'normal range' and interobserver error. Only 50% of SFD fetuses are recognised as such. However, routine antenatal practice still includes assessment of the symphyseal – fundal height as a screening test for uterine size which indirectly also measures the contents, i.e. fetus and liquor.

After 20 weeks the fundal height should be the same number of centimetres as weeks gestation ± 3 cm.

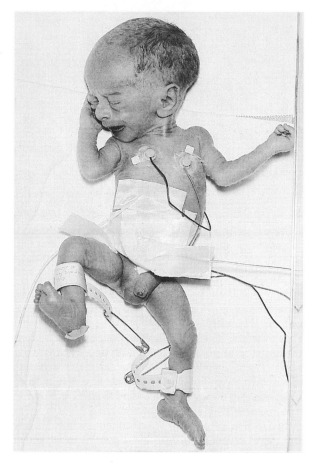

Fig 34.1 *Neonatal picture of growth-retarded baby. Reproduced, with the author's permission, from N.A. Beischer, E.V. Mackay, P.B. Colditz, Obstetrics and the Newborn, 3rd edn, 1997, W.B. Saunders.*

Making the Diagnosis

It is essential to establish the correct gestational age prior to any other investigation. You must establish the gestational age from dates or an early scan as reliably as possible, and if there is any doubt then use the scan dates.

Relevant History

Presenting Complaint

Small for dates is usually a clinical finding, and there is usually no presenting complaint as such, unless the relatives pass comment on the small size of the mother!

Obstetric History

INDEX PREGNANCY – The LMP should be carefully documented together with details of the cycle. Up to 40% of mothers cannot remember their last menstrual period or subsequently their recollection proves to be inaccurate; therefore, ultrasound estimation of gestational age is often used where there is any doubt.

Details of pre-pregnancy contraception can be helpful, particularly the oral contraceptive pill because regular ovulatory cycles may not immediately return and there may be a variable period of 'post-pill amenorrhoea' after discontinuation of the pill. A history of decreased fetal movements is important, as this can be a sign of fetal compromise. A history of any maternal viral illnesses early in pregnancy is important, as intrauterine infection with cytomegalovirus can impair fetal growth. Any history of fluid loss per vaginam should be elicited to exclude ruptured membranes.

OBSTETRIC HISTORY – The largest single risk factor for the delivery of a SFD infant is a previous history; therefore it is important to document previous birth weights. Similarly, birth order is important: a woman who is clinically small after previous well-grown babies should alert suspicion.

Medical History

There is an increased risk of both oligohydramnios and growth retardation with hypertensive disease. Chronic illness, e.g. renal failure or inflammatory bowel disease, can also predispose to IUGR.

Drug History

DRUGS – IUGR is strongly associated with drug use. Some drugs directly reduce placental perfusion through vasoconstriction e.g. cocaine, whereas others indirectly contribute to IUGR through the poor nutrition, etc., associated with the chaotic life led by many drug abusers.

CIGARETTES – Heavy smoking is associated with small babies, probably because smoking reduces placental perfusion.

ALCOHOL – Drinking in excess of 2 standard measures daily throughout pregnancy is associated with developmental abnormalities, and heavier drinking can also lead to growth retardation.

Social History

Low socioeconomic class correlates with small babies.

Relevant Clinical Examination

General Features

GENERAL – Small mothers have small babies; indeed there are physiological, maternal constraints placed on intrauterine growth to ensure 'normal' delivery, and therefore it is important to note the maternal size. Features of predisposing causes should also be sought, e.g. hypertensive disease as well as evidence of heavy smoking, etc.

Abdomen

PREGNANCY – The symphyseal–fundal height will be less than expected (3 cm or more less than expected). Oligohydramnios can be suspected where the fetal parts are very easily felt, i.e. the normal 'cushion' of liquor is absent. Breech presentation is more common in the SFD pregnancy though the exact mechanism is unclear. Various theories have been proposed: it may be more difficult to rotate to cephalic where there is oligohydramnios, a compromised baby may move less, or abnormal babies may not move around properly; it is not clear.

Pelvis

VAGINAL EXAMINATION –

Speculum: A speculum examination may identify liquor in the vagina after rupture of membranes.

Vaginal examination: Vaginal examination should be avoided where there is a possibility of ruptured membranes. After ROM has been excluded and induction of labour is contemplated, then the cervical state can be assessed to aid decision making.

Relevant Investigations

Haematology and Biochemistry

Serological investigations are rarely useful except where investigation of concurrent complications is required, e.g. PET. Biochemical investigation of fetal wellbeing (oestriol and human placental lactogen) is not useful and no longer undertaken except in a research context.

Cytology

Chromosomal abnormalities are associated with IUGR, and a cordocentesis can be undertaken to obtain fetal blood for cytology.

Microbiology

Fetal blood obtained at cordocentesis can be examined serologically for intrauterine viral infection.

Diagnostic Imaging

USS – Ultrasound scanning is essential for the diagnosis, investigation and management of the SFD uterus. Indeed, they most commonly refute a diagnosis of small for dates.

LIQUOR VOLUME – There are a number of different methods used to measure liquor volume. Most commonly the deepest pool is measured (see Figure 34.2) and should normally be between 2 and 8 cm. Liquor volumes do change with gestation but the above general limits apply throughout. Occasionally the deepest pool is measured in 4 quadrants and the depths averaged. There appears to be no added advantage gained by using the latter, more complicated method.

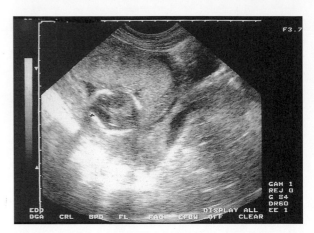

Fig 34.2 *USS demonstrating oligohydramnios. With kind permission of Dr Heather Andrews, Bristol.*

GROWTH – Classically, the estimated fetal weight, and therefore size, is calculated from two different fetal parameters: abdominal circumference and biparietal diameter, but the abdominal circumference alone is often used in clinical practice. Babies with an estimated fetal weight < 10th centile are defined as small. However, it is important to remember that growth is different from size, and at least two measurements of size are required to measure growth velocity: see IUGR.

ANOMALIES – Major structural and chromosomal anomalies are more common in the presence of both oligohydramnios and small babies; see below for details. Therefore it is important not just to make the diagnosis but also to identify any potential causes, e.g. renal agenesis for oligohydramnios.

BIOPHYSICAL PROFILE – The biophysical profile comprises four different ultrasound parameters: fetal movements, fetal breathing movements, fetal tone and liquor volume, and a CTG trace. These parameters have been combined in an attempt to improve the predictive value of the individual measurements for impending fetal doom. It is used though it is not 100% accurate.

DOPPLER – Doppler ultrasound is used to measure blood flow in fetal arteries. Alterations in blood flow can be an early indication of fetal compromise, because part of the normal fetal response to inadequate nutrition is to redistribute blood flow from peripheral viscera to the brain. Therefore, where there is an increase in blood flow to the head and a decrease more peripherally, then compromise can be suspected.

Also, particular waveforms can be seen which are suggestive of compromise (see Figure 34.3). Doppler ultrasound has been shown to be useful in managing

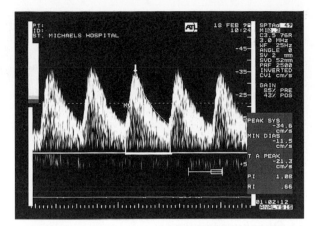

Fig 34.3 *Doppler ultrasound of the umbilical cord demonstrating normal wave forms. With kind permission of Dr Heather Andrews, Bristol.*

pregnancies complicated by IUGR but not as a screening test in a low-risk population.

CTG

The CTG is commonly used to assess immediate fetal condition, and the interpretation of traces uses similar criteria to those for intrapartum traces (see Chapter 39). However, the value of these tests is not well established. There are problems with interpretation of preterm traces, and CTGs appear to be better at identifying acute hypoxia – i.e. secondary to an acute event, abruption – rather than the chronic hypoxia more commonly found in IUGR. These problems notwithstanding, CTGs are commonly employed throughout the UK.

DETAILS OF INDIVIDUAL CONDITIONS

1. Small Fetus/Intrauterine Growth Retardation

Background

DEFINITION – It is important to understand or at least recognise the distinction between fetal size and fetal growth. Babies below the 10th centile, or > 2 standard deviations below the expected mean for the gestation, are defined as small though not necessarily growth retarded. IUGR is a reduction of growth velocity and therefore the diagnosis can only be made after estimating size on at least two occasions: characteristically 2 weeks apart. The estimated fetal weight will not follow the projected growth pattern, i.e. the baby is not fulfilling its growth potential (see Figure 34.1).

AETIOLOGY – Small babies are usually genetically small.

There is an intrinsic cause (low growth potential): e.g. babies of Asian mothers or mothers of small stature themselves, though babies compromised by a very early insult such as viral infection or congenital defects can also be small.

In contrast, the main aetiology of growth retardation is extrinsic: inadequate nutrition often secondary to poor placental function. The fetus responds to this hostile environment by invoking physiological changes to maximise its survival chances: redistributing blood flow from peripheral viscera to the brain and reducing fetal movements. These changes form the basis of the tests used for fetal assessment.

Maternal:
- **Socioeconomic factors** – mothers from socio-economic groups IV and V are often lighter, less well nourished and smoke more than their counterparts in higher socioeconomic groups.
- **Smoking** – it is clear that maternal smoking reduces birth weight, probably by reducing placental perfusion.
- **Drug abuse** is associated with growth retardation. This may be a direct effect, e.g. crack and cocaine will both reduce placental perfusion, or an indirect one through drug addict lifestyle.
- **Medical complications** – hypertensive disease is associated with reduced placental perfusion and subsequently IUGR. Diabetes mellitus can similarly cause IUGR as well as the more obvious macrosomia. Antepartum haemorrhage is also associated with IUGR. Antiphospholipid antibodies can cause placental infarction, which will reduce the surface area of functioning placenta therefore causing IUGR.

Fetal:
- **Congenital anomalies** – babies with an abnormal karyotype are characteristically small.
- **Intrauterine viral infection** also can cause early IUGR.
- Siblings from **multiple pregnancies** are characteristically smaller than their singleton counterparts.

MAIN COMPLICATIONS –
Maternal: The main maternal complications are from any precipitating causes of the IUGR, e.g. PET.
Fetal: There can be a significant fetal morbidity and mortality. The perinatal mortality is higher for growth-retarded babies: they are more likely to be delivered prematurely, suffer from perinatal asphyxia and can be stillborn.

There is a neonatal morbidity: hypoglycaemia secondary to poor nutrition, and polycythaemia secondary to chronic intrauterine hypoxia. This polycythaemia subsequently results in hyperbilirubinaemia. Birth asphyxia and its consequences are also more common as there is less physiological reserve.

Treatment Options

Once a diagnosis has been made, it is important to exclude any treatable causes – stop smoking, manage any medical causes, e.g. PET, and rule out any intrinsic fetal conditions such as chromosomal abnormality. Subsequently, as in all high-risk pregnancies, the management is surveillance followed by pre-emptive delivery. Supportive treatment until fetal maturity allows delivery, ideally > 37 weeks gestation, or the IUGR compromises fetal health.

CONSERVATIVE AND REASSURANCE – The methods of surveillance have been previously discussed in the Investigations section. However, there is no ideal method of assessing fetal wellbeing; consequently, a battery of tests are frequently employed, including ultrasound estimation of weight and growth, Doppler examination of the umbilical artery flow, and CTGs of the fetal heart rate. Timing of delivery can therefore be difficult, particularly for severely premature babies.

Intrauterine growth retardation can be managed on an outpatient basis with regular hospital visits. Admission to hospital is sometimes recommended, particularly where there is an underlying medical complication such as PET. However, there is no evidence that bed rest improves outcome.

Where early delivery is anticipated, steroids should be administered to enhance fetal lung maturity.

MEDICAL – There have been attempts to directly feed the growth-retarded fetus by infusing glucose and/or amino acids either indirectly intravenously via the mother or directly using cordocentesis into the baby. Unsurprisingly, these methods have been unsuccessful: poor placental function is a barrier, and, where glucose was administered directly to the baby, the baby became more acidotic because of the necessarily anaerobic metabolism demanded by a hypoxic fetus.

The main medical treatment is therefore induction of labour. However, induction of labour is often unsuccessful in severely affected fetuses because they have insufficient physiological reserve for labour at gestations of less than 37 weeks.

SURGICAL – Surgical intervention is delivery by caesarean section, and this is favoured where induction of labour is unlikely to be successful, as described above.

Information for Patients

PROGNOSIS – The prognosis for growth-retarded fetuses is generally good, particularly for those where placental dysfunction is the primary problem. They often exhibit 'catch up' growth after delivery. However, other causes such as chromosomal abnormality and intrauterine viral infections have a less optimistic outlook.

Follow-up

SHORT TERM – Routine management does not require hospital admission. Kick charts can be useful for the mother. Facilities for the necessary surveillance are often accommodated in a Day Assessment Unit with twice weekly visits for CTGs and Doppler examination as well as fortnightly growth scans.

LONG TERM – There is an increased recurrence risk after IUGR and also some of the causes, e.g. PET, and therefore careful follow-up is often required in ensuing pregnancies.

2. Oligohydramnios

Background

DEFINITION – Oligohydramnios is said to be present when the largest pocket of liquor is < 2 cm depth, measured at ultrasound scan. The diagnosis of oligohydramnios is important as a marker of high-risk pregnancy, particularly fetal abnormality and/or fetal hypoxia.

AETIOLOGY – From the second trimester, one of the main components of liquor is fetal urine. Therefore conditions that reduce, or impede, fetal urine output can result in oligohydramnios:

Maternal:
- Direct causes: rupture of membranes.
- Indirect causes: secondary to poor placental perfusion.
- Drugs: drugs that reduce fetal urine output directly, e.g. NSAIDs and ACE inhibitors, will reduce liquor volume.

Fetal:
- Anomalies: renal agenesis, without kidneys no urine will be produced at all, producing very early, severe oligohydramnios.
- Renal dysplasia and cystic kidneys impair fetal urine output.
- Urethral valves block the urethra, impairing urine output into the amniotic cavity. Note that because voiding of the urine is impeded, the bladder, and later the upper urinary tract, become distended.
- Hypoxia: chronic fetal hypoxia invokes various fetal compensatory changes, including a reduction in visceral blood flow; the decrease in renal blood flow reduces urine output, and consequently the liquor volume is similarly reduced.

MAIN COMPLICATIONS –

Maternal: There are few direct maternal complications of oligohydramnios except perhaps ascending infection after prolonged rupture of the membranes.

Fetal: Oligohydramnios is a marker of high-risk pregnancy: the incidence of major lethal abnormalities and the perinatal mortality rates are both increased almost forty fold by oligohydramnios. Indirect risks associated with oligohydramnios include IUGR, chronic intra-uterine asphyxia and intrauterine death. More directly, oligohydramnios reduces the 'room' inside the amniotic cavity and this can impair fetal movement: reduced fetal breathing movements allow lung fluid to egress and thence pulmonary hypoplasia. Similarly, a lack of room can directly compress the baby, resulting in fixed flexion deformities including talipes.

Treatment Options

The management of oligohydramnios requires the exclusion of fetal anomalies, growth retardation and ruptured membranes, followed by supportive measures until the fetus is mature enough for delivery.

Amnio-infusion has been advocated to reduce some of the direct fetal complications of intrauterine compression, though this has been largely unsuccessful. It is more commonly used in early pregnancy to visualise the fetus properly, in particular to diagnose renal agenesis.

Termination of pregnancy can be offered in severe, early oligohydramnios or where there is a major lethal abnormality, as the prognosis is extremely poor. Otherwise the management is as for specific conditions: IUGR and fetal growth retardation.

Information for Patients

PROGNOSIS – The prognosis is generally good except where there is severe, early oligohydramnios or where there is a major lethal abnormality as above. The prognosis after rupture of membranes is dependent upon the gestation, and likewise the prognosis with IUGR.

Follow-up

SHORT TERM – Women with uncomplicated oligohydramnios and those where the liquor is reduced secondary to poor placental perfusion can be followed as for IUGR. Women with severe, early oligohydramnios can also be followed up as outpatients until a definitive cause is identified, and they can be counselled about the potentially poor outcomes, usually by a multidisciplinary team.

LONG TERM – A 'debriefing' visit may be required after a complicated postnatal period, usually scheduled for 6 weeks.

3. Other Causes

The management of the other causes of small for dates is problem specific, though it is largely conservative.

Rupture of Membranes

Please refer to Chapter 37.

Incorrect Dates

Correct the dates.

GOLDEN POINTS

1. Small for dates is a clinical finding which should alert the clinician to the possibility of fetal compromise.

2. The majority of women deemed small for dates are subsequently found to be normal after appropriate investigation.

3. The distinction between size and growth is important, as there are different causes: intrinsic and extrinsic, respectively.

4. Oligohydramnios can be a manifestation of both fetal compromise and fetal anomaly.

5. The management of small for dates is surveillance followed by preemptive delivery.

6. Fetal assessment is an imprecise art, and therefore a combination of ultrasound, Doppler and heart rate monitoring is used.

7. Consider steroids where appropriate.

35 Multiple pregnancy

CLINICAL SIGNIFICANCE

All complications of pregnancy and labour are increased with multiple pregnancy.

The perinatal mortality of twins and triplets is correspondingly higher than for singleton pregnancies. The increase is mainly due to the high rate of preterm delivery (> 25% are delivered < 37/40), but there are other aetiologies too: increased rates of congenital abnormality, asphyxia and problems at delivery.

The problems of multiple pregnancy do not stop at delivery. The problems of looking after two or more small babies should not be underestimated – it is very hard work indeed! These problems are compounded where there have been complications through congenital abnormality or prematurity. Not surprisingly, women report higher rates of anxiety and depression after multiple pregnancy. Community support and follow-up should be available.

The incidence of twin pregnancy is classically quoted as 1:80, and higher multiples follow Hellin's law, i.e. triplets $1:80^2$ and quads $1:80^3$. However, the incidence of multiple pregnancy has been increased by assisted conception techniques.

The incidence of monozygotic twins is virtually constant at 30% of the total. It is the incidence of dizygotic twins that varies with maternal age and across national boundaries. The excess mortality of multiple pregnancy is increased still further in monozygotic twins because of the extra problems specific to monozygous twins: for example, malformation, i.e. conjoined twins, and abnormal placental connections resulting in twin–twin transfusion, etc.

DIFFERENTIAL DIAGNOSIS

Multiple pregnancy	Assisted conception
	Natural cycle
Other causes of 'large for dates'	
Main categories	
1. *Fetal macrosomia*	
2. *Polyhydramnios*	
3. *Uterine abnormalities*	Fibroids

CLINICAL ASSESSMENT

In the UK the vast majority of women routinely have a scan as part of their screening programme for congenital pregnancy either in the first or second trimester. Therefore, undiagnosed multiple pregnancies are rare. However, there are some women who do not book and who decline an ultrasound scan, and a clinical diagnosis can be required.

Rapid Emergency Assessment

Is rarely required unless the woman is labouring and the administration of Syntometrine for the third stage would be a disaster for any subsequent fetus. An ultrasound scan should be performed where there is any suspicion of undiagnosed twins.

Relevant History

Commonly Associated Symptoms

SYMPTOMS OF PREGNANCY – The physiological changes of pregnancy are exaggerated by multiple pregnancy: there is an increase in the plasma volume, a lesser increase in the red cell mass and an increase in all the pregnancy-related hormones. These changes contribute to an increase in the normal symptoms of pregnancy: e.g. hyperemesis gravidarum is increased in the first trimester secondary to the increased levels of β-hCG. All minor symptoms of pregnancy are also increased: back pain, reflux, insomnia, etc.

Gynaecological History

SUBFERTILITY – Assisted reproduction techniques increase the risk of multiple pregnancy. Even in the best centres, 10–15% of pregnancies after gonadotrophin stimulation are multiple, and up to one quarter of those will be triplets or more. The risks are reduced with other methods of ovulation induction, e.g. clomiphene.

Obstetric History

DELIVERIES – A history of multiple pregnancy increases the likelihood of multiple pregnancy in subsequent pregnancies.

Social History

AGE – The risks of multiple pregnancy are increased with maternal age, though the aetiology is unclear. A family history of multiple pregnancy increases the incidence of multiple pregnancy, and again the aetiology is unclear, though most of the excess twinning is dizygotic. Similarly, the increased rates of multiple pregnancy seen in Afro-Caribbeans are dizygotic.

Relevant Clinical Examination

General Features

GENERAL – The normal findings of pregnancy are exaggerated. There may be more oedema, but apart from looking larger than expected for a singleton pregnancy there are few general physical findings characteristic of multiple pregnancy.

Abdomen

GENERAL – Check for abdominal scars, including laparoscopy scars, as treatment for subfertility will predispose to multiple pregnancy.

PREGNANCY – The uterus is larger than expected. The palpation of > 2 fetal poles suggests a diagnosis of multiple pregnancy in a woman who is large for dates. By contrast, in pregnancies complicated by polyhydramnios, the cushion of extra fluid and tight abdominal skin prevents palpation at all. However, polyhydramnios is more common in twin pregnancies, and the two may coexist.

Pelvis

VAGINAL EXAMINATION –

Vulva/vagina: The extra burden of multiple pregnancy increases the risk of vulval varicosities.

Cervix: In continental Europe most women undergo a vaginal examination to assess the cervix as part of a screen for premature labour; bed rest can be recommended for those women whose cervix is showing early signs of labour, i.e. softening, effacement or dilatation. Although women with multiple pregnancies are at increased risk of premature labour, routine examination of the cervix is not performed in the UK.

Uterus: The uterus is larger than expected at all gestations.

Relevant Investigations

The booking investigations should be completed as normal. However, there are problems specific to multiple pregnancy.

Haematology

Anaemia complicates approximately 3% of singleton pregnancies and 15% of multiple pregnancies. The increase is partly as a result of dilution secondary to an increased plasma volume and partly because of the increased nutritional requirements of multiple pregnancy. Routine iron and folate supplementation has therefore been advocated for women with multiple pregnancy.

Serum Screening

Biochemical screening for chromosomal abnormality is

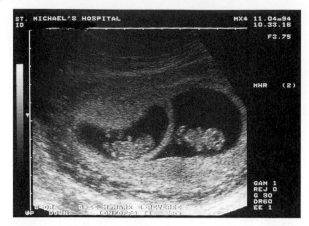

Fig 35.1 *Twin pregnancy. With kind permission of Dr Heather Andrews, Bristol.*

difficult in multiple pregnancy. There are normal ranges available for twin pregnancies; however, if once there is a positive test result, there is a dilemma as to further investigation. Amniocentesis can be employed to identify any abnormal karyotypes, but identifying the abnormal twin afterwards can be difficult, and even where this is possible there are obvious difficulties with termination of the pregnancy. Fetocide of the one abnormal twin can be performed, but there is an increased risk of miscarriage and possibly neurological deficit in the remaining twin. Serum screening is not available for higher multiples.

Diagnostic Imaging

Ultrasound scanning is the most useful of all investigations in multiple pregnancy. Ultrasound is used initially to make or confirm the diagnosis of multiple pregnancy (Figure 35.1). Ultrasound in the first trimester can also be used to determine the zygosity of multiple pregnancy. Previously this was performed by measuring the thickness of the membrane dividing the twins; thicker membranes are found in dichorionic and diamniotic twins than in monochorionic or mono-amniotic twins. More recently, the chorionicity has been determined using the lambda sign on ultrasound scan. This is important, as there is an increase in the rate of complications for monozygotic pregnancies, and increased surveillance is required.

Anomaly scanning is performed as routine. There are a number of anomalies specific to multiple pregnancies, all of which are specific to monozygotic twins:

* conjoined twins
* twin–twin transfusion
* acardiac twin.

These will be discussed in more detail in the section on complications.

Many obstetricians routinely offer scans at regular intervals throughout the third trimester for multiple pregnancy: to identify growth problems in one or more fetuses, to identify any polyhydramnios and to determine presentation prior to decision regarding the optimal mode of delivery.

Antenatal Schedule

Because the incidence of complications is increased, women with multiple pregnancy are offered more antenatal visits to their healthcare professional. This is particularly important for screening for hypertension.

POTENTIAL COMPLICATIONS

First Trimester

Maternal

Maternal complications in the first trimester are limited to an increase in the symptoms of pregnancy and an increase in the miscarriage rate (see fetal complications). Hyperemesis gravidarum is more common in multiple pregnancy, as there is an increased circulating β-hCG hormone.

Fetal

MISCARRIAGE – Miscarriage is more common in multiple pregnancy and it is a function of the pregnancy order, i.e. miscarriage is more common in quadruplet pregnancy than twin pregnancies. The risks are so high in pregnancies with > 3 fetuses - only 20% of quadruplet pregnancies will progress past 20 weeks gestation - that many centres offer selective reduction. This has the benefit of increasing the chance of the pregnancy progressing to viability, but often presents a huge dilemma to the prospective parents.

It is possible to miscarry one or more of the fetuses naturally and for the pregnancy to progress normally afterwards - the so-called vanishing twin phenomenon. Otherwise miscarriage is managed as described in Chapter 6.

ANOMALIES – The measurement of the fetal nuchal fat pad by ultrasound, in the first trimester, can provide a risk assessment for chromosomal abnormalities. This method has the advantage over serum screening that it can provide a risk for individual fetuses from a multiple pregnancy and therefore it can be used more easily in higher-order pregnancies

Second Trimester

Fetal

ANOMALIES – The risk of anomalies is increased in multiple pregnancy. This is a function both of the increase in the number of fetuses and also the extra problems specific to twin pregnancies.

Conjoined twins result from the incomplete division of the embryo after formation. It is rare, approximately 1:500 twin pregnancies. It is commonly diagnosed by ultrasound scan and requires delivery by caesarean section followed by surgical attention.

Twin–twin transfusion is also a complication of monozygotic pregnancies, severe in 1%. The problems arise because there are communicating vessels in the placenta connecting the twin circulations. The exact mechanism is unknown but characteristically one twin becomes the donor twin and one the recipient. The recipient twin becomes polycythaemic and the donor anaemic. The anaemic twin is hypovolaemic and develops IUGR. The recipient twin is hypervolaemic and develops heart failure with subsequent polyhydramnios.

There is a very high mortality (> 70%). The main risks are premature labour secondary to the polyhydramnios and/or death of the donor twin from hypoxia. The polyhydramnios can be reduced by serial amniocentesis, though this is not always successful, or the aberrant communicating vessels can be divided using a laser. Unfortunately, there is a high procedure-related loss rate with both methods.

Third Trimester

Maternal

All complications are increased in multiple pregnancy. Remember the components of pregnancy to remember the potential complications: i.e. mother (medical), uterus, liquor and placenta.

MEDICAL –

- **Pre-eclampsia** occurs in approximately 15% of multiple pregnancies (3% of all singleton pregnancies). Also, the risk of eclampsia is increased six-fold in multiple pregnancies complicated by pre-eclampsia compared with singletons. For management, see Chapter 31.
- **Diabetes** is also increased in multiple pregnancy, partly because of the increased diabetogenic steroid load of the pregnancy. Refer to Chapter 32 for management details.

PREGNANCY-RELATED –

- **APH** is increased both by abruption and placenta praevia. This is due to the increased placental surface area and also an increase in other predisposing causes, i.e. pre-eclampsia and abruption.
- **Premature rupture of the membranes** is more common, which predisposes to preterm labour and increased infectious morbidity.

- **Polyhydramnios** is also more common. The increase is due to problems specific to multiple pregnancy, i.e. twin–twin transfusion, and also indirectly due to the associated increase in other disorders such as maternal diabetes.
- **Premature labour** is one of the most important potential complications of multiple pregnancy, therefore prevention of prematurity or optimal management of unavoidable premature labour is imperative. See Chapter 29 for details of management. In particular, there should be arrangements for the early use of steroids and early transfer for tertiary SCBU facilities. The fetal outcome is related to its gestation rather than its size.

Fetal

- **IUGR** is increased in multiple pregnancy. Regular growth scans are employed routinely in the third trimester to investigate both discordance between fetuses and asymmetry in individuals. See Chapter 34 for further details on management.
- **Antenatal death of one twin** increases the risk for the other twin. The risks are death of the second twin or cerebral palsy if the twin survives. This is due to septic thrombi crossing the placentae from the dead twin to the living one. The risks therefore are increased in monozygotic twins.

Intrapartum

Once again, all complications are increased, maternal and fetal. Twins may deliver vaginally supervised by an experienced obstetrician supported by the appropriate facilities. However, there is an increased risk of intervention, and the second twin is at greater risk of asphyxia due to premature placental separation and cord prolapse.

Higher-order pregnancies and pregnancies complicated by malpresentation, i.e. first twin presenting other than by the vertex, and/or other maternal or fetal complications, e.g. IUGR or PET, are usually delivered by caesarean section.

The position of the leading twin should be checked on admission: 45% of twins are both cephalic; cephalic and breech occur in 25% and other presentations (requiring consideration of elective LSCS) occur in the remaining 30%.

Labour should be managed normally for the first twin. There is one first stage and two second stages. Following delivery of the first twin and prior to rupture of the membranes, an abdominal examination must be performed to ensure the second twin is longitudinal. Where the second twin is transverse, it can be corrected using external version and the membranes of the second amniotic sac ruptured allowing the presenting part to descend into the pelvis. The delivery of the second twin can then be managed as normal. The contractions can diminish during delivery of the second twin, and Syntocinon may be required. Where correction of transverse lie is unsuccessful, a caesarean section should be performed. The third stage should be managed actively to reduce the risk of PPH.

There are a number of intrapartum complications specific to multiple pregnancies. Although failure to diagnose multiple pregnancies is less common now that most women are scanned routinely in pregnancy, **undiagnosed twins** are occasionally discovered in unbooked women. If Syntometrine is administered then the uterus contracts tonically without relaxing, which reduces fetal blood flow. Delivery should be expedited by LSCS.

The other main complication specific to twins is **locked twins**. This is very rare complication, where the first twin presents by the breech and the second twin is cephalic. As the first twin descends, the underside of its chin becomes entangled with the underside of the chin of the other twin. Delivery is difficult, even by LSCS, and both twins may not survive.

Postpartum

All complications are increased. Consider both the mother and the fetus.

Maternal

PPH is increased. This is due both to increased rates of uterine atonia secondary to overdistension and also to increased obstetric trauma.

Other complications are also increased, resulting in an increased morbidity and mortality: pulmonary embolus, infectious morbidity, depression, etc. Refer to Chapter 45 for further details.

Fetal

Hypoxia is increased for the second twin as outlined above. The risks increase exponentially after a delay in delivery of more than 5 minutes.

Puerperium

The problems of coping with two or more babies simultaneously should not be underestimated. These problems are often exacerbated by both maternal and fetal complications, e.g. maternal morbidity associated with operative delivery or the problems of premature or abnormal babies. Increased support is essential, and this should be made available to the parents.

Information for Patients

Prognosis

The risks are not increased for mothers who receive appropriate obstetric care; however, information should be provided about the excess maternal morbidity and the extra demands of caring for multiple babies after delivery.

However, the fetal risks are greatly increased, as detailed above. These predominantly relate to prematurity, and close collaboration with the paediatricians is essential. Antenatal education about the risks is imperative.

Self-help groups

There are many self-help groups for multiple pregnancy e.g. TAMBA (Triplets and Multiple Births Association); and contact should be encouraged.

Follow-up

Short term

Antenatal visits are scheduled more frequently as part of the increased surveillance for problems, e.g. PET and preterm labour. Women should also have a low threshold for seeking medical advice during the pregnancy.

Long term

Post-delivery follow-up is perhaps best provided by the community, as they are better placed to provide long-term support.

GOLDEN POINTS

- All complications of pregnancy and labour are increased in multiple pregnancy.

- To remember the potential complications consider the components of a pregnancy: mother, babies, amniotic fluid, placenta, uterus and cord.

- Careful antenatal care and increased surveillance are necessary to reduce the excess mortality and morbidity to a minimum.

- Do not underestimate the burden of caring for multiple babies after multiple pregnancy.

36 Abnormal lie or presentation

CLINICAL SIGNIFICANCE

The fetal lie is usually longitudinal after 32 weeks gestation in line with the growing uterus. However, in 1:200 pregnancies the lie can be transverse, i.e. across the main axis of the uterus. With a transverse lie there is obviously no fetal pole in the pelvis and therefore there is an increased risk of cord prolapse during labour or ruptured membranes.

Face and brow presentations are diagnosed in labour, often as a result of a delay in the first stage. Because of this association, they are discussed in more detail in Chapter 40.

Breech presentation occurs in 2% of deliveries at term but it is more common preterm: 20% at 28 weeks and 15% at 32 weeks. There is an increasing trend towards caesarean section, but breech presentation is associated with an increased perinatal mortality irrespective of the mode of delivery. In several large and uncontrolled studies, vaginal delivery was associated with an excess risk. However, breech presentation is a heterogeneous group, and a blanket LSCS policy is not appropriate. The baby can often be turned – external cephalic version (ECV) – to a cephalic presentation obviating the need for caesarean section.

DIFFERENTIAL DIAGNOSIS

MAIN CATEGORY

1. Breech presentation

2. Face presentation

3. Brow presentation

4. Transverse lie

5. Oblique lie

CLINICAL ASSESSMENT

It is essential to identify any underlying causes after discovering a transverse lie/breech, etc., because turning the baby, version, is contraindicated in the presence of many of the underlying causes.

Anything that prevents the head entering the pelvis predisposes to transverse or oblique lie and breech presentation:

* **Fetal**
  – Multiple pregnancy
  – Prematurity
  – Hydrocephalus
* **Liquor**
  – Polyhydramnios
* **Pelvic**
  – Pelvic contractures
  – Cervical fibroid
* **Placenta**
  – Placenta praevia
* **Uterus**
  – Abnormality, e.g. single uterine horn.

Remember that breech presentation, or an abnormal lie, may complicate other obstetric problems such as PET, and the treatment of each condition is affected by the other.

Rapid Emergency Assessment

There is an increased risk of cord prolapse with abnormalities of lie, and therefore it is important immediately to exclude cord prolapse after rupture of the membranes.

Relevant History

Presenting Complaint

MAIN COMPLAINT – There is usually no specific complaint with either abnormalities of lie or breech presentation. They are most commonly discovered during routine abdominal palpation during antenatal visits. Some women do describe feeling a 'hard' lump in the upper abdomen, particularly with a breech presentation – the fetal head!

COMMONLY ASSOCIATED SYMPTOMS – There may, however, be symptoms associated with some of the predisposing causes. Polyhydramnios and multiple pregnancy may present with the pain of uterine overdistension. Different conditions may also coexist – fetal hydrocephalus can cause polyhydramnios.

Obstetric History

INDEX PREGNANCY – Breech presentation is more common in premature labour, and it is important to establish the gestation carefully. Multiple pregnancy is associated with breech presentations and abnormal lies. A history of a normal fetal anomaly scan with normal placental site is important, as both fetal anomalies and placenta praevia are associated with breech presentation and abnormal lie.

OBSTETRIC HISTORY – Grand multiparity and/or a lax abdominal wall also predisposes to abnormal lie. It is important to elicit any history of previous caesarean section, as both ECV and trial of vaginal delivery in a breech presentation are contraindicated after a caesarean section. Some of the causes of breech presentation are potentially recurrent, e.g. abnormal uterine shape, and there may be a previous history of breech presentation.

Relevant Clinical Examination

General Features

GENERAL – Abdominal wall laxity can be readily apparent.

Abdomen

PREGNANCY – The symphyseal–fundal height may be higher than expected with polyhydramnios and multiple pregnancy. The fetus may be difficult to palpate where there is coexisting polyhydramnios.

The abdomen may be abnormally wide in transverse lie.

In a transverse lie the main body can be palpated running transversely across the abdomen. The head is again ballotable. It is important to establish where the fetal back is, because caesarean section is difficult where the fetal back is down.

Classically, in a breech presentation, the lie is longitudinal and the head is palpable at the fundus as a ballotable hard lump, i.e. feels like an apple bobbing in water. However, the breech (bottom) is also occasionally ballotable, and identification of a breech presentation can be difficult.

When the main axis of the fetus is palpated obliquely then there is an oblique lie. The fetus may be either oblique breech or an oblique cephalic presentation.

OTHER – A single uterine horn or abnormal uterine shape can be palpated.

Pelvis

VAGINAL EXAMINATION – Cervical fibroids or other obstructing pelvic tumours can be identified by vaginal examination. The main feature of vaginal examination in an abnormal lie is an empty pelvis, as there is no fetal pole in the pelvis. A breech may be diagnosed in labour when the breech is palpated vaginally – it is softer than a head and the usual suture lines cannot be palpated. The feet may be palpated in a footling breech.

Exclude cord prolapse. Clinical pelvimetry, i.e. using vaginal examination to measure the capacity of the pelvis, is useless.

Relevant Investigations

Ultrasound is the key investigation; it is used to confirm the lie and the presentation as well as to identify potential predisposing causes.

Diagnostic imaging

USS – The lie and presentation can be confirmed. With a breech presentation it is important to identify the type of breech presentation – extended, flexed or footling – as there are different management options for each (see section on breech presentation). Notice that the type of breech is classified by the knees: extended or flexed (see Figure 36.1).

Estimation of fetal weight (EFW) is important; where the EFW is > 3.5 kg there is an increased risk of delay in labour and therefore an elective caesarean section should be considered. The attitude of the fetal head is also important, as hyperextension of the fetal head (so-called star gazing) predisposes to difficulty with delivery of the head and is therefore a contraindication to vaginal delivery.

Ultrasound can also be used to exclude placenta praevia, fetal anomalies and polyhydramnios.

X-RAY – Although x-ray/CT pelvimetry has featured prominently in protocols for vaginal breech delivery, no

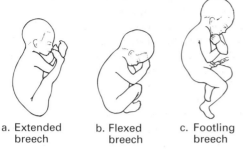

a. Extended breech   b. Flexed breech   c. Footling breech

Fig 36.1 *Types of breech presentation: (a) breech with extended legs; (b) breech with flexed legs; (c) footling. Reproduced from E. Symonds,* Essential Obstetrics & Gynaecology, *3rd edn, 1997, Churchill Livingstone.*

studies have confirmed this procedure in selecting those women who are more likely to succeed in a vaginal breech birth, or in improving the perinatal outcome. Therefore pelvimetry is not routinely used.

DETAILS OF INDIVIDUAL CONDITIONS

1. Breech Presentation

Background

DEFINITION – The breech is the baby's bottom, and therefore a breech presentation is where the baby's bottom, foot, or feet present instead of the head. Although breech presentation is associated with uterine and fetal abnormalities, it is usually simply a question of orientation.

As mentioned previously, there are three different types of breech defined by the flexion/extension of the knees; the hips are flexed in all three presentations.

* An extended breech (extended knees) is the most common (65%) and the best presentation for trial of vaginal breech because it is the most streamlined shape through the pelvis. However, the extended legs can impede ECV because they splint the fetus, making flexion of the baby prior to turning more difficult.
* A flexed breech (flexed knees) is slightly less common (25%) and most amenable to ECV.
* A footling breech is the least common (10%) and also the most dangerous type of breech. The feet are below the breech, which therefore prevents a snug fit of the breech, predisposing to cord prolapse.

AETIOLOGY – See general aetiological factors at start of chapter.

MAIN COMPLICATIONS –

Fetal: There is an increased perinatal mortality associated with breech delivery. This is predominantly because of the association with fetal anomaly and prematurity.

Whilst there are a number of fetal complications specific to vaginal breech delivery, e.g. entrapment of the after-coming head, the outcomes for babies after vaginal delivery appear no different from those delivered by caesarean section.

Maternal: The main maternal risks are related to the increased risk of caesarean section in labour with breech delivery. 50% of women undergoing a trial of vaginal breech delivery will have an emergency caesarean section, and the risks of infection, thromboembolism, etc., are increased by an emergency caesarean in labour compared with both vaginal delivery and elective CS.

Treatment Options

CONSERVATIVE AND REASSURANCE – There is no evidence that the use of maternal posture during pregnancy (the mother kneeling on the floor with the pelvis elevated) encourages a breech to turn. Acupuncture, homeopathy and moxibustion have all been used to turn babies, but no research has investigated these methods.

MEDICAL – External cephalic version (ECV) – the baby can be converted to a cephalic presentation by external manipulation on the women's abdomen – has attracted increasing interest over recent years, particularly because of the increasing caesarean section rate for breech presentation. After 36 weeks gestation in an uncomplicated pregnancy, ECV can be attempted. The abdomen is covered in talcum powder or gel, a hand cups and lifts the breech, and the baby is encouraged into a forward or backward roll, whichever is easiest.

The success of ECV varies considerably depending on the skill of the operator, but the conversion rate can be as high as 50%, and the caesarean section rate is also reduced. There appear to be very few risks associated with ECV, especially when attempted > 36 weeks gestation. There is a risk of rhesus isoimmunisation, and anti-D should be administered to rhesus negative women.

The Royal College of Obstetricians and Gynaecologists now recommends that, 'all women with an uncomplicated pregnancy and breech presentation should be offered ECV'. ECV has been carried out in early labour with some success, providing the breech has not already engaged.

SURGERY – Where ECV fails, or is not undertaken in line with the woman's wishes, there is a choice of trial of vaginal delivery or elective caesarean section.

Vaginal delivery – selection criteria have been used to identify those women most likely to successfully deliver vaginally. USS is used to estimate the fetal weight, and those babies > 3.5 kg appear more likely 'to get stuck' and therefore routinely should be offered caesarean section. Pelvimetry is not useful.

Epidural anaesthesia is not routinely required; indeed it may increase the caesarean section rate by 10%.

A vaginal breech delivery is not just a vertex delivery in reverse. There are a number of specific manoeuvres required to deliver the breech in the least traumatic manner possible. As the breech descends onto the perineum an episiotomy may be performed if deemed potentially useful, though it should not be routine, and the breech should deliver spontaneously. The breech should be gently held over the bony prominences with the forefingers in the groins and the thumbs over the sacrum, and the breech should be encouraged to rotate until the back is uppermost. Then the breech should be allowed to descend until the scapulae are visible, and then the arms can be delivered by sweeping them forward and out over the chest. The breech should continue to descend until the nape of the neck is visible and therefore the head is in the pelvis. The baby is born by raising the body upwards with neck flexion (chin on the chest) maintained by either forceps or the Mauriceau-Smellie-Veit manoeuvre.

Caesarean section – The main benefits of elective caesarean section are to reduce the excess risks of emergency caesarean section. The morbidity and mortality of emergency section is up to 10 × that of a normal vaginal delivery, whereas the perinatal morbidity and mortality of an elective section is only 1.5 × that of a normal vaginal delivery.

Between 26 and 32 weeks gestation there is some tenuous evidence that caesarean section is the safest mode of delivery because of the risks of head entrapment in a partly dilated cervix. However, caesarean section can be difficult, and a classical caesarean may be necessary with significant repercussions for subsequent pregnancies. After 32 weeks gestation there appears little benefit in caesarean section.

OVERVIEW – A woman with a breech presentation at term, in the absence of complications, should be offered ECV. Otherwise there should be a frank and fair discussion of the pros and cons of elective caesarean section and vaginal breech delivery. There appears to be little to choose between them as far as fetal morbidity is concerned, but the excess maternal risks of an emergency caesarean in labour for 50% of women may justify elective caesarean for all. Women should be able to make an informed choice.

Information for Patients

PROGNOSIS – The prognosis is generally excellent irrespective of the mode of delivery. There is, however, an increased recurrence risk of breech presentation in future pregnancies.

Follow-up

SHORT TERM – Women with a breech presentation should be followed routinely until 36–37 weeks gestation, whereupon the chance of spontaneous version is low and they should be counselled about their options, i.e. ECV and mode of delivery.

LONG TERM – There is a recurrence risk in subsequent pregnancies, and women with a breech presentation should be carefully followed in future pregnancies. Women in whom a pelvic or uterine abnormality is suspected can also be thoroughly investigated outside pregnancy using x-rays, etc.

2. Transverse Lie

Background

DEFINITION – A transverse lie is where the baby lies transversely across the abdomen (Figure 36.2). It is abnormal after 32 weeks gestation, and underlying causes should be sought.

AETIOLOGY – A transverse lie results when the normal forces that usually maintain a longitudinal lie fail. Causes include grand multiparity, abdominal laxity, uterine or fetal abnormalities, and conditions that inhibit engagement of the presenting part, e.g. placenta praevia. See above.

MAIN COMPLICATIONS –

Fetal: The main fetal complication is cord prolapse after rupture of the membranes, as there is no presenting part filling the pelvis and stopping the cord prolapsing. There is also a risk of obstructed labour should labour be allowed to proceed, as the longitudinal axis of the baby cannot pass through the pelvis.

Maternal: The main maternal risk is obstructed labour.

Treatment Options

CONSERVATIVE – Before labour and in the absence of complications, ECV can be attempted.

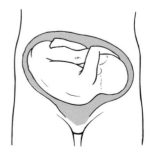

Fig 36.2 *Transverse lie. Reproduced from E. Symonds,* Essential Obstetrics & Gynaecology, *3rd edn, 1997, Churchill Livingstone.*

MEDICAL – Some obstetricians, in the presence of intact membranes, use Syntocinon to induce labour. The majority will become longitudinal as the uterine tone increases, and the membranes can be ruptured with engagement of the presenting part. This strategy is particularly useful for an oblique lie and will reduce the caesarean section rate.

SURGICAL – Once labour has started or a decision has been made to deliver, then the baby should be delivered by caesarean section. After ruptured membranes, and particularly where the baby is transverse and back down, a classical caesarean (longitudinal incision on the uterus) may be required, as a transverse incision may permit insufficient access to the fetus.

Follow-up

SHORT TERM – There is a significant risk of cord prolapse in labour or after rupture of the membranes. Rupture of the membranes may be completely unheralded, and therefore women may be offered admission 'just in case'. This is an individual decision and should be discussed with the potential parents.

LONG TERM – Long-term follow-up is rarely necessary, though there is a recurrence risk in subsequent pregnancies.

3. Oblique lie

Background

DEFINITION – The baby lies across the abdomen at an oblique angle. The presentation can be either cephalic or transverse.

Oblique lies can be transitory and are more likely to undergo spontaneous version. Note the use of Syntocinon to correct the lie during induction of labour. However, in all other respects the aetiology and management are identical to those in a transverse lie.

GOLDEN POINTS

1. Abnormal lie and presentations are more common the earlier the gestation.

2. Underlying causes should be excluded.

3. Women with either a breech presentation or an abnormal lie should be offered external cephalic version. This can obviate the need for caesarean section.

4. Where ECV fails then the parents should be counselled about the mode of delivery. The main advantage of an elective section is that it reduces the excess morbidity for the 50% of women who would have had a caesarean section in labour.

5. Selection criteria for breech vaginal delivery are not completely reliable.

6. There is an increased risk of cord prolapse in women with a transverse lie.

7. If ECV fails then delivery should be expedited by caesarean section for transverse lie.

37 Pre-labour rupture of membranes

CLINICAL SIGNIFICANCE

Spontaneous rupture of membranes precedes labour by an interval of more than 4 h in 10% of cases, more for preterm labours. After the membranes have ruptured the main risk is ascending infection from the non-sterile vagina, leading to chorio-amnionitis which is a significant cause of mortality and morbidity for both mother and baby – in particular, infection of the fetal lungs. The other risks are related to the reduced amniotic fluid volumes, oligohydramnios (see Chapter 34), and the open cervix, which predisposes to cord prolapse particularly with preterm infants. Therefore the main aim of treatment is pre-emptive delivery with a minimum of intervention.

Pre-labour rupture of membranes (PROM) is an umbrella term, which includes three very different groups defined by gestation: non-viable, < 24 weeks; preterm, 24–37 weeks; and term, > 37 weeks. The management of each group is different because the risks of prematurity must be weighed against the risk of infection. The risks of prematurity are obviously increased at earlier gestations, particularly < 34 weeks, and therefore the management is predominantly observation until maturity or infection intervenes, and then delivery.

The diagnosis of SRM can be difficult. The classical symptom of sudden loss of fluid from the vagina can be due to urinary incontinence (common in pregnancy) or vaginal discharge as well as SRM, so accurate diagnosis is essential.

DIFFERENTIAL DIAGNOSIS

MAIN CATEGORY	DIAGNOSIS
1. *Pre-labour rupture of membranes*	Before viability < 24 weeks gestation Preterm 24–37 weeks gestation Term > 37 weeks gestation
2. *Urinary incontinence*	
3. *Vaginal discharge*	

CLINICAL ASSESSMENT

Rapid Emergency Assessment

SRM is rarely an emergency, though the complication of chorio-amnionitis and cord prolapse can be. These potential complications should be excluded on admission as detailed below.

Relevant History

Presenting Complaint

MAIN COMPLAINT – The presenting complaint is classically a sudden loss of fluid from the vagina.

The normal history for SRM is a sudden, unprovoked, large loss that subsequently has become a trickle, but hasn't stopped altogether. There may be some uterine tightenings or contractions, but otherwise the loss is painless. Although liquor is clear, occasionally it can be bloodstained by the mucus plug of the cervix, which is normal, but heavy bloodstaining requires further investigation – see Chapter 30. Also it can be meconium stained, which can be normal post-term but is a sign of fetal distress and/or chorio-amnionitis at earlier gestations, and assessment for immediate delivery is required.

In contrast, the loss of urinary incontinence is caused by coughing, sneezing, etc., and it is a discrete loss without the subsequent continuous trickling. There may also be symptoms of UTI, and the fluid smells of urine!

Vaginal discharge produces a feeling of continuous wetness, and there may be some vulval irritation. Usually there is no gush of large quantities of fluid.

GESTATION – Accurate estimation of the gestation is essential to the management of PROM. Most women will have had a scan, at least at 18 weeks, from which the gestation can be accurately determined. Where the dates by LMP and scan differ by more than 1 week, the scan dates should be used.

OTHER SYMPTOMS – A history of flu-like symptoms should also be elicited, which would indicate a possible ascending infection.

Obstetric History – Index Pregnancy

ANTENATAL – There is increasing evidence that bacterial vaginosis (BV) is associated with preterm SRM, and therefore previous symptoms of BV are important. The symptoms of bacterial vaginosis are classically a thin, grey vaginal discharge with an ammoniacal smell, particularly after intercourse.

Preterm SRM is also related to uterine overdistension, and therefore a history of polyhydramnios, macrosomia or multiple pregnancy increases the risk of preterm SRM.

OBSTETRIC HISTORY – The risk of pre-labour rupture of membranes, especially preterm, is increased by a previous pre-labour SRM.

Relevant Clinical Examination

General Features

GENERAL – Signs of infection should be excluded, particularly tachycardia and pyrexia. The patient's temperature and fetal heart rate are two of the most accurate predictors of intrauterine infection and therefore should be monitored regularly.

Abdomen

PREGNANCY – On abdominal examination reduction in the liquor volume may be clinically obvious, i.e. the fetal parts are easy to palpate and the symphyseal–fundal height will be less than expected. The presence of uterine contractions should also be determined because they indicate impending labour and also the possibility of intrauterine infection. Uterine tenderness may indicate an intrauterine infection.

FETUS – A fetal tachycardia is a sinister finding, as it can reflect intrauterine infection with fetal involvement. However, it is important to remember that the fetal heart rate may be faster at early gestations than at later, but it should always be below 160 beats per minute.

The fetal presentation should be determined, as abnormal presentation is more common in preterm labour. Transverse lie increases the risk of cord prolapse, particularly where labour ensues, and always requires delivery by LSCS at any gestation. Transverse lie with SRM at less then 34 weeks may require a classical section, as it can be difficult to deliver the baby through a transverse incision.

Pelvis

VAGINAL EXAMINATION – **Vulva/vagina** – a sterile speculum examination should be undertaken to look for amniotic fluid draining through the cervix. The presence of vernix (> 32 weeks) would help confirm the source of the fluid. In reality there rarely is a large pool of liquor, and if there is then the diagnosis is self-evident.

There are a number of stick tests to help confirm whether or not fluid is in the vagina. Nitrazine sticks are pH sensitive and turn black in the low pH of the amniotic fluid; however, they are not very specific. More-specific sticks are available that measure amniotic fluid proteins, i.e. AFP and insulin growth factor 1; however, they are expensive and not yet in routine use in the UK. Liquor ferns, i.e. produces a ferning pattern on a slide, if allowed to dry.

Ensure there is no umbilical cord in the vagina!

Cervix – do not digitally examine the cervix unless you are concerned about the possibility of labour or are actively considering delivery soon, as examination may increase the risk of ascending infection.

Relevant Investigations

The investigations are primarily used as part of the monitoring, though they are fairly non-specific markers of infection.

Haematology

A raised white cell count (WCC) and ESR can be measured serially as markers of infection, though they may rise late in the natural history of chorio-amnionitis. Negative results should not therefore be relied upon for reassurance. A sample for Group and Save should be taken if delivery by LSCS is anticipated.

Biochemistry

C-reactive protein is often measured serially as a non-specific marker of infection. Fibronectin has been used as a marker for preterm labour.

Microbiology

A swab should be taken from the vagina and sent for culture. The aim is not to elucidate the aetiology of the PROM but to identify potentially dangerous fetal pathogens. β-haemolytic Streptococcus is particularly dangerous to the fetus, with a 50% mortality after pneumonia. Treatment of the mother with antibiotics will both prevent ascending infection and treat any fetal infection present.

In the USA, amniocentesis, followed by microbiological culture of the liquor, is commonly undertaken after premature SRM to identify occult infection. Where there are bacteria or an elevated WCC in the liquor, delivery should be expedited. This technique is not routine in the UK.

Diagnostic Imaging

Ultrasound scans can be used to measure the liquor volume, which may be reduced, and also to guide any amniocentesis needles. Scanning can also determine fetal presentation more accurately than palpation. The presence of fetal breathing movements on scan has been proposed as being a reassuring sign to mark a sterile environment for the fetus; however, it suffers from the same problem as all the other serum markers in that it is not very specific.

DETAILS OF INDIVIDUAL CONDITIONS

1. Pre-Labour Rupture of Membranes

Background

DEFINITION – Rupture of the membranes without establishment of labour.

AETIOLOGY – There is a decrease in the collagen content of the membranes as pregnancy advances towards term, and this is thought to be, at least in part, the normal mechanism of membrane rupture. This decrease in collagen is mirrored in those pregnancies where the PROM is thought to be related to overdistension of the uterus, e.g. polyhydramnios.

Abnormal bacterial colonisation of the vagina during pregnancy is related to PROM. In normal pregnancy the increase in oestrogen encourages the growth of lactobacilli which reduce the pH of the vagina through their production of lactic acid. Abnormal colonisation, particularly with BV, increases the pH of the vagina, and this weakens the cervical mucus and permits dissolution of the membranes, especially as some of these bacteria produce phospholipase A_2, which can stimulate cervical effacement via stimulation of prostaglandins.

MAIN COMPLICATIONS –

Maternal: The main maternal complications are related to ascending infection and an increase in the intervention rates associated with pre-labour rupture of membranes.

Fetal: The main fetal risks are ascending infection and prematurity. Long-term risks include lung hypoplasia and fixed flexion deformities secondary to oligohydramnios.

PREVENTION – Antibiotics have been proposed for prophylaxis against ascending infection after PROM, but no benefit has been demonstrated thus far. A large multicentre study is currently under way to investigate this further – Oracle. The results are awaited.

There are screening tests available for BV, and these are appropriate for women with a previous history of preterm PROM. Swabs are taken at 14 and 20 weeks gestation and metronidazole prescribed for those who are positive. This can reduce the recurrence risk by up to 30%.

Treatment Options

The treatment options vary according to the gestation, but the principles of treatment are to minimise the risk of prematurity by expectant management until delivery is possible because the pregnancy has reached a sufficient maturity or because the risks of continuing the pregnancy, i.e. ascending infection, outweigh the risks of prematurity.

NON-VIABLE (< 24 WEEKS) – The prognosis for pregnancies with PROM at less than 24 weeks gestation is extremely poor. Even should the pregnancy continue to viability the risks of ascending infection are compounded by the complications of oligohydramnios, i.e. lung hypoplasia. The chances of the pregnancy resulting in an alive or developmentally normal child are very small indeed.

The prospective parents should be counselled about the risks and their two treatment options: delivery or expectant management. Some parents choose the former option, and labour is induced usually with prostaglandin pessaries.

Those women who opt for expectant management are monitored by measuring the maternal temperature. An increase in the temperature is one of the most specific signs of ascending infection. There is a lot of debate about the optimum place for observation, but when the fetus is less than 22 weeks then home may be appropriate with twice-weekly review at the hospital and home monitoring of the temperature.

Prophylactic antibiotics can be used, but there is no proven benefit as yet. If the pregnancy progresses to 24 weeks then it can be managed as below.

PRETERM (24–37 WEEKS) – All women should be managed expectantly with monitoring for intrauterine infection: usually maternal temperature and the fetal heart rate. An increase in the fetal heart rate is a reasonably specific indicator of intrauterine infection and should be auscultated twice per day. It is important to note that the fetal heart rate is normally slightly faster at gestations less than 34 weeks compared with term. However, it should always be below 160 beats per minute, and an upward trend in the rate over time is sinister.

Serial estimation of serum markers of infection: WCC, ESR and CRP are often used, although the benefit is disputed. They are non-specific and rise late in the natural history of chorioamnionitis, therefore a normal result can be falsely reassuring.

Prophylactic antibiotics are not used routinely. The necessity for hospitalisation is also controversial; after 32 weeks some patients may be allowed home with monitoring and regular hospital review. Monitoring should include twice-daily measurement of maternal temperature.

Uterine irritability or labour can indicate chorioamnionitis, and therefore tocolysis is inappropriate, as it can increase the risk of intrauterine infection for the baby.

The pregnancy should otherwise be managed as if labour is imminent: transfer the mother to a hospital with suitable SCBU facilities and administer steroids for pregnancies < 34 weeks gestation. Consultation with the neonatal team is helpful. The neonatal benefits of steroids outweigh the potential risks of masking sepsis.

Active consideration should be given to delivery between 35 and 37 weeks gestation as the risks of prematurity are similar to term.

TERM (> 37 WEEKS) – The decision to be made at these gestations is when to deliver rather than if. The rate of ascending infection is very low within 24–36 h of rupture of membranes, and up to 70% of women will labour spontaneously in that time. Induction of labour increases the duration of labour and rates of intervention. However, recent evidence from the USA suggests that the intervention rates are similar for induced or not, and indeed conservative management may result in an increased perinatal mortality, partly because of an excess risk of cord prolapse.

The routine management of PROM at term in the UK consists of diagnosis, followed by immediate induction or initial conservative management depending on the woman's choice.

OVERVIEW – The management of PROM is a balance of the risks of delivery, usually prematurity, versus the risks of ascending infection as a result of expectant management. Monitoring is not perfect and there should be a low threshold for delivery where there is an increase in maternal temperature, symptoms of infection or an increase in the fetal heart rate. Antibiotics or tocolysis should not be routinely employed for women after PROM.

Information for Patients

PROGNOSIS – As labour ensues commonly within 1 week of membrane rupture the prognosis is almost entirely dependent on the gestation. The neonatal prognosis for PROM at less than 24 weeks is almost universally gloomy, whereas the prognosis at term is excellent. The paediatricians can be consulted for an accurate prognosis after preterm SRM.

Follow-up

SHORT TERM – Follow-up is essential for those women allowed home. The community team can monitor the maternal temperature and fetal heart rate closely at home with regular hospital attendance at the day assessment unit and antenatal clinic. There should be early recourse to hospital assessment for symptoms of chorioamnionitis.

LONG TERM – Follow-up is essential for women after a poor outcome, i.e. extreme prematurity or death related to intrauterine infection, to 'debrief' and explain the recurrence risks. An early visit to an antenatal clinic in any future pregnancy for BV screening would be appropriate after a poor outcome in the index pregnancy.

GOLDEN POINTS

- The diagnosis of PROM can be difficult.

- A low vaginal swab should be undertaken to exclude β-haemolytic Streptococcus colonisation of the genital tract.

- The prognosis after PROM depends on the gestation.

- Management of PROM is a balance between the risks of ascending infection and prematurity.

- Serum markers of infection are not as reliable as maternal temperature and fetal heart rate for the prediction of ascending infection.

- Tocolysis should not be routinely employed after PROM.

- Women may be offered immediate induction or a limited trial of conservative management at term.

38 Prolonged pregnancy

CLINICAL SIGNIFICANCE

Prolonged pregnancy – gestation lasting more than 42 weeks – complicates between 5% and 10% of normal pregnancies. There are a variety of different euphemisms used for prolonged pregnancies: post-dates, post-maturity, post-term etc. However, all of them mean slightly different things. For the purposes of this chapter, post-term means > 294 days (42 weeks) gestation.

It is a cause of concern for both mothers and their doctors. At its simplest, late pregnancy is uncomfortable and therefore continuation past the EDD is not desirable. Furthermore the risk to the fetus increases post-term: the incidence of unexplained stillbirths after 42 weeks is up to three times that at 39–40 weeks.

Unfortunately, there are no screening tests available to monitor the fetus accurately and absolutely safely post-term.

Delivery may be an obvious solution, but induction of labour is associated with increased intervention and may be unacceptable to the mother.

Optimal management is not year clear, but the risks of continuation of the pregnancy must be balanced against the risks of induction.

DIFFERENTIAL DIAGNOSIS

1. *Prolonged pregnancy*
2. *Wrong dates*

CLINICAL ASSESSMENT

Expectant management of prolonged pregnancy can only be considered where the pregnancy is 'low risk', i.e. there are no fetal or maternal problems that should prompt delivery. Therefore the pregnancy should be carefully assessed to exclude any maternal and fetal risks that would compromise the pregnancy as well as to ensure accurate dating.

Relevant History

Presenting Complaint

MAIN COMPLAINT – Women are routinely booked for a hospital antenatal clinic visit at 41 weeks gestation, and this is the ideal opportunity for review of the pregnancy and counselling about their options should they not spontaneously labour.

COMMONLY ASSOCIATED SYMPTOMS – The most common symptoms are those of late pregnancy, i.e. insomnia, reflux oesophagitis and generally feeling very uncomfortable!

Obstetric History

OBSTETRIC HISTORY – A history of stillbirth or other adverse outcome should preclude expectant management.

Prolonged pregnancy has a recurrence risk of 30–40%, therefore a previous history can be a good indicator of the likely length of the index pregnancy. Previous delivery outcomes are also important; some women may have suffered a prolonged labour or difficult delivery, and this may colour their views of one particular management option.

INDEX PREGNANCY – Accurate dating of the pregnancy is essential. Menstrual dating is notoriously inaccurate because of irregular cycles or difficulty in remembering the exact date of the last menstrual period. Therefore it is often prudent to check the dates by scan, though this should have been done earlier in pregnancy.

Hypertension and diabetes should also preclude expectant management, as well as other medical conditions that impair fetal or maternal outcome.

FETAL – Good fetal movements are reassuring.

Relevant Clinical Examination

Abdomen

PREGNANCY – IUGR and oligohydramnios can both indicate fetal compromise. They will both reduce the symphyseal–fundal height, and therefore the SFH should be determined. The amount of amniotic fluid can be also determined clinically – see Chapter 34. The lie and presentation of the fetus should be accurately determined.

Pelvis

VAGINAL EXAMINATION – Vaginal examination can be performed prior to discussion of management options to determine the 'ripeness' of the cervix – induction of labour is more likely to be successful where the cervix is 'favourable', i.e. Bishop's score > 5 – and also to perform a membrane sweep. The examining finger is inserted through the cervix and swept around between the amniotic membranes and the top of the cervix. This releases endogenous prostaglandins leading to onset of labour within 48 hours in 50% of multiparous women. It is less successful for primigravidae.

Relevant Investigations

There are no specific diagnostic tests for prolonged pregnancy. However, a wide variety of investigations are employed to assess fetal wellbeing.

Tests of Fetal Wellbeing

Biochemical tests are no longer routinely employed to assess placental function. Although there are a plethora of tests available, very few of them have been validated. There is no single test that accurately predicts fetal compromise in a low-risk population, and perhaps more importantly there is no test that absolutely excludes poor neonatal outcome.

Fetal Kick Charts

Fetal kick charts are commonly utilised to monitor fetal health. The fetus is expected to move 10 times in 12 h on the 'count to ten' chart. Most mothers find this reassuring, though it is a source of anxiety for some because movements can be difficult to feel.

Fetal movements correlate well with fetal health, but they are not diagnostic and there is no evidence that routine formal fetal movement counting reduces the incidence of stillbirth in late pregnancy. Overall, a fetal movement chart alone is probably not sufficient to monitor fetal wellbeing.

Cardiotocography

A 20–40 min CTG is one of the most popular methods of fetal surveillance. A CTG with normal baseline (120–160 bpm) and normal variability (> 10–15 bpm) with two or more accelerations is reassuring. 'Reassuring' means that only 7 in 1000 babies will die within 1 week of a normal test! It is therefore not perfect.

A non-reactive (low baseline variability) CTG or one that demonstrates decelerations is abnormal and should prompt intervention.

Ultrasound Scan

AMNIOTIC FLUID VOLUME – Oligohydramnios can indicate fetal compromise (see Chapter 34). Amniotic fluid volume is commonly measured using ultrasound either by measuring the maximum vertical depth of amniotic fluid – normal > 3 cm – or by measuring the amniotic fluid depth in four different quadrants and summing to give the Amniotic Fluid Index (AFI) – normal > 5 cm. The AFI is a better predictor of perinatal outcome, but it is not a perfect test either. Amniotic fluid volume can decline over a period of 3–4 days, and therefore twice-weekly assessment is required.

GROWTH SCAN – Fetal growth retardation indicates a high-risk pregnancy, and delivery should be contemplated.

BIOPHYSICAL PROFILE – Scores that combine ultrasound evaluation of fetal movement (including gross movements, breathing movements and fetal tone), amniotic fluid volume and CTGs – biophysical profile – may be useful, but five inaccurate tests do not necessarily make an accurate one, and therefore further confirmatory tests are needed.

DOPPLER – Abnormal or poor blood flow in the umbilical artery is related to poor placental function and identifies a high-risk pregnancy. Nevertheless this test is only as accurate as the previous ones: an abnormal Doppler merits delivery, but a normal Doppler does not exclude poor perinatal outcome.

In clinical practice a 'belt and braces' approach is commonly employed and a CTG, AFI and/or Doppler examination are performed twice weekly, usually where the appropriate facilities are available in one place, i.e. Day Assessment Unit.

DETAILS OF CONDITION
Prolonged Pregnancy

Background

DEFINITION – Prolonged pregnancy is a pregnancy lasting more than 42 weeks gestation or 294 days from the first day of the LMP. Prolonged pregnancy is analogous to post-term whereas post-mature or postmaturity describes a newborn infant with meconium-stained skin, minimal subcutaneous fat and long nails, etc. This appearance is not confined to prolonged pregnancies and therefore should not be used to describe prolonged pregnancy.

AETIOLOGY – The aetiology of prolonged pregnancy is unknown, partly because the mechanism of labour initiation is also unknown; however, pregnancy up to 42 weeks is probably in the normal range. There is a recurrence rate in subsequent pregnancies of up to 30–40%. There is also an association with placental sulphatase deficiency, an extremely rare condition where the woman never labours spontaneously.

MAIN COMPLICATIONS – There is an increased perinatal fetal mortality and morbidity associated with prolonged pregnancy. The increased risks of antepartum stillbirth are well described: up to three times the risk compared with 39 weeks. However, the increase in perinatal morbidity is less well known. There is an increase in hypoxia, shoulder dystocia and birth injuries even after spontaneous delivery. Moreover, neonatal convulsions and cerebral palsy are increased in babies delivered after 41 weeks. Remember to keep these risks in perspective; three times a very small risk is still a very small risk.

PREVENTION – There are no effective clinical interventions to prevent postmaturity. There are commonly held beliefs that sex, a curry or the No. 73 bus may all help precipitate labour. There are no data supporting the efficacy of these interventions, though suffice it to say that the 5% of women who present with prolonged pregnancy will have tried all of them! A policy of routinely sweeping the membranes may reduce the induction rate, with little excess risk.

Treatment Options

EXPECTANT AND REASSURANCE – Expectant management is less invasive and more natural, in theory, though the extra monitoring required seems rather intrusive, to me at least! Expectant management is where the pregnancy is allowed to continue with extra fetal surveillance until the woman labours spontaneously or complications develop which merit induction of labour. The woman should be counselled that she should attend the hospital, usually the DAU, twice weekly until 43 weeks when the situation can be reviewed by her obstetrician.

INDUCTION – Induction of labour decreases the risk of perinatal death (500 inductions would be needed to prevent 1 perinatal death) and also the incidence of meconium-stained liquor. There is a two-fold increase in the LSCS and instrumental delivery rate in some studies after induction of labour for prolonged pregnancy, though there is an increase in operative delivery after expectant management also. This may be in the nature of the pregnancy itself. Induction of labour is probably cheaper as there are no extra costs for monitoring.

The methods of induction and subsequent risks for an individual woman are dependent on her parity and the state of the cervix, or the Bishop score. Amniotomy and/or Syntocinon are commonly used for women with a ripe cervix (Bishop score > 5) whereas prostaglandin preparations are used for those with a less ripe cervix. Induction with prostaglandin preparations is associated with a lower rate of operative delivery, compared with Syntocinon, although, overall, the rate of operative delivery is increased in primigravidae and women with an unripe cervix.

The risks of PPH and infection are increased only where the labour is prolonged – see Chapters 40 and 43.

OVERVIEW – An analysis of all the research on prolonged pregnancy suggests that for a low-risk woman there is little to choose between the two options. Induction of labour is probably safer and cheaper, but it is more intrusive. Expectant management is less invasive, though the woman should be counselled that the methods of fetal surveillance are less than perfect.

Overall, after counselling about the risks and benefits of each option, the woman and her partner should be allowed to choose. It is interesting that in one study where pregnant women were surveyed, the percentage who favoured expectant management dropped dramatically between 37 and 41 weeks!

Information for Patients

PROGNOSIS – The prognosis is generally good for all low-risk women with prolonged pregnancy irrespective of the management. There are extra risks of perinatal death associated with expectant management, whilst induction of labour is associated with increased intervention.

Follow-up

SHORT TERM – Women with prolonged pregnancy should

be reviewed at 41 weeks gestation and counselled about their options. For women who choose induction of labour, this can be arranged at term + 12 days. Women who opt for expectant management should be reviewed twice weekly for assessment of fetal wellbeing and also to exclude other complications.

GOLDEN POINTS

1. Prolonged pregnancy complicates 5–10% of pregnancies.

2. There is an increased risk of perinatal death after 42 weeks gestation.

3. 500 inductions are needed to prevent 1 fetal death.

4. Induction of labour is associated with increased intervention.

5. The methods of fetal surveillance during expectant management are not perfect.

6. Ensure accurate dating of the pregnancy, usually by second trimester ultrasound.

7. Exclude possible contraindications to expectant management, e.g. maternal hypertension or fetal compromise.

8. Counsel for risks/benefits of expectant management and induction of labour.

39 Abnormal fetal heart pattern in labour

CLINICAL SIGNIFICANCE

There remains considerable debate about the role of 'routine' continuous electronic fetal heart monitoring with the cardiotocograph.

The fetal heart rate is monitored in all labours by regular auscultation using a pinard stethoscope or a Doppler instrument.

Recent large-scale studies have shown that, whilst continuous fetal heart monitoring is indicated in high-risk pregnancies and those where a complication develops during labour, the situation in normal, low-risk labours is not proven. There is, therefore, no need to continuously monitor the fetal heart in the majority of labours.

Continuous electronic fetal monitoring should be used in all twin pregnancies and in singleton pregnancies if intermittent auscultation reveals:

- *a bradycardia of less than 110 beats per minute;*
- *a tachycardia of greater than 150 beats per minute;*
- *the appearance of fresh meconium in the amniotic fluid;*
- *the occurrence of decelerations following contractions;*

or in the presence of bleeding per vaginam during labour.

Further indications will depend upon the policy of individual units.

DIFFERENTIAL DIAGNOSIS

MAIN CATEGORY	DIAGNOSIS
Maternal	Hypotension
	Pyrexia
	Haemorrhage
	Tachycardia
Fetal	Cord compression
	Hypoxia
	Congenital abnormality
	Placental accident

The features of a cardiotocograph (CTG) are as follows.

COMPONENTS OF A CARDIOTOCOGRAPH

A cardiotocograph is made up of two components.

- The first component is a continuous reading of the fetal heart rate. The heart rate of the fetus at any given time will depend on interplay between the sympathetic and parasympathetic nervous systems. It can be recorded in two ways: either by use of an external Doppler probe or by the use of an internal fetal scalp electrode. Clearly, the latter can only be used once the membranes have ruptured and the patient is in labour. However, once these criteria have been satisfied, a scalp electrode is usually to be preferred since it provides more information regarding the baseline variability of the cardiotocograph trace and generally avoids problems

Box 39.1 Normal CTG patterns

Baseline rate	110–150 bpm
Beat-to-beat variability	± 5 bpm May be reduced for up to 30 min
Accelerations	> 15 bpm above baseline
Tocograph	Contractions

with loss of contact which is common with external monitoring. The use of a fetal scalp electrode is, however, contraindicated in cases where the fetus is thought to have a coagulation defect or in certain cases of intrauterine infection.

- The second component is a tocograph or measurement of uterine contractions.

CARDIOTOCOGRAPH PATTERNS

Correct interpretation of a cardiotocograph requires knowledge of whether or not the woman is in labour, and the stage of labour which has been reached. As well as this, knowledge of the gestational age, presence of sedative drugs in the maternal blood or intercurrent maternal disease is also necessary. Box 39.1 gives normal values of some CTG parameters.

Baseline Rate

A normal fetal heart rate lies between 110 and 150 bpm at term. Since the sympathetic nervous system matures more rapidly than the parasympathetic nervous system, preterm fetuses may tend to have slightly higher heart rates. The baseline rate may be altered by hypoxia, maternal disease (thyrotoxicosis, fever), congenital heart block or drugs such as caffeine, nicotine, beta-blockers, sedatives and narcotics.

Baseline Variability

A normal cardiotocograph has a baseline variability of at least 5 bpm, which occurs in cycles of 3–5 per min. Baseline variability may be reduced in the 'sleep' phase of a cardiotocograph, in fetal hypoxia and in the presence of drugs such as beta-blockers. Occasionally, baseline variability may be greatly increased. This may indicate fetal hypoxia. In addition, there is a sinusoidal pattern which may indicate hypoxia, fetal anaemia or may indeed be quite normal.

Generally speaking, a fetus 'sleeps' for only about 20–30 min at a time. Any period of reduced variability that continues beyond this should therefore be viewed with suspicion.

As external heart rate monitors generally average the fetal heart rate over 3 beats, the term 'beat-to-beat variation' is best reserved for those CTGs obtained by the use of an internal fetal scalp electrode.

Periodic Changes

The maternal blood flow to the uterus is reduced during a contraction, producing a mild hypoxic stress to the fetus. How the fetus reacts to this tells us something of the oxygen reserve of the fetus.

ACCELERATIONS – This is the normal response of a fetus to a mild stress. They may occur in response to a contraction or fetal movement. An acceleration, by definition, must rise to at least 15 bpm above the baseline rate and last for at least 15 s. The presence of accelerations implies good fetal oxygen reserve. Their absence in an antenatal trace may imply hypoxia. If there are 3 or more accelerations within a 20 min period of continuous fetal heart rate monitoring, the CTG can be said to be normal or 'reactive'.

EARLY DECELERATIONS – A deceleration (Table 39.1) can be said to be early if its onset occurs at the onset of a contraction and the nadir of the deceleration coincides with the peak of the contraction. These are due to increased vagal tone secondary to fetal head compression. They are a normal response and are not indicative of hypoxia. They occur most commonly in the second

Table 39.1 Types of decelerations

	Early	Variable	Late
Onset	Starts with contraction	Starts with contraction	Starts after contraction
Nadir	At peak of contraction	Variable	After peak of contraction
Shape	'V' shaped	'M' shaped or 'V' with shouldering	Shallow
Aetiology	Fetal head compression increases vagal tone	Cord compression	Mild fetal hypoxia
Significance	Normal finding, especially in the second stage	Usually normal; less so if combined with other CTG abnormalities	Sinister finding – demands further action

stage of labour as the fetal head traverses the pelvis but may occur in the first stage or occasionally antenatally. When they occur in the early stages of labour, close observation is recommended, as other abnormalities may develop later in pregnancy which may have more significance on the fetal prognosis.

LATE DECELERATIONS – In late decelerations the onset of the deceleration is after the onset of the contraction, and the nadir of the deceleration occurs after the peak of the contraction. These are an abnormal response to mild hypoxic changes and may be indicative of reduced fetal oxygen reserve. They may not necessarily predict poor fetal outcome but suggest hypoxia secondary to uteroplacental insufficiency. It is when the decelerations are combined with other abnormalities in the fetal heart rate pattern that the fetal prognosis worsens significantly.

MIXED OR COMBINED DECELERATIONS – A combination of head compression and decreased oxygen reserve such as may occur in labour can produce decelerations with an early onset but which continue after the contraction has ceased.

VARIABLE DECELERATIONS – Variable decelerations are always early in onset, but they may be variable in shape; they are best recognised by their characteristic 'M' shape. They may in fact be stereotyped and are

classically due to cord compression. As such, they are not necessarily sinister unless the compression is severe enough to compromise the fetus. Generally, severe variable decelerations are defined as those which fall to a rate of less than 60 bpm, fall by more than 60 bpm from the baseline, or last for more than 60 s. Variable decelerations associated with any other fetal heart rate abnormality are significant and demand closer observation of the fetus.

SPORADIC DECELERATIONS – These are usually of short duration, 'spike' shaped in appearance and are not of immediate significance but suggest the need for further observation, as other abnormalities may develop. These decelerations can occur secondary to episodes of supine hypotension associated with epidural anaesthesia; relevant treatment is usually associated with a prompt return to a normal fetal heart rate pattern.

Normal Cardiotocographic Patterns

In labour, accelerations may normally be absent, but to be acceptable the cardiotocograph should still have a normal baseline, normal variability and no late or severe variable decelerations. Early decelerations are acceptable in labour, especially in the second stage.

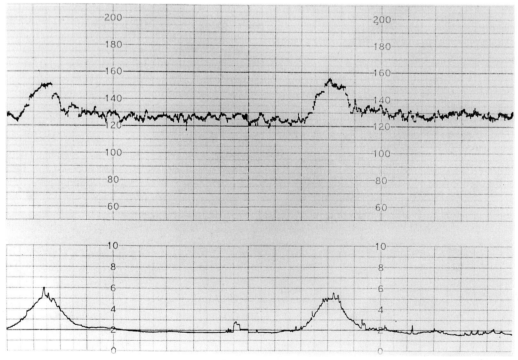

Fig 39.1 *A reassuring fetal heart rate trace demonstrating a normal baseline, normal beat-to-beat variability and accelerations. Reproduced, with permission, from M.D. Read, D. Welby,* A Practical Guide for the Obstetric Team, *Wiley.*

Reassuring Patterns

I. Normal

The baseline is between 110 and 150 bpm with either transient accelerations or no change with contractions, and a baseline variability of between 5 and 25 bpm. See Figure 39.1.

II. Uncomplicated Baseline Bradycardia

The baseline rate is between 100 and 120 bpm; otherwise it is the same as the normal pattern above. This pattern represents good vagal tone in the fetus.

A normal fetal heart rate pattern within 30 min of delivery is associated with satisfactory Apgar scores in 99% of cases.

Non-reassuring Patterns

I. Uncomplicated Baseline Tachycardia

The baseline rate is over 150 bpm; otherwise it is as for the normal pattern. This may be due to maternal ketosis or pyrexia.

II. Uncomplicated Variable Decelerations

There is a normal baseline and variability, with decelera-

tions starting early but which are irregular and variable in amplitude and duration. See Figure 39.2.

III. Uncomplicated Loss of Baseline Variability

The baseline variability is less than 5 bpm; otherwise it is as for the normal trace above. This may be due to maternal sedation. See Figure 39.3.

IV. Presence of Atypical Variable Decelerations

It is important to remember that a suspicious pattern must be reviewed carefully and frequently, as it may lead to a definitely abnormal pattern.

Unsafe Patterns

I. Late Decelerations

Any trace where there are decelerations with a definite time lag.

II. Any Trace Showing Multiple Abnormalities or a Further Complication Arising in one of the Suspicious Patterns

The most sinister patterns are a complicated baseline tachycardia, e.g. a baseline greater than 150 bpm with poor variability (Figure 39.4), and also a progressive

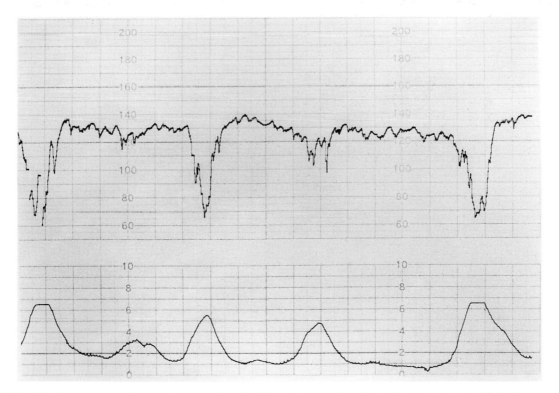

Fig 39.2 *A fetal heart rate trace demonstrating uncomplicated variable decelerations. Reproduced, with permission, from M.D. Read, D. Wellby,* A Practical Guide for the Obstetric Team, *Wiley.*

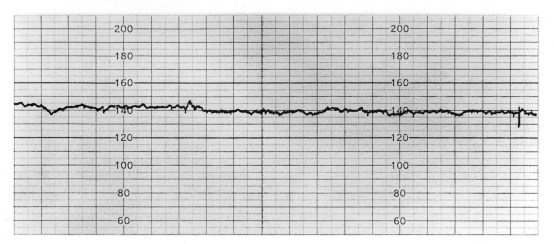

Fig 39.3 *A fetal heart rate trace demonstrating decreased beat-to-beat variability from a normal baseline. Reproduced, with permission, from M.D. Read, D. Wellby,* A Practical Guide for the Obstetric Team, *Wiley.*

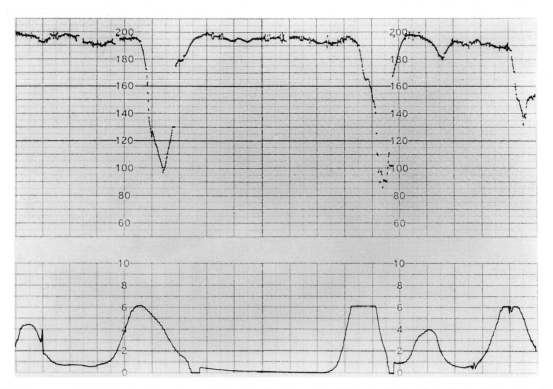

Fig 39.4 *A non-reassuring fetal heart rate trace demonstrating a baseline tachycardia with late decelerations. Reproduced, with permission, from M.D. Read, D. Wellby,* A Practical Guide for the Obstetric Team, *Wiley.*

bradycardia with a fixed baseline or sinusoidal oscillations. In other circumstances the significance of a sinusoidal pattern is uncertain.

TREATMENT

If an abnormal pattern persists then a fetal scalp blood sample should be taken to measure the fetal acid base status. The currently used index of fetal acid base status is the measurement of the pH of a sample of capillary blood obtained from the fetal scalp. Clearly this is only possible when the cervix is sufficiently dilated (> 4 cm in practice) and the vertex has descended into the pelvis. It is only rarely performed on breech presentations and is contraindicated if there is any possibility that the fetus may have a coagulation defect or in cases of intrauterine infection.

The action taken depends on the pH value.

- If the pH >7.25, this is a normal result and labour should be allowed to progress, provided there is no further deterioration in the cardiotocograph.
- If the pH <7.20, this is clearly abnormal and the fetus should be delivered immediately.
- If the pH is between 7.20 and 7.25 the sample should be repeated in 30–60 min provided that there is not further deterioration in the cardiotocograph, in which case it should be repeated immediately.

GOLDEN POINTS

1. Cardiotocography is a very indirect method of assessing fetal wellbeing.

2. Even in the presence of the most severely abnormal cardiotocograph, the fetus will in fact be hypoxic in only about half the cases.

3. Judicious use of cardiotocography during labour, careful and accurate interpretation of the trace obtained and, where possible, the use of fetal scalp blood sampling to support the diagnosis of fetal hypoxia will minimise unnecessary intervention.

4. The baseline, beat-to-beat variability, presence of accelerations and the nature of decelerations are all important.

5. The CTG should be interpreted taking the whole pattern of labour into account, rather than in isolation.

40 Delay in the first stage of labour

CLINICAL SIGNIFICANCE

Delay or difficulty in labour (dystocia) is a common complication, particularly in primigravidae. Prolonged labour is defined as a labour lasting more than 12 h after the onset of active labour – defined as regular uterine contractions with cervical change, dilatation and effacement. The incidence is 5–8%, and prolonged labour is twice as common in primigravidae than in multiparous women.

Prolonged labour is associated with increased maternal and fetal morbidity as well as an increase in the rate of intervention. The risks of fetal distress, maternal dehydration, exhaustion and PPH are all increased by prolonged labour. Prolonged labour can also be psychologically quite traumatic. In third-world countries, without ready access to obstetric care, severely prolonged labour (> 48 h) can lead to more serious complications, i.e. uterine rupture, vesicovaginal fistula and even maternal death.

True cephalopelvic disproportion (CPD) is rare in the UK, although it is a common diagnosis particularly after a prolonged first labour. Even where a first labour ended with a LSCS for CPD there is an 80% chance of a normal delivery subsequently, often with a larger baby. Therefore the main problem appears not to be that the baby is too large for the pelvis but that the uterine contractions are ineffective in primigravidae.

There are maternal and fetal causes, which are similar for delay in both the first and second stages of labour. However, the treatment options are different.

DIFFERENTIAL DIAGNOSIS

Maternal	
1. *Pelvis*	Abnormal shape Abnormal size
2. *Uterus*	Inefficient uterine action Uterine rupture
3. *Other*	Exhaustion Obstruction: fibroids in the birth canal
Fetal	
1. *Position*	Malposition: occipitotransverse (OT)/occipitoposterior (OP)
2. *Presentation*	Malpresentations: transverse lie/face/brow/shoulder
3. *Other*	Macrosomia Fetal abnormality

CLINICAL ASSESSMENT

The progress of labour is measure by cervical dilatation and descent of the presenting part, charted using a partogram. The cervix should dilate by at least 1 cm per hour in the first stage, though there is a wide variation in normal labours. The routine schedule for vaginal examinations in the UK is three-hourly, and therefore, if in that time the cervical dilatation is less than 3 cm, a diagnosis of prolonged or abnormal labour can be made.

The management of prolonged labour relies on diagnosis of the underlying cause prior to any intervention.

Relevant History

Presenting Complaint

MAIN COMPLAINT – The main complaint is an abnormally long labour, i.e. > 12 h. In order to pre-empt a long labour, vaginal examination is performed every 3 h to determine the progress of labour. The pattern of the partogram is helpful to elucidate the cause of the prolonged labour, as detailed below and in Figure 40.1.

Long latent phase: A long latent phase is the time from the onset of uterine contractions to cervical dilatation and is a feature of primigravid labours with hypoactive uterine contractions. Intervention at this stage is not always warranted and can precipitate more problems.

Prolonged active phase: A prolonged active phase is a pattern where the cervix dilates, but slowly. This is classifically a feature of inefficient uterine action in a primigravid labour.

Secondary arrest of cervical dilatation: The labour initially progresses normally and then the progress tails off and perhaps stops. Although this can be due to inefficient uterine action, obstruction of labour should be excluded, particularly in multiparous labours.

COMMONLY ASSOCIATED SYMPTOMS –

Vaginal bleeding: Uterine rupture is characterised by a sudden cessation of contractions, fetal distress and vaginal bleeding. There should be a low threshold of suspicion in multips, particularly after augmentation with Syntocinon or after a previous LSCS.

Backache: Backache can be a feature of a labour complicated by an occipitoposterior position.

EFFECT ON PATIENT – Maternal exhaustion and fetal distress are more common in prolonged labours. Epidural anaesthesia is more common in women with prolonged labour, and there is a lot of debate about whether or not epidural anaesthesia contributes to prolonged labour, as women who are tired and suffering a prolonged labour are more likely to resort to an epidural. However, a review of the effect of epidural anaesthesia on labour concluded that there is a tendency for the first stage to be longer, and, where the epidural is maintained beyond the first stage, there is an increase in malrotation of the presenting part and consequently operative delivery. The effect is exaggerated with an early epidural. The exact mechanism for this is not clear.

Maternal exhaustion is more significant in the second stage where the mother's expulsive efforts contribute to delivery. Maternal anxiety can reduce uterine contractility, as the increased levels of adrenaline are tocolytic.

Obstetric History

INDEX PREGNANCY –

Antenatal: The presenting part usually engages in the pelvis at term. Failure to engage may indicate impending CPD and should be regarded as suspicious. Please note that in Afro-Caribbean patients the fetal head can be high because of the increased angle of inclination of the pelvis. Fetal abnormality, e.g. hydrocephaly, can interfere with a normal labour, and this is often diagnosed on routine anomaly scanning early in the second trimester.

Intrapartum: The partogram is often revealing, as detailed above. Epidural anaesthesia can prolong labour, particularly when it is sited early. Primigravid labours are characteristically longer than multiparous labours, and this is a reflection of the improved efficiency of the uterine contractions. Indeed babies are usually larger after the first pregnancy, and, contrary to popular belief, there is no difference in the birth canal.

OBSTETRIC HISTORY – A thorough history of any previous labour problems is essential. Whatever the outcome, the duration and maximum cervical dilatation should be documented for all previous labours. Women who have laboured at all, i.e. > 4–5 cm, should be treated as multiparous. Women delivered by LSCS before labour, e.g. primigravid breech, can be treated as a primigravida in the subsequent pregnancy, though extra care is required when using Syntocinon. A previous history of LSCS is important as a risk for uterine rupture.

Previous malposition in labour is important, as there are some women who have a pelvic shape that predisposes to recurrent malposition, e.g. an android pelvis is funnel shaped and this inhibits the rotation of the fetal head, predisposing to OT or OP positions.

Grand multiparity can produce a lax abdomen and uterus that predisposes to an abnormal lie.

Gynaecological History

A history of fibroids is important, as low cervical fibroids can obstruct labour.

Medical History

OPERATIONS – Previous pelvic fractures or congenital deformities can contribute to an abnormal pelvic shape, which can obstruct labour.

MEDICAL CONDITIONS – Diabetes mellitus predisposes to fetal macrosomia.

Social History

HEIGHT – Most people under 1.5 m will deliver normally because there are maternal constraints on fetal intrauterine growth, so that most women have the right-sized baby for them. However, 30% of women < 1.5 m have a straight sacrum (rather than the more favourable curved sacrum), and this may contribute to prolonged labour.

Shoe size has no prognostic value.

Relevant Clinical Examination

General Features

GENERAL DEMEANOUR – Maternal exhaustion and anxiety may be self-evident.

BODY-MASS INDEX – Maternal body-mass index is a useful predictor of fetal weight. Short, fat women are at highest risk of CPD.

Abdomen

CONTOUR – Inspection and palpation of the gravid abdomen is essential. A scaphoid abdomen is characteristic of an OP position where the fetal back is posterior. Palpation of the strength and frequency of uterine contractions is important and should be documented on the partogram.

The lie must be determined to exclude a transverse or oblique lie that would require immediate LSCS. The uterus is characteristically wide with a tranverse lie, and the lower pole is empty. The presentation should also be determined to exclude a breech presentation, which is associated with prolonged or abnormal labour. The head can be ballotable and the breech cannot.

OLD SCARS – LSCS scars are important to note.

TENDERNESS – Tenderness over a previous LSCS scar may suggest a dehiscence underlying it, but it is very non-specific.

Pelvis

VAGINAL EXAMINATION – Vaginal examination is the keystone of both the diagnosis and management of prolonged labour. There are a number of different parameters that should be measured during the examination, as follows.

Pelvis: Clinical pelvimetry – the measurement of internal pelvic diameters is no longer undertaken routinely during the antenatal period, as it is very poorly predictive of labour outcome.

Cervix: Failure of cervical dilatation is the sine qua non of prolonged labour, and accurate measurement of cervical dilatation is essential.

Membranes: Rupture of the membranes is one of the therapeutic interventions for prolonged labour in the first stage, and therefore the presence of intact membranes should be documented.

Presenting part: Station, presentation, position, moulding and caput formation should all be determined, particularly in the second stage prior to operative delivery – see Chapter 41. There may be nothing in the pelvis for a transverse or oblique lie, or a hand/shoulder may be palpable. See Chapter 36.

Determining the position of the fetus is particularly important in the second stage – OA, OP or OT. In the first stage of labour there are no therapeutic interventions that can alter the fetal position, but it is worth noting; it is discussed further in Chapter 41.

Relevant Investigations

Haematology

FBC and Group & Save should be taken where there is a possibility of LSCS or PPH. It is often prudent to take the samples at the time of venflon insertion, i.e. prior to an epidural.

Diagnostic Imaging

USS – Ultrasound estimation of fetal weight can be used antenatally for suspected fetal macrosomia; although babies with an estimated weight > 4000 g are more likely to get stuck in labour, the test is extremely non-specific – most women will deliver normally. USS estimation of fetal weight is not used in labour.

LATERAL X-RAY – Lateral pelvimetry was previously used antenatally as a two-dimensional measurement of the pelvic inlet and outlet. It has been used both in labour and also after LSCS for previous CPD. However, it delivers a significant dose of radiation to the fetus (increased risk of childhood leukaemia), and recent studies have demonstrated no discriminatory value at all in predicting those that will require LSCS in any future pregnancy. Therefore most units have stopped using X-ray pelvimetry routinely.

CT SCAN – CT scans deliver a much smaller dose of radiation, but they too have not been shown to predict CPD with sufficient accuracy to justify routine use even after delivery. X-rays and CT scans are not used in labour.

CTG

Fetal distress is more common during a prolonged labour, and therefore auscultation or electronic fetal heart rate monitoring is essential. Electronic fetal monitoring also allows simultaneous monitoring of the uterine contractions, though it is important to note that there is no quantitative measurement of uterine power; frequency of contractions is useful, however.

Intrauterine Pressure Monitoring

Intrauterine pressure monitoring has been used to measure the efficiency of uterine action but, outside of research programmes, there is no indication for its use.

DETAILS OF CONDITION

Background

Definition

The first stage of labour starts with the onset of uterine contractions and ends at full cervical dilatation. Slow progress in the first stage of labour occurs in either the latent phase prior to progressive cervical dilatation or in the active phase.

The duration of the latent phase is so variable that a normal range is difficult to define. However, slow progress in the active phase of labour is easier to define both as a total duration of labour – 12 h – or rate of cervical dilatation < 0.5 cm/h. See Figure 40.1.

Aetiology

Cephalopelvic disproportion is defined as the failure of the fetal head to pass through the pelvis safely because the pelvis is too small and/or the head is too large. CPD must be considered when the labour is slow, but the diagnosis can only be made by excluding functional causes, e.g. uterine hypotonia. In primigravidae this must be assured using stimulation.

Rickets and polio were important causes of abnormal pelves in the past but less so now; indeed, any abnormal pelvis is rare in modern UK practice. There are a variety of normal pelvic shapes, some more favourable than others, but they are largely irrelevant in clinical practice. Obstruction of the birth canal by fibroids, etc. can obviously hinder labour in the first stage.

Inefficient uterine activity is a common cause of slow progress in labour, complicating 3% of all pregnancies, 6% of primigravidae, but the aetiology is unclear.

Poor application of the presenting part can also contribute to slow progress in labour – malpresentations. The flexion of the fetal head is also important. Occipitoposterior positions are characteristically less flexed, which increases the diameter of the presenting part, slowing labour – malpositions (see Chapter 41).

MALPRESENTATIONS – There are a number of different aetiologies, which apply to all the malpresentations, with one common theme: interference with engagement or descent of the presenting part:

Liquor
- polyhydramnios

Placenta
- placenta praevia

Uterus
- laxity – secondary to multiparity or abnormalities
- incoordinate uterine activity

Pelvis
- pelvis abnormalities and obstructing tumours

Fetus
- anatomical abnormalities, e.g. anencephaly – characteristically a face presentation
- abnormal muscle tone – myotonic dystrophy
- multiple pregnancy.

There may be no predisposing factors
Examples of malpresentations are as follows.

Transverse lie is an important complication of labour occurring in 1 in 400 deliveries. The risk of cord prolapse is high, and the woman should be delivered by LSCS immediately.

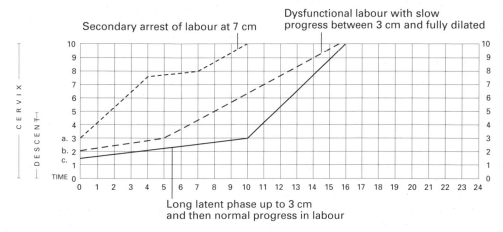

Secondary arrest of labour at 7 cm

Dysfunctional labour with slow progress between 3 cm and fully dilated

Long latent phase up to 3 cm and then normal progress in labour

Fig 40.1 *Partogram demonstrating: leftmost line, secondary arrest of labour at 7 cm; middle line, dysfunctional labour with slow progress between 3 cm and fully dilated; rightmost line, long latent phase up to 3 cm and then normal progress in labour.*

Face presentation (Figure 40.2) Has an incidence of 1 in 500 women. 15% are due to congenital abnormality, anencephaly or tumour of the fetal neck muscles. Most occur by chance after the head extends rather than flexes in labour. Mentoanterior presentations may deliver vaginally by flexion, but in a mentoposterior position the chin (mentum) gets stuck in the sacral hollow and LSCS is obligatory.

Brow presentation (Figure 40.3) is rare – 1 in 2000 deliveries – and it is associated with large babies and/or small pelves. A brow presentation is mentovertical, the largest presenting cephalic diameter being 13.5 cm, and therefore requires delivery by LSCS. It should be excluded particularly after secondary arrest in labour in multiparous women.

Main Complications

MATERNAL – Ascending infection is an important cause of maternal morbidity after prolonged labour because of both the duration and also the increased number of vaginal examinations and other interventions.

One of the primary aims of active management of labour is to prevent the maternal exhaustion characteristic of slow progress in labour. The exhaustion is psychologically traumatic and reduces the satisfaction of the birth experience, but it also can reduce the ability to push in the second stage of labour, which increases the risk of operative delivery.

The risk of PPH is increased – see Chapter 43.

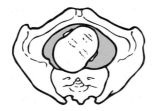

Fig 40.2 *Face presentation.*

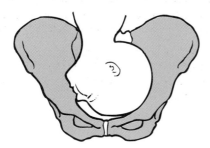

Fig 40.3 *Brow presentation.*

FETAL – There is also an increase in fetal morbidity and mortality, particularly fetal distress and ascending infection, during a prolonged labour.

Prevention

'Active management' of labour was first proposed in Dublin in the 1960s to reduce the incidence of prolonged labour and subsequently the rate of operative delivery, particularly LSCS. A rigid scheme was proposed, of early amniotomy and liberal use of oxytocin in slow primigravid labours: i.e., where the labour was not progressing by at least 0.5 cm/h, an ARM was performed, followed by oxytocin where the former alone was not sufficient to augment or speed up the labour.

However, since its first introduction there have been a number of trials that have failed to demonstrate any benefit for active management, although the results in the parent hospital in Dublin are still excellent. Therefore the benefits of such a scheme may lie in the peripheral parts of the protocol, i.e. excellent antenatal education, almost continuous care by a single midwife and very strict audit by senior consultants.

Treatment Options

Perhaps the only parameters of the first stage of labour that can be controlled or altered are the force of uterine contractions and the cervical resistance. Certainly the shape of the pelvis cannot be changed, nor can the fetus. Therefore, clinical treatment options rely on increasing the force of uterine contractions using oxytocin, or decreasing cervical resistance usually by endogenous release of local prostaglandins after amniotomy.

Conservative

Many factors affect myometrial contractility and the progress of labour. Consideration of more conservative measures first may obviate the need for clinical intervention in some cases.

COMPANION AND BIRTH ATTENDANT – The presence of a supportive companion and mobilisation have both been shown to shorten labour and reduce intervention. Moreover, women who are allowed to eat and drink in labour require less analgesia and progress more quickly in labour. As stated previously, maternal anxiety can decrease uterine contractility, and this can be allayed by good antenatal education and pleasant surroundings with supportive staff. Indeed, the proponents of home delivery would suggest that these are the benefits of home delivery. They probably are!

Medical

ARM – Amniotomy can reduce the length of labour by between 1 and 2 h. However, there does not seem to be any difference in outcome, i.e. you get to the same place quicker. There do not appear to be any direct adverse effects of ARM in labour, but it is an intervention that proponents of 'natural' labour criticise. Nonetheless it is frequently used in clinical practice in the UK.

SYNTOCINON – Intravenous Syntocinon is routinely used to improve uterine contractility. However, it is important to exclude other causes of slow labour before use. This is particularly important for secondary arrest in labour and in multiparous labours because the risk of a significant underlying pathology is increased, i.e. malpresentation, CPD.

Intravenous Syntocinon is infused at an increasing rate until there are three uterine contractions in every 10 min. Uterine hyperstimulation is a common complication and can precipitate fetal distress because there is insufficient time between contractions for feto-maternal oxygen transfer. Syntocinon also increases the subjective assessment of the pain of labour and therefore other measures should be used first. Despite all of these problems, Syntocinon is widely used, though this may be more a reflection of the paucity of other medical agents rather than the efficacy of syntocinon.

Syntocinon should be used with caution after previous LSCS or in multipara. Seek senior help.

Surgical

CAESAREAN SECTION – There are some women who will require abdominal delivery despite adequate uterine contractions. There may be CPD, a malpresentation or no obvious reason.

There are two main types of caesarean section defined by the uterine incision: lower segment and classical. In the lower segment caesarean section the uterus is opened transversely in the lower segment. In the classical version the uterus is opened longitudinally, but there is an increase in the complication rate and uterine rupture in subsequent labours. Therefore classical sections are reserved for women with a poorly formed lower segment, i.e. prematurity, or where the lower segment is inaccessible, i.e. secondary to adhesions, etc.

Overview

Prolonged labour is a common and potentially distressing complication. It usually, though not necessarily, results from inefficient uterine action. It may be due to CPD or abnormal fetal presentation. Where malpresentation has been excluded, it will often be necessary to ensure adequate uterine action with oxytocics before resorting to abdominal delivery for dystocia.

Information for Patients

Prognosis

The prognosis after prolonged labour is generally good: there is an 80% likelihood of vaginal delivery after even a LSCS for CPD in a first pregnancy. However, the experiences of a prolonged difficult labour may be sufficiently psychologically traumatic for women to ask for an elective LSCS in future pregnancies. They should be counselled that all complications of the puerperium are increased after LSCS compared with vaginal delivery, and 80% of women will deliver vaginally after a previous LSCS. Therefore a trial of vaginal delivery is in their best interests.

Follow-up

Short term

A longer postnatal hospital stay may be necessary after a prolonged labour, particularly after delivery by LSCS. Early ambulation is encouraged, and a stay of 2–5 days is routine. A 'debriefing' visit may be appropriate after a difficult labour.

GOLDEN POINTS

1. Dystocia is one of the most common complications of labour, particularly in primigravidae.

2. The incidence of ascending infection, maternal exhaustion, PPH and fetal distress are increased after prolonged labour.

3. Malpresentation and other causes requiring immediate delivery by LSCS should be excluded.

4. Mobilisation, eating in labour and a birth companion can all reduce the incidence of intervention in labour.

5. Most primigravidae will require at least an ARM and trial of oxytocics to ensure sufficient uterine contractions before delivery by LSCS for CPD.

6. The prognosis after prolonged labour is generally good: there is an 80% likelihood of vaginal delivery after even a LSCS for CPD in a first pregnancy.

41 Delay in the second stage of labour

CLINICAL SIGNIFICANCE

The second stage of labour is that time from full cervical dilatation to delivery of the baby. It is in some ways artificial to separate the first and second stages, as they are a continuum and some factors that contribute to a prolonged first stage of labour can also prolong the second stage, notably inadequate or incoordinate uterine contractions, malpresentation or, more commonly in the second stage, malposition and cephalo-pelvic disproportion.

A prolonged second stage carries similar risks to a prolonged first stage, and although early resort to surgical intervention (i.e. instrumental delivery) is tempting, it is not without risk, and other less invasive interventions should be tried first. Although instrumental delivery is one of the commonest obstetric interventions, the skill required to use the instruments safely and effectively should not be underestimated.

The instrument of choice for delivery is now the ventouse. There is a three-fold decrease in maternal trauma compared with forceps, with similar fetal outcomes, and less maternal analgesia is required.

There is no place for brave deliveries these days, and where a difficult instrumental delivery is anticipated then a caesarean section may be most appropriate.

DIFFERENTIAL DIAGNOSIS

Maternal

1. *Pelvis*	Abnormal shape Abnormal size
2. *Uterus*	Inefficient uterine action Uterine rupture
3. *Other*	Exhaustion Obstruction: fibroids in the birth canal

Fetal

1. *Position*	Malpositions: occipitotransverse (OT) / occipitoposterior (OP)
2. *Presentation*	Malpresentations; transverse lie / face / brow / shoulder
3. *Other*	Macrosomia Fetal abnormality

CLINICAL ASSESSMENT

A slow first stage of labour often heralds delay in the second stage, and, like the management of prolonged first stage, the management of a prolonged second stage requires an accurate diagnosis of any underlying causes prior to any intervention.

In the second stage, up to 1 h of active pushing is deemed normal, although it may be appropriate to allow some time in the second stage prior to pushing. Women should therefore be assessed by a senior obstetrician/midwife after 1 h of pushing.

Rapid Emergency Assessment

A prolonged second stage is rarely an emergency unless there is concurrent fetal distress, but it should not be ignored, as maternal exhaustion is often a feature.

Relevant History

Presenting Complaint

MAIN COMPLAINT – There are two distinct parts of the second stage: a passive stage where the head descends without pushing, and an active or expulsive phase with pushing. There is no strict definition of a prolonged second stage, though 1 h pushing is considered 'enough' by most (mothers!).

It is important to understand that the second stage is not a race that starts as soon as the cervix is fully dilated; equally, pushing is not synonymous with the second stage. Sufficient time should be allowed for the presenting part to descend passively, without pushing, particularly where the presenting part is initially high or there is an epidural in situ. Therefore, although pushing should be limited to approximately 1 h, the total second stage may last up to 3 h without undue problems.

COMMONLY ASSOCIATED SYMPTOMS –

Maternal exhaustion: Maternal exhaustion can be very significant in the second stage of labour. The effects are often cumulative through the labour: a prolonged first stage causes maternal exhaustion, which impairs the maternal expulsive effort, which then contributes to a prolonged second stage.

Fetal distress: Fetal distress can be a feature of a prolonged second stage, as the fetal pH falls more rapidly in the second stage than the first, i.e. the baby becomes more acidotic and more hypoxic. In normal labours this is rarely problematical, but, where the fetus is already bordering on hypoxia, a long second stage can exacerbate the problem and precipitate fetal distress.

Obstetric History

INDEX PREGNANCY – Features of the first stage, such as a prolonged active phase suggestive of inefficient uterine action and secondary arrest, which should alert the accoucheur to the possibility of a malposition, also hold true for the second stage.

A long first stage, particularly delay between 7 cm and fully dilated, can indicate that expediting delivery with either forceps or ventouse may be difficult. Therefore, in this event, a trial of instrumental delivery in theatre with recourse to caesarean section in the event of failure may be appropriate.

Epidural anaesthesia can prolong the second stage of labour as well as the first.

OBSTETRIC HISTORY – A thorough history of any previous labour problems is essential. A previous history of LSCS is important as a potential risk factor for uterine rupture. Previous malposition in labour is important, as there are some women who have a pelvic shape that predisposes to recurrent malposition: an android pelvis is funnel shaped and this inhibits the rotation of the fetal head, predisposing to OT or OP positions.

Gynaecological History

Low cervical fibroids can obstruct labour, as they take up valuable room within the fixed confines of the pelvis, preventing the presenting part from descending.

Medical History

OPERATIONS – Previous pelvic fractures or congenital deformities can contribute to an abnormal pelvic shape, which can obstruct labour.

MEDICAL CONDITIONS – Fetal macrosomia secondary to maternal diabetes can result in a slow second stage and even an obstructed labour. In the presence of a large baby, a slow labour should alert the obstetric team to the possibility of shoulder dystocia, and the birth should be attended by senior obstetricians/midwives.

Relevant Clinical Examination

General Features

GENERAL DEMEANOUR – Maternal exhaustion is usually self-evident. Both the mother and her partner may be tired, and this can increase the anxiety in the birth room as well.

BODY-MASS INDEX – Maternal body-mass index is a useful predictor of fetal weight. Short, fat women are at highest risk of CPD.

Abdomen

The abdomen should be palpated in a similar fashion to that in the first stage of labour. Palpation of the strength and frequency of uterine contractions is important and should be documented on the partogram. The presentation should also be determined to exclude an abnormal presentation – see Chapter 36.

However, most importantly of all, the descent of the presenting part should be palpated abdominally. Instrumental delivery must not be attempted where there is any head palpable abdominally. This is because moulding of the fetal head during a prolonged labour can confuse the unwary; the presenting part may feel below the ischial spines on vaginal examination, but it may not be wholly in the pelvis, and this would preclude a vaginal delivery.

OLD SCARS – LSCS scars are important to note.

TENDERNESS – Tenderness over a previous LSCS scar may suggest a dehiscence underlying it, but it is very non-specific.

Pelvis

VAGINAL EXAMINATION – Again, vaginal examination is the keystone of both the diagnosis and management of a prolonged labour, including delay in the second stage. The following should be assessed during the examination.

Pelvis: A brief assessment can be made of the 'room' inside the pelvis, i.e. the sacral curve, ischial spines and the distance between the pubic rami. A narrow pelvis is more likely to cause CPD and therefore should prompt more careful evaluation if operative vaginal delivery is anticipated. Any soft tissue obstruction can also be determined, e.g. cervical fibroids.

Cervix: Full dilatation of the cervix defines the second stage and is also a prerequisite for consideration of instrumental delivery.

Membranes: Any intact membranes should be ruptured in the presence of delay in the second stage.

Presenting Part

The main difference between assessing the presenting part in the first and second stages of labour is the detail required. For delay in the second stage, it is essential to be able to accurately determine the station, presentation and, if it is cephalic, the position, as these are all important factors in determining whether or not instrumental delivery should be attempted. Moulding and caput are also important, but it is determination of the position and the station that is the key to successful delivery.

STATION – The ischial spines are easily palpable at vaginal examination and are used as a marker to determine how low the presenting part is inside the pelvis. Where the presenting part is at, or, better still, below the spines then it is reasonable to attempt vaginal delivery – with the caveat that there is no head palpable abdominally as can be the case with excessive moulding.

Although assessment of station is an inexact science, there is a scoring system: above the spines (–1), at the spines (0), 1 cm below the spines (+1), and 2 cm below the spines (+2).

PRESENTATION – One hopes that the presentation will be cephalic. Instrumental delivery is contraindicated for all other presentations, including face and brow presentations; caesarean section is required should there be delay in the second stage.

POSITION – Determining the position of the fetal head can be difficult, but it is all important prior to instrumental delivery. Different positions require different instruments and different techniques.

There are basically only four positions, and each is defined by the position of the occiput: occipitoanterior (OA), occipitotransverse (OT), occipitoposterior (OP) and oblique.

Occipitoanterior – the occiput is at 12 o'clock, i.e. the baby is looking down towards the rectum.

Occipitioposterior – the occiput is at 6 o'clock, i.e. the baby is looking up towards the symphysis pubis.

Occipitotransverse – the occiput is at either 3 o'clock (left OT) or 9 o'clock (right OT). (Remember that the left and right are maternal left and right.)

Oblique can be predominantly OA (10 and 2 o'clock) or OP (4 and 8 o'clock).

MOULDING – The fetal skull bones are joined by sutures and these can be displaced in labour so that one bony plate can ride over another in order to reduce the diameter for delivery. This can be palpated as a ridge. Extensive moulding should suggest a degree of cephalopelvic disproportion – think of an egg in an eggcup!

CAPUT FORMATION – In labour the dilating cervix may press on the fetal scalp, reducing venous and lymphatic return. This causes oedema, palpable as a soft swelling on the baby's head, and it is called caput.

In labour a brow presentation is characteristically high, the anterior fontanelle is central because the head is very deflexed, and the supraorbital ridges can be palpated as well as the closed eyes.

A face presentation is diagnosed from the malar prominences, the mouth and nose. During the labour the face can become very oedematous, and a breech may be diagnosed inadvertently.

Relevant Investigations

Haematology

As previously in the first stage, a FBC and G&S should be taken where there is a possibility of LSCS or PPH. It is often prudent to take the samples at the time of venflon insertion, i.e. prior to an epidural.

CTG

Auscultation of the fetal heart can be difficult in the second stage, and therefore electronic fetal monitoring can be used in preference. Some form of monitoring is important lest the fetus become hypoxic unnoticed.

Compression of the fetal head can give rise to variable decelerations in the second stage, and it is important to appreciate that these are normal, otherwise unnecessary intervention may result. (See Chapter 39.)

DETAILS OF INDIVIDUAL CONDITIONS

1. Maternal Exhaustion/Inefficient Uterine Action

Background

DEFINITION – Maternal exhaustion and inefficient uterine action often, though not necessarily always, coexist. An efficient labour is a slow labour and therefore more likely to cause exhaustion.

AETIOLOGY – The most common cause of inefficient uterine action is the incoordinate action of the primigravid uterus. Other related causes include malposition, especially OP positions (see below).

MAIN COMPLICATIONS – The main maternal risks are prolonged labour leading to increased intervention rates as well as an increase in ascending infection febrile morbidity, etc., as described after a prolonged first stage. A prolonged second stage can also result in urinary retention, as the bladder base is traumatised by prolonged pressure by the fetal head in the vagina.

There is also an increase in fetal morbidity and mortality, particularly fetal distress and ascending infection, with the additional inherent risks of instrumental delivery.

Treatment Options

CONSERVATIVE – The presence of a supportive companion and mobilisation may once again be useful. Adequate analgesia may reduce exhaustion to a minimum (see Chapter 42).

MEDICAL – Syntocinon can correct inefficient uterine action and should be used early in the second stage if a prolonged second stage is anticipated. There is no point starting Syntocinon after the poor woman has pushed for an hour, as she will be both unwilling and probably unable to push for another hour.

SURGICAL – Episiotomy can be used to expedite delivery if the head is well down on the perineum and it appears that the perineum is delaying delivery. Although selective episiotomy can be useful, it should not be used in a cavalier fashion and certainly not routinely. Adequate analgesia should also be used.

Instrumental deliveries are one of the commonest interventions in obstetrics, and maternal exhaustion is one of the commonest indications for their use. There are a number of prerequisites to check before assisted delivery, assuming a valid indication for intervention:

- The presentation should be cephalic
- There should be no evidence of CPD or excessive moulding
- The head should be engaged and none of the head should be palpable abdominally
- The position of the head should be known
- Analgesia should be adequate
- The obstetrician should be sufficiently skilled and experienced.

There are two main groups of instruments used to expedite delivery: obstetric forceps and the ventouse cup. Until recently, forceps were the most commonly used of the two, but now there is increasing evidence to support the ventouse cup as the instrument of first choice (see Table 41.1).

Instrumental delivery of a fetus in the **occipitoanterior position** is as follows.

Forceps (non-rotational): Forceps consist of two blades joined at the handle. The blades have a curve that fits around the fetal head (cephalic curve) and a curve that fits the inside curve of the sacrum and therefore the internal contours of the pelvis (pelvic curve) – see Figure 41.1. A pudendal nerve block may be required. A guarded needle is placed in the vagina, and 10 ml of lignocaine is injected at the ischial spines bilaterally. This anaesthetises the pudendal nerve as it curls around the ischial spine, resulting in an anaesthetised vulva and perineum.

The blades are placed into the vagina, separately, around the baby's head. The direction of traction is 'J' shaped to mimic the normal direction of travel, i.e. down until the occiput descends and then up as the baby's head is born by extension using the pubic arch as a fulcrum. An episiotomy is often indicated to reduce the risk of anal sphincter trauma.

Table 41.1	Advantages and disadvantages of forceps and ventouse	
	Forceps	Ventouse
Maternal trauma	Three-fold increase in maternal trauma	Significantly less anal sphincter trauma
Episiotomy	Recommended	Not required routinely
Analgesia requirement	Pudendal block and perineal infiltration	Perineal infiltration
Marginal CPD	Forceps exacerbate marginal CPD, as they add width to the fetal head	
Fetal trauma	Facial bruising and occasionally facial nerve palsy secondary to compression	Cephalohaematoma and increased caput (chignon).
	Rarely, skull fracture and tentorial vein tears	Rarely, retinal haemorrhages (significance unknown)
Success rates	There is no difference in well-trained hands	

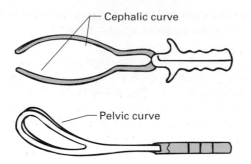

Fig 41.1 *Non-rotational forceps demonstrating cephalic and pelvic curves.*

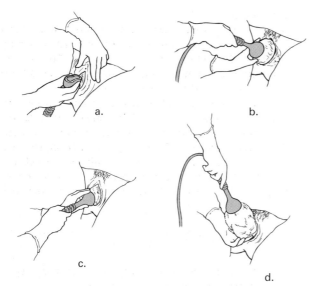

Fig 41.2 *Delivery by ventouse.*

Ventouse: The cup is placed in the vagina and thence over the posterior fontanelle (Figure 41.2). The suction tubing is attached, and a vacuum of 0.8 kg/cm² is used to attach the cup to the fetal scalp. The direction of traction is similar to that for forceps, but the ventouse cup also encourages flexion so that the smallest possible diameter is presented. This and the fact that the ventouse sits on top of the fetal head and not around it is therefore probably why there is less maternal trauma. Less analgesia is routinely required.

2. Fetal Malposition

Background

DEFINITION – Position other than occipitoanterior, i.e. occipitoposterior or occipitotransverse.

AETIOLOGY – In a number of women the fetus starts off in labour with its back to the maternal back. In a normal labour the uterine contractions will push the head down onto the gutter-shaped pelvic floor and the head flexes (chin to chest) with the increased resistance. The gutter of the pelvic floor tilts forward from posterior to anterior, and therefore the head should rotate to OA. However, where there are insufficient uterine contractions to flex the fetal head or the pelvis is slightly funnel shaped, which reduces the room for rotation, it can fail to rotate, resulting in an OP position.

MAIN COMPLICATIONS –

Maternal:

Prolonged first and second stages of labour: A number of features about an OP position contribute to a prolonged first and second stage. Because the head is less flexed in an OP position (chin not on chest, as if baby looking upwards) then the presenting diameter is not reduced to its minimum as it would be if it were completely flexed (chin on chest). The less flexed head with its larger presenting diameter make its passage through the pelvis more difficult, which prolongs the labour.

Back pain: When the baby is in the OP position then the presenting part presses more towards the back, causing back ache, and the pressure over the rectum induces bearing down (wanting to push) sensations prior to full cervical dilatation.

Fetal: The main fetal complications are increased moulding and the consequences of a prolonged labour, increased rates of hypoxia and potential injury during instrumental delivery.

Treatment Options

The majority of fetuses in an OP position will rotate spontaneously during labour to an OA position (75%) and deliver relatively easily. 5% will continue to descend without further rotation and require an assisted delivery or deliver 'face to pubes' where the pelvis is large enough to accommodate the larger diameter of the presenting part. The remaining 20% will begin to rotate to OA and get stuck half way in an OT position – classically, a deep transverse arrest. The treatment is similar for both OT and OP positions.

CONSERVATIVE – Again, the presence of a supportive companion and mobilisation can improve the contractility of the uterus and therefore encourage flexion and therefore rotation of the fetal head. However, intervention is often required.

MEDICAL – Intravenous oxytocin is routinely used to improve uterine contractility, and where there is evidence of poor or inefficient uterine action this would be appropriate to try, particularly in a primigravid labour. Even if the woman has reached full cervical dilatation spontaneously, it is worth considering judicious use of Syntocinon in the second stage.

An epidural is often recommended in tandem with Syntocinon, as this will reduce the premature bearing-down sensation, backache and potentially the maternal exhaustion. Especially where there is an epidural in situ, sufficient time should be allowed for the head to descend prior to commencing pushing.

SURGICAL – Where the head is above the spines or there is some head palpable abdominally, there should be early resort to caesarean section rather than instrumental delivery.

It is sometimes possible to hold the baby's head in the vagina and manually rotate it to an OA position, though this is rare, and more often instrumental delivery is required. The same principles and caveats apply to instrumental delivery as noted above. However, in both OP and OT deliveries the instruments are slightly different.

Ventouse: The ventouse cap can also be used to deliver babies in both OP and OT. The cap is again applied over the occiput, but in an OP position the occiput lies inside the vagina along the posterior wall (6 o'clock). Traction on the ventouse encourages flexion, reducing the presenting diameter and encouraging rotation on the pelvic floor. There is no directly applied rotation force; the baby rotates on the pelvic floor as normal.

Forceps: The type of forceps also differs. Rotational, or Kjelland's, forceps do not have a pelvic curve like non-rotational forceps, as this would increase the rotating diameter of the forceps and could result in maternal trauma. Kjelland's forceps are applied to the fetal head, and the baby is physically rotated to OA from either an OP or an OT position. There is some evidence that Kjelland's forceps are associated with an excess maternal and fetal trauma, and therefore only experienced operators should use them.

OVERVIEW – Fetal malposition is a common complication of labour and often resolves spontaneously. Judicious use of Syntocinon, where there is evidence of inefficient uterine action, and an epidural may encourage rotation in as many of the rest as possible. However, where this

fails then a careful and skilled instrumental delivery may be required, probably with the ventouse.

Information for Patients

PROGNOSIS – The prognosis after a prolonged second stage is good even after an instrumental delivery. The chance of a repeat instrumental delivery is small. However, the effect of a painful difficult instrumental delivery should not be underestimated; many women have nightmares about them afterwards!

SELF-HELP GROUPS – Self-help groups are useful, particularly for those whose birth experiences have left them psychologically traumatised. Postnatal counselling and support can be very helpful.

Follow-up

SHORT TERM – Women rarely require follow-up, though women with postoperative complications such as urinary retention should be seen at 6 weeks or so. Women who have endured a difficult delivery should also be offered a 6 weeks visit to discuss the delivery.

LONG TERM – Long-term follow-up is rarely necessary, though an early antenatal visit is recommended to discuss future plans for delivery. Some women are so traumatised after a difficult delivery that they may request delivery by caesarean section. Full discussion of the delivery can identify the precise area of anxiety with a view to allaying specific fears and encouraging a vaginal delivery.

GOLDEN POINTS

1. Delay in the second stage is a common and distressing complication of pregnancy.

2. It is essential to be able to determine the position and the station of the fetus as part of the assessment of delay in the second stage.

3. Instrumental delivery should not be considered lightly; other interventions may be offered first.

4. The ventouse is the instrument of first choice.

5. An OP position should be treated with respect; do not deliver vaginally at all costs!

42 Maternal distress in labour

CLINICAL SIGNIFICANCE

Some degree of maternal distress almost always occurs in labour because labour is accompanied by pain, an acute concern about the mother and her baby, as well as tiredness. Distress can be detrimental to the progress of labour and fetal wellbeing as well as ruining the birth experience and possibly leading to increased rates of depression, which can have a profound effect both on the patient and her family.

Support is essential in labour, and the simple expedient of providing a sympathetic companion has been shown to reduce the requirement for intervention in labour. Support may include helping the woman to choose among pharmacological and non-pharmacological methods of pain relief. There are many different methods of pain relief, each with different advantages and disadvantages. The woman should be provided with information about each one such that she can make her decision.

Most commonly a pain relief ladder is used: non-pharmacological methods initially, followed by drugs and finally an epidural should the others prove insufficient. However, whilst drugs can be used to provide analgesia, they should not be used in isolation to overcome maternal distress in normal labour.

DIFFERENTIAL DIAGNOSIS
METHODS

Non-pharmacological

1. *Support*
2. *Natural childbirth*
3. *Bath*
4. *Acupuncture*
5. *Transcutaneous electrical nerve stimulation (TENS)*

Pharmacological

1. *Inhalational*
2. *Opiates*
3. *Regional analgesia - epidural*
4. *General anaesthesia*

CLINICAL ASSESSMENT

An important feature in decreasing maternal distress is giving the mother the freedom to conduct labour in the way she feels most comfortable.

Assessment of others' distress can be difficult. Women experience a wide variety of pain in labour, and an equally wide range of responses to it. Ideally the woman will have been well enough briefed antenatally to make her own decisions. However, where there is obvious distress, it may be appropriate to counsel the woman about her options.

The detrimental effects of stress and anxiety are mediated through the (fight or flight) sympathetic nervous system. Adrenaline and noradrenaline are released which have direct effects on the uterus and its blood flow. Stimulation of the β-2 receptors by adrenaline relaxes the pregnant uterus (note the use of β-2 agonists to suppress preterm labour) and also reduces the uterine blood flow. Together these actions can directly prolong labour and precipitate fetal distress.

Relevant History

There are a number of important features of the history and examination that merit special attention prior to commending particular methods of analgesia.

Presenting Complaint

MAIN COMPLAINT – The main complaint is obviously pain. The experience of pain is affected by the labour; women who are well supported and making good progress are more likely to 'put up with the pain' whereas women suffering longer labours may feel less able to cope.

Obstetric History

INDEX PREGNANCY – An epidural is recommended for women with PET to reduce the blood pressure and also for women at high risk of intervention, e.g. twins or breech, though this is not mandatory.

OBSTETRIC HISTORY – A previous poor outcome may increase anxiety. A good or bad experience with methods of analgesia in previous pregnancies may colour the choice in the index pregnancy.

Medical History

A history of thrombocytopaenia is important, as low platelets increase the risk of an epidural haematoma, which can cause adverse neurological effects. Thrombocytopaenia is more common in pregnancy – usually idiopathic. Very low levels of platelets ($< 50 \times 10^9$/L) also preclude the use of intramuscular injections, e.g. opiates, as there is an increased risk of haematoma.

There are also some other rare conditions in which regional anaesthesia is contraindicated, e.g. aortic stenosis – if in doubt consult the anaesthetist for advice.

Drug History

Previous opiate abuse can make the prescription of narcotics in labour difficult.

Social History

A supportive partner is probably the single most effective method of reducing maternal distress to a minimum. The partner need not necessarily be the husband; other family members or friends may be just as effective.

Relevant Clinical Examination

Cardiovascular System

The blood pressure is important. Regional anaesthesia reduces the blood pressure by dilating the capacitance vessels (veins) in the legs. Therefore it can be useful with high blood pressure, whilst low blood pressure should prompt further thought.

Relevant Investigations

Haematology

An epidural is contraindicated with a platelet count of $< 100 \times 10^9$/L.

Prevention

Antenatal education can help reduce some of the anxiety inevitably associated with childbirth and therefore reduce maternal distress. Information about methods of analgesia can also be provided 'cold'.

TREATMENT OPTIONS

Conservative and Reassurance

A wide variety of non-pharmacological methods have been and are employed.

Support

Simple measures such as adequate explanation of procedures, mobilisation and companionship can decrease maternal fear and stress. This should not be the sole preserve of natural childbirth; all health professionals must endeavour to meet these expectations.

Baths

Baths have been used for centuries, and there is some evidence that immersion in water can reduce pain and distress. There has been a recent upsurge in interest in water births for this reason. Although immersion in water is generally extremely safe, absolute safety has been questioned. Very high water temperatures may cause fetal overheating, possibly causing fetal death or brain damage, and moreover the baby may begin to gasp after birth, prior to reaching the surface of the water, causing problems. However, with a few simple precautions, sitting in a bath should be very safe.

Acupuncture

There are no controlled trials of acupuncture in labour, though there are a number of proponents who suggest that it might provide good analgesia.

Transcutaneous Electrical Nerve Stimulation (TENS)

The TENS unit consists of a portable battery-powered generator of electrical impulses. A low-voltage electric current is transmitted to the skin via surface electrodes placed over the lumbar region. These electrical currents are supposed to partially block the cutaneous pain fibres, thus decreasing the sensation of labour pain. Although many women try a TENS machine because there are no side effects for the mother or baby, its efficacy remains in doubt.

Food and Drink

Maternal distress can be aggravated by hunger. In previous years, food and liquid intake was limited in labour because the risks of aspiration of stomach contents during general anaesthesia were significant. However, emergency general anaesthetics are less commonly used now as spinal anaesthesia is more commonly used, and therefore women may be allowed a light diet throughout labour.

Medical

The benefits of pain relief are obvious, but most women really want to know which method will achieve an acceptable degree of pain relief whilst least compromising themselves or their baby. The answer is necessarily an individual one, and compromises must be made.

Inhalational Analgesia – Entonox

Nitrous oxide in a 50/50 mixture with oxygen (Gas & Air) is an effective analgesic in labour. The woman inhales the mixture on demand, and it is popular at least partly because of this element of control. It also has a very rapid onset of action and it alleviates the pain rather than eliminates it. It has an equivalent analgesic effect to pethidine.

MAIN COMPLICATIONS –
Maternal: Some women complain of nausea and vomit with Entonox, though this is rare. More commonly, women complain of feeling giddy or lightheaded Serious side effects are rare. It does not affect labour directly.
Fetal: There are no reported fetal side effects.

Opiates

Systemic narcotics can provide reasonable pain relief, and pethidine is the most commonly used analgesic in obstetric units. However, it is not a perfect analgesic, and indeed there is a dearth of evidence to suggest that it is even better than Entonox. Again it will reduce pain, not eliminate it, and mothers should be made aware of this. Intramuscular pethidine is often combined with an antiemetic to reduce the maternal side effects.

Other opiates, e.g. diamorphine, are used in other countries but are rarely used in routine practice in the UK.

MAIN COMPLICATIONS –
Maternal: Nausea and vomiting is the most commonly encountered side effect. Opiates also delay gastric emptying and therefore increase the risk of aspiration should an emergency CS be required. There is also a risk of depression of both the levels of consciousness and respiration at high doses of pethidine. There is no effect on labour.
Fetal: Opiates readily cross the placenta and therefore can depress the fetus. This most commonly manifests as a decrease in the baseline variability of the CTG. Fetal oxygenation is unaffected.
Neonatal: Fetal depression by opiates translates into neonatal depression after delivery, particularly respiratory depression, low apgar scores and decreased muscle tone. These effects can be minimised by keeping the dose to a minimum and avoiding pethidine within 3 h of delivery.

Regional Analgesia

Regional analgesia, particularly epidural analgesia, has increased in popularity in recent years. The increase in use is not just for labour; spinal anaesthetics, in particular, are increasingly being used for operative procedures also.

Epidural Analgesia

Epidural anaesthesia is undoubtedly the most effective method of analgesia in labour, completely relieving the pain of labour for >95% of women without fetal or maternal depression. However, it requires skilled anaesthetic cover.

Local anaesthetic is injected into the epidural space,

Table 42.1	Advantages/disadvantages of pain relief in labour		
	Entonox	Pethidine	Epidural
Analgesia	Partial	Partial	Complete
Maternal effects	Occasionally, nausea and vomiting	Depression of consciousness/respiration	Very occasional epidural haematoma
Effect on labour	None	None	Prolongs labour and increases intervention rates
Neonatal effects	None	Significant risk of depression	None
Advantages	Patient controlled	Easy to administer	Good analgesia
Disadvantages		Neonatal effects	Requires anaesthetist

producing a very effective nerve blockade. Unfortunately the local anaesthetic action is not confined to the pain fibres, and there is often a degree of motor and sensory block which limits mobility and can be an uncomfortable sensation in itself. Epidural opioids have recently been introduced to reduce this problem: injection of opioids, mixed with local anaesthetic, into the epidural space reduces the requirement for local anaesthetic and consequently results in reduced motor blockade.

Epidurals can be intermittently topped up to provide analgesia over a variable period of time and a variable block sufficient for labour or operative delivery.

MAIN COMPLICATIONS –

Maternal: Epidural analgesia is not without problems. Hypotension is a common side effect due to venous dilatation. This can be avoided in the majority of women by preloading with intravenous fluids. Hypotension can also complicate top-ups.

The effect of epidurals on labour remains a contentious area. Women with epidurals do tend to have a longer first stage of labour, and oxytocin is more commonly used. The second stage is also characteristically longer with increased intervention, especially instrumental delivery, after malrotation of the fetus. The exact mechanisms underlying these changes are unknown, though relaxation of the pelvic floor may contribute to malrotation.

There have been a number of recent reports concerning backache after epidural analgesia. In well controlled trials, backache appears to be just as common in women who did not have an epidural.

Where the dura is inadvertently punctured during the insertion of the epidural catheter the loss of CSF drags on pain-sensitive structures in the brain, causing a severe headache. This is a rare complication in skilled hands.

Very rarely, an epidural haematoma can form, with resultant neurological sequelae.

Fetal: Prolonged maternal hypotension can reduce placental perfusion, leading to fetal hypoxia. Otherwise there are very few direct fetal side effects.

Spinal Analgesia

Local anaesthetic is injected directly into the dural space. It provides a very rapid, dense blockade that lasts for 2–3 h. Its use is therefore limited to operative procedures with a finite time span. It is not routinely used in labour.

It is the preferred anaesthetic method for caesarean section, as it is safer than general anaesthesia for both the mother and baby.

OVERVIEW – Maternal distress is a common and complex problem. Antenatal education and adequate support in labour by both companions and health care professionals are the most effective solutions to maternal distress.

Adequate analgesia is a useful adjunct to support in labour but should not be used in isolation as a treatment for maternal distress. There is a wide choice of analgesia available to labouring women, and they should make an informed choice about the method that best suits them.

GOLDEN POINTS

1. Maternal distress is common but not inevitable in labour. It can result in prolonged labour, fetal distress and a poor 'birth experience'.

2. Antenatal education and support in labour can ameliorate maternal distress.

3. A light diet should be permitted in labour.

4. The choice of analgesia in labour is a personal one, and a compromise is often required between analgesic effect and side effects.

5. Non-pharmacological agents can be very effective.

6. Opiate analgesics can result in neonatal depression.

7. Epidural analgesia is very effective, but there can be problems with maternal hypotension and increased intervention in labour.

43 Bleeding after delivery

CLINICAL SIGNIFICANCE

Postpartum haemorrhage (PPH) is the largest cause of maternal death worldwide – 125 000 deaths per annum – which translates into a 1 in 1000 risk for pregnant women in the developing world.

The risk in the UK is 1 in 100 000, although it is interesting to note that these risks increase to third-world levels where blood transfusion is refused. Therefore, it is perhaps the availability of relatively safe transfusion, rather than improved maternal health and obstetric care, that has greatly reduced mortality. However, PPH remains a common obstetric emergency (approx 1% of deliveries are subject to major haemorrhage) with potential mortality and morbidity; therefore vigilance and prompt, accurate management are required.

Postpartum haemorrhage is traditionally defined as bleeding > 500 ml after delivery of the fetus. Blood loss after delivery is often underestimated and it may be concealed, i.e. broad ligament haemorrhage. Severe blood loss can also precipitate clotting abnormalities, e.g. DIC, and therefore prompt action is essential. Prevention is important: the routine use of oxytocic drugs for the third stage of labour will reduce the risk of PPH by up to 40%. Anticipation of PPH through the identification of known risk factors is also important, particularly for primary PPH.

DIFFERENTIAL DIAGNOSIS

1. *Primary PPH* (occurs within 24 h of delivery)	Uterine atony (90% of cases) Trauma Coagulation disorders
2. *Secondary PPH* (occurs between 24 h and 6 weeks after delivery)	Poor epithelialisation of the placental site (80% of cases) Retained placental fragments Injection – often complicating retained products

CLINICAL ASSESSMENT

PPH is the commonest cause of severe hypotension – 'shock' – in clinical obstetric practice. However, hypotension is often a late sign of blood loss in fit young women (normal obstetric population) and should not be relied upon. Do not wait for hypotension when you otherwise suspect PPH. A tachycardia and an increase in pulse pressure, i.e. difference between diastolic and systolic blood pressures, are more reliable. A difference > 10 mmHg between lying and sitting diastolic blood pressures is especially significant.

Rapid Emergency Assessment

It is important to assess the blood loss and make arrangements for rapid fluid replacement. Therefore, all women with any signs of shock should be aggressively resuscitated: large-bore intravenous access, cross-match 4 units of blood, start colloid fluid replacement, call for senior help and make arrangements for theatre.

After resuscitation it is important to elucidate the cause of the bleeding. Has the placenta been delivered? The fundus of the uterus should be palpated; this in itself can promote a contraction. The fundus of an atonic uterus will be higher than expected. In severe cases an EUA is required. At the time of EUA, bleeding from trauma can be identified, or excluded, and any remaining fragments of placenta removed manually.

Relevant History

Main Complaint

Most commonly you will be called to a delivery room by a midwife to assess a woman with heavy bleeding post delivery. However, the presentation can vary: sudden collapse, shock or continuous oozing post delivery. It is important not to underestimate the total loss.

Pain and offensive lochia can indicate endometrial infection, and whilst this can rarely lead to primary PPH, it is a more common finding in, and association with, secondary PPH.

Obstetric History - Index Pregnancy

ANTENATAL – Features predisposing to uterine atonia can present antenatally. Uterine atonia is more common after uterine overdistension; for further details see Chapter 33. Common causes include polyhydramnios and multiple pregnancy.

Previous APH also predisposes to PPH. This may be directly, e.g. placenta praevia may stop the lower segment contracting after delivery, or indirectly, e.g. an acute coagulopathy after a placental abruption.

INTRAPARTUM – Prolonged labour predisposes to uterine atonia, partly because prolonged labour may be a marker of poor uterine contractility, and prolonged use of Syntocinon will exacerbate this. Prolonged labour also predisposes to instrumental delivery, with an increase in trauma and consequent PPH.

A history of sudden-onset fetal distress, intrapartum vaginal bleeding and reduction in contraction frequency suggests uterine rupture. Look for other features, e.g. previous LSCS and the use of Syntocinon in a multiparous woman. Assisted delivery also predisposes to secondary PPH.

THIRD STAGE – Physiological management of the third stage is associated with an increase in PPH, as no oxytocics are used routinely. The cord is cut once pulsation has ceased, and the placenta is delivered by maternal effort without controlled cord traction.

In the UK, Syntometrine (Syntocinon 5 units; ergometrine 0.5 mg) is routinely administered with the delivery of the anterior shoulder of the baby, and the placenta is delivered by controlled cord traction after separation.

A retained placenta can cause PPH, though, in the absence of heavy bleeding, the placenta can be left for up to 1 h before a manual removal of placenta is required under anaesthetic. Retained placental fragments may not cause an immediate PPH, but they can predispose to secondary PPH.

Obstetric History

A previous history of PPH predisposes to PPH again. This may be because there is an underlying coagulopathy or because the uterus is poor at contracting post delivery. Grand multiparity is no longer considered a risk factor for PPH, either in the UK or in the developing world.

Medical History

MEDICAL CONDITIONS – A history of coagulopathies is also important and will obviously predispose to PPH, both primary and secondary. The most common coagulopathies in young women are Von-Willebrand's and idiopathic thrombocytopaenia purpura; however they are very rare.

Social History

Maternal obesity predisposes to PPH. This effect may be mediated through the link between maternal obesity and fetal macrosomia, leading to overdistension of the uterus and consequently an atonic PPH. Maternal age may also predispose to PPH, and it certainly affects the ability to withstand acute volume loss.

Relevant Clinical Examination

General Features

GENERAL – Remember that most women who present will be haemodynamically stable. However, be aware of these more sinister findings. Sweating and pallor are characteristic of shock. Check the pulse and BP for the features noted above. Signs of PET should alert the clinician to avoid the use of drugs which can exacerbate hypertension, e.g. ergometrine – Syntocinon should be used instead.

Abdomen

GENERAL – Is the placenta delivered? If not, then deliver it. Check for signs of peritonism indicative of a peritoneal bleed, particularly after LSCS and where the external blood loss does not correlate with the haemodynamics.

PREGNANCY – The fundus of an atonic uterus is classically higher than expected, as it has not contracted. The umbilicus is a handy landmark; a normally contracted uterus will be lower than the umbilicus after delivery (20 weeks size). An atonic uterus also feels 'boggy' and soft rather than firm. A broad ligament haematoma will displace the uterus towards the opposite side, and the fundus can be palpated to one side. The uterus can also be less well contracted than expected for secondary PPH.

TENDERNESS – Tenderness over a previous LSCS scar is associated with scar dehiscence or uterine rupture, though it is not a very specific finding, as women are abdominally tender after delivery, particularly over a previous LSCS scar. Uterine tenderness can be indicative of infection.

Pelvis
VAGINAL EXAMINATION –
Vulva/Vagina: The vagina can accommodate a significant volume of blood and clot (> 500 ml) after delivery, and it is imperative that the vagina is evacuated, particularly again where the observed loss does not match the expected loss. The vagina, vulva and perineum should also be examined for trauma and evidence of bleeding thereof. High posterior vaginal tears may not be visible without an EUA.
Cervix: The cervix can be traumatised during delivery, particularly after injudicious use of forceps when the cervix is not fully dilated. Examination of the cervix requires an anaesthetic and can be difficult – it should be undertaken methodically, a bit at a time.

The cervix should close in the week following delivery if the uterus is empty, and therefore a secondary PPH with an open cervix may indicate RPoC.
Uterus: After an EUA the interior of the uterus can be palpated to exclude any retained fragments of placenta or membrane and remove them manually. The interior of the uterus can also be checked for signs of uterine rupture.

Relevant Investigations

Haematology
Full blood count and clotting are necessary as part of the baseline investigations. Cross-matched blood is essential. Group O, rhesus D positive, Kell negative blood can be used if necessary before the cross-matched blood is available. The blood tests should be repeated regularly during the PPH and particularly where a coagulopathy develops.

Diagnostic Imaging
Ultrasound scans can be used for the identification of RPoC in the uterus in the presence of a secondary PPH, though the ultrasound findings are not 100% specific.

DETAILS OF INDIVIDUAL CONDITIONS

1. Primary PPH

Background
DEFINITION – Blood loss > 500 ml within 24 h of delivery. With this definition, primary PPH complicates up to 5% of all deliveries. Blood loss > 1000 ml is probably more

significant and complicates 1–2% of all deliveries.
AETIOLOGY – It is important to understand the normal mechanism of haemostasis after delivery, as this will facilitate understanding of the pathophysiology of PPH. After delivery, it is essential that the uterus contracts very firmly. Strong uterine contractions and retraction kink and shorten the uterine arterioles running through the myometrium, 'nipping' them off. There is also a retraction of the placental bed, all of which contributes to the normal haemostasis. Therefore, factors which prevent uterine contraction, e.g., uterine atonia and/or retained placental fragments, will lead to failure of the normal haemostatic mechanism and subsequently PPH. Aetiological factors are:

Uterine atony (90% of cases)
- Uterine overdistension
- Antepartum haemorrhage
- Prolonged labour
- Assisted delivery
- History of PPH
- Retained products

Trauma
- Vulva/vaginal, including episiotomy
- Cervix – tears
- Uterus – rupture

Coagulation disorders
- Pre-existing – Von Willebrand's disorder/idiopathic thrombocytopaenia purpura
- Acute – DIC.

MAIN COMPLICATIONS – There is a significant maternal morbidity and even mortality associated with primary PPH.
PREVENTION – As detailed above, the routine use of oxytocics can reduce the PPH rate by up to 40% compared with physiological management. Syntometrine is marginally more effective than oxytocin but causes more nausea and vomiting. It is also contraindicated with pregnancies complicated by hypertension.

Misoprostol is a PGE analogue that is effective orally; it has great potential, particularly for the third world, as it is cheap and stable at room temperature. Further trials are awaited.

Treatment Options – Delivery of the Placenta
The treatment of primary PPH depends on whether or not the placenta has been delivered – the placenta must always be delivered first. If all attempts at delivery fail using controlled cord traction then arrangements can be made for a manual removal of the placenta (Figure 43.1).
MANUAL REMOVAL OF THE PLACENTA – Under anaesthetic – regional or GA – a gloved hand is placed into the vagina

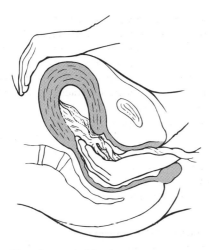

Fig 43.1 *Manual removal of the placenta.*

and through the dilated cervix into the uterine cavity. The cervix sometimes needs to be carefully dilated with the fingers of the exploring hand. The cord can be followed up to the placenta and a lateral edge identified. The exploring hand then attempts to identify a plane of cleavage between the placenta and the uterus; the other hand is employed abdominally to stabilise the uterus by holding the fundus. The placenta is then separated off the uterus by the intrauterine hand and then removed. It is prudent to check the placenta and then the cavity to ensure complete removal. A further dose of Syntometrine and a single dose of intravenous antibiotics can be administered as cover.

Occasionally, the placenta may be impossible to remove – morbidly adherent. This is usually due to a placenta accreta (see Chapter 30) and may require hysterectomy to arrest the bleeding.

Treatment options – after delivery of the placenta

CONSERVATIVE - It is possible to 'rub up' a uterine contraction by massaging the uterine fundus, and this may help until more effective measures can be employed. There are other emergency techniques that can be employed, particularly where there is very heavy loss, as first aid measures: for example, bimanual compression of the uterus can reduce the blood loss temporarily. A gloved hand is inserted into the vagina and the uterine body is pushed upwards to the other hand which is pressing down on the fundus.

The bladder should be emptied.

MEDICAL - If the uterus is atonic and continues to relax, despite attempts to 'rub up' a contraction, then an oxytocic

should be used. There are a variety of agents that can be employed, and they are often used in a stepwise fashion, after checking that the uterus is empty:

1. intravenous Syntometrine or Syntocinon 10 u as a bolus, repeated once more if necessary
2. an intravenous infusion of Syntocinon 10 u/h
3. intramuscular Haemabate, which is a 15MPGF$_2$ analogue that causes intense smooth-muscle contraction; it has also been given intramyometrially with good effect by injecting directly into the fundus through the anterior abdominal wall.

The development of an acute coagulopathy is extremely sinister and requires expert help – involve senior haematologists early. Fresh frozen plasma (FFP) contains a lot of clotting factors and is used to replace those lost by the consumption in a DIC. Platelets are used similarly.

SURGICAL – An examination under anaesthetic is often required in the event of a severe PPH. The uterine cavity can be checked for retained fragments, and the genital tract can be examined for trauma (Figure 43.2). Trauma to the perineum, vulva, vagina and cervix can often be repaired under direct vision whereas uterine trauma can require laparotomy.

Surgery is sometimes necessary for the treatment of PPH from an atonic uterus that doesn't respond to medical treatment as outlined above. A panoply of measures have been proposed for this life-threatening situation, including: uterine packing, using a sengstaken tube (usually used for oesophageal varices), direct ligation of the uterine arteries (NB: uterine viability is maintained by extensive collateral circulation – normal menses and pregnancy are possible afterwards), tying off the internal iliac arteries and, finally, hysterectomy.

OVERVIEW – Primary PPH is an important cause of maternal mortality. Active management of the third

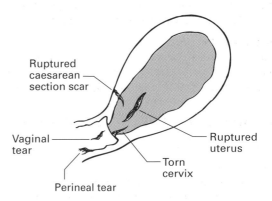

Fig 43.2 *Traumatic causes of postpartum haemorrhage.*

stage using oxytocic drugs routinely reduces the risk of PPH. Aggressive resuscitation is required for PPH, with early resort to an EUA followed by accurate and problem-specific management.

Information for Patients

PROGNOSIS – The prognosis for most women after a PPH is good, but the women should be informed of the recurrence risk. However, the psychological sequelae should not be underestimated, particularly after a hysterectomy or a spell on ITU. Prolonged follow-up and counselling are often required.

SELF-HELP GROUPS – There are no self-help groups for PPH in particular, though there are a number of groups which deal with traumatic delivery experiences.

Follow-up

SHORT TERM – The follow-up depends, to some extent, on the severity of the PPH. However, all women who have experienced a traumatic delivery should be followed up at 4–6 weeks to ensure that wounds, etc., are healing normally but more importantly for a 'debriefing' where they can ask their own questions.

LONG TERM – Prenatal counselling is often useful, as there is a recurrence risk, and a plan can be formulated for the pregnancy.

2. Secondary PPH

Background

DEFINITION – Secondary PPH is defined as loss > 500 ml between 24 h and 6 weeks postnatally. The prevalence is 0.5–1.5%, and, although it is not usually a life-threatening complication, there can be a significant associated morbidity.

In continental Europe it is standard practice to routinely administer oral ergometrine to all women as prophylaxis against secondary PPH. There is no evidence to support this practice.

AETIOLOGY – The exact aetiology is uncertain. In the majority of cases there is a failure of involution and epithelialisation of the placental site, and, although this can undoubtedly be caused by infected RPoC, their presence is almost certainly overdiagnosed. This can lead to unnecessary curettage. Postnatal curettage should be avoided where possible, as the endometrium is friable and overzealous treatment can produce an Ashermann's syndrome.

It is important to note that irregular bleeding vaginal bleeding and oligomenorrhoea are features of breast-feeding; therefore secondary PPH should be a new loss > normal period.

Aetiological factors are:

- poor epithelialisation of the placental site – > 80% of cases
- retained placental fragments

Rarely,

- rupture of a vulval haematoma
- the development of choriocarcinoma/placental site tumour.

Treatment Options

Treatment is as conservative as possible.

MEDICAL – Broad-spectrum antibiotics can be used where infection is suspected, e.g. bulky tender uterus with an open cervical os. Some authors also advocate intra-muscular oxytocics, e.g. ergometrine 0.5 mg, to promote uterine involution.

SURGICAL – Curettage is rarely required; it carries a significant risk of uterine perforation and subsequent Ashermann's syndrome. Curettage should only be performed where medical treatment has failed and placental fragments are seen on ultrasound scan. The curettings should be sent for histological analysis to exclude choriocarcinoma.

GOLDEN POINTS

1. PPH is an important health problem both in the UK and worldwide.

2. Active management of the third stage reduces the risk of PPH.

3. The blood loss is often underestimated, and hypotension is a late finding of acute blood loss, therefore resuscitation should be prompt and aggressive.

4. The most common cause of primary PPH is an atonic uterus. The management requires oxytocics, and surgery where these measures fail, following the exclusion of RPoC.

5. The management of secondary PPH should be conservative where possible, with resort to ERPC only where these measures fail and RPoC are definitely identified.

44 Maternal collapse after delivery

CLINICAL SIGNIFICANCE

Sudden postpartum collapse often precedes maternal death. Rapid, accurate management is required to minimise morbidity and mortality.

Fortunately, this is a rare complication. There are a number of conditions which can cause sudden collapse, which show common clinical features of hypotension, cyanosis, apnoea and sometimes tonic-clonic seizures. Massive haemorrhage is another cause of collapse that will be considered separately.

DIFFERENTIAL DIAGNOSIS

1. *Amniotic fluid embolus*
2. *Pulmonary embolus*
3. *Eclampsia*
4. *Myocardial infarction*
5. *Regional anaesthetic complications*
6. *Major obstetric haemorrhage*

CLINICAL ASSESSMENT

It is essential that appropriate help is summoned immediately. Senior anaesthetic and obstetric help should be summoned, and, as many conditions can be associated with coagulation defects, the haematologists can be very helpful. ITU facilities are often required.

Rapid Emergency Assessment

Rapid resuscitation and accurate management is essential. An airway must be established and ventilation maintained. Intravenous lines with wide-bore cannulae should be set up to maintain the circulation, initially with isotonic crystalloids.

Relevant History

Presenting Complaint

There is often a sequence of events which have a common presentation: precipitating cause → hypotension → +/- apnoea → circulatory collapse → loss of consciousness and collapse. Accurate diagnosis of the underlying problem can therefore be difficult, but it is vital. Remember that a history is often unavailable from the patient. The partner or midwife should be asked for relevant information.

PAIN – Sharp pleuritic pain, worse on inspiration, is a feature of pulmonary embolus. Features of myocardial infarction usually resemble those in the non-pregnant patient, with substernal pain, radiating to neck and the left arm.

DYSPNOEA – Amniotic fluid embolism and pulmonary embolism can be very difficult to differentiate. In both there is a rapid collapse, with apnoea, cyanosis and loss of consciousness.

FITTING – With eclampsia there may be warning clues, e.g. hypertension, hyperreflexia, visual disturbances and headaches, but seizures may be the first sign. A focal seizure is usually followed by a generalized tonic-clonic seizure and apnoea.

Obstetric History

INDEX PREGNANCY – A rapid labour predisposes to amniotic fluid embolism. Eclampsia is preceded by proteinuric hypertension (PET) in approximately 65% of cases.

Timing after potential precipitants is important: problems associated with regional anaesthetic administration usually occur within 20 min of administration. There may be prodromal symptoms, e.g. a metallic taste in the mouth, tinnitus, confusion and dyspnoea. Involvement of respiratory muscles will give rise to apnoea and cyanosis. Seizures and possible cardiac arrest can then follow.

Operative delivery increases the risk of pulmonary embolus. See Chapter 43 for features of PPH.

OBSTETRIC HISTORY – A previous CS or other uterine operation predisposes to uterine rupture.

Medical History

MEDICAL CONDITIONS – A history of thromboembolism is important. Atherosclerotic heart disease, hypertension, insulin-dependent diabetes and hyperlipidaemia all predispose to MI.

Social History

SMOKING – Smoking predisposes to both myocardial infarction and thromboembolism.

OBESITY – Obesity increases the risk of MI.

AGE – Increasing maternal age increases the risk of both PE and MI.

Relevant Clinical Examination

General Features

GENERAL DEMEANOUR – Cyanosis is common to many of the precipitating causes, after collapse. However, it is characteristically an early feature of amniotic fluid embolus and pulmonary embolus, sometimes preceding collapse.

CARDIOVASCULAR SYSTEM – Tachycardia is not common after MI, but can be a feature of the other causes of collapse. Hypotension is a feature of circulatory collapse, e.g. MI. Hypertension is a characteristic feature of eclampsia.

RESPIRATORY SYSTEM – Left ventricular failure is a feature of amniotic fluid embolus and MI. Crepitations may be heard at the base of the lungs. A pleural rub, splitting of the second heart sound, an increase in the prominence of the pulmonary valve closure and an S3 gallop are features of pulmonary embolus.

ABDOMEN – There may be abdominal distension and signs of peritonism with incidental abdominal haemorrhage, e.g. splenic artery aneurysm.

Relevant Investigations

Haematology

Check clotting profile, looking for signs of a disseminated intravascular coagulation, particularly after amniotic fluid embolus. Thrombocytopaenia and clotting abnormalities are also a feature of eclampsia. Red cells and fresh frozen plasma should be requested where DIC is diagnosed.

Biochemistry

Enzyme studies are not useful acutely but may help where the patient survives.

- CPK rises within 4–6 h of the infarct, reaching a maximum level at 24 h.
- STPT/SGOT rise within 6–8 h of the infarct, to a maximum between 24 and 48 h.
- LDH starts to rise at 12 h, with a peak between 3 and 6 days.

Blood Gases

Blood gases should be performed (a normal pO_2 is not compatible with massive pulmonary embolus).

ECG

ECG may show right axis deviation, p pulmonale and an S1, Q3, T3 complex after pulmonary embolus. A raised ST segment is a feature of an acute MI.

Diagnostic Imaging

X-RAY – Chest x-ray is often normal but can show pleural effusion or thickening. In cases of doubt a ventilation perfusion scan can be performed. Right heart catheterization may be appropriate, which will show an increased pulmonary artery pressure and pulmonary capillary wedge pressure with raised central venous pressure.

DETAILS OF INDIVIDUAL CONDITIONS

1. Amniotic Fluid Embolus

Background

DEFINITION – Until recently, it was hard to make the diagnosis without a postmortem, but recently the diagnosis may be made with a triad of features: collapse, cyanosis and DIC.

INCIDENCE – The incidence may be higher than the previously published figure of less than one in four thousand deliveries.

AETIOLOGY – Amniotic fluid gains access to the circulation and is carried to the lung, where it lodges in the capillary network. There is an anaphylactic type reaction which produces pulmonary vasoconstriction and an increase in pulmonary artery pressure. Subsequent activation of the complement cascade gives rise to a leakage of intravascular fluid into the intra-alveolar and interstitial spaces. This results in hypoxia and left ventricular failure. See Figure 44.1 Disseminated intravascular coagulation occurs in the majority of women surviving the initial episode.

MAIN COMPLICATIONS – The clinical features of amniotic fluid embolism usually develop without any warning. There is dystonia, often with production of a pink frothy

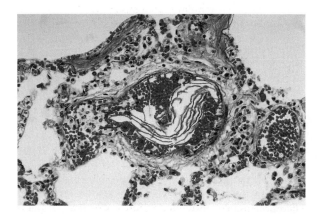

Fig 44.1 *Fetal squames in the maternal circulation, characteristic of amniotic fluid embolism.*

sputum and cyanosis. Apnoea rapidly follows with loss of consciousness. Convulsions can occur in up to 20% of cases. 20% of women do not survive the acute episode. Overall mortality rate is approximately 85%, death being due to the complications of coagulopathy and left ventricular failure.

Treatment Options

Treatment requires resuscitation (ABC) followed by problem-specific management. Adequate ventilation will require intubation. Circulation should be maintained, and shock should be treated.

PROBLEM-SPECIFIC – Left ventricular dysfunction will require digitalisation, and vasopressor therapy may be required. Dopamine or dobutamine are preferable, as they are associated with increased perfusion and myocardial contractility. Disseminated intravascular coagulation should be treated with red cells, platelets and fresh frozen plasma as directed by the haematologist.

2. Pulmonary Embolus

Background

INCIDENCE – Postpartum pulmonary embolus occurs in approximately 1 in 3500 pregnancies and accounts for 75% of all pregnancy-related pulmonary emboli. It is a significant cause of maternal mortality.

AETIOLOGY – Pregnancy is associated with an increased predisposition to thromboembolic phenomena. There is an increase in hepatic production of factors I, VII, VIII, IX and X. The distension of the uterus increases venous pressure in the pelvis and causes a relative stasis in the lower limbs. At delivery there is trauma to the vascular endothelium which actuates a coagulation cascade. Any pre-existing affection can exert effects on the vascular endothelium.

The majority of pulmonary emboli can be traced to thrombosis in calf or iliofemoral veins. Risk factors for pulmonary embolus include increasing age, obesity, a history of deep vein thrombosis, operative delivery and immobility.

MAIN COMPLICATIONS – Pulmonary embolus is one of the most common causes of maternal mortality, though the exact risk is unclear.

Treatment Options

Treatment requires resuscitation (ABC) followed by problem-specific management. Adequate ventilation will require intubation. Circulation should be maintained, and shock should be treated.

PROBLEM-SPECIFIC – Anticoagulation is essential. A bolus of heparin 5–10 000 units should be given followed by an infusion according to haematology results. Where

there is a massive embolus in the proximal part of the main pulmonary artery, surgery may have to be considered where the condition deteriorates despite adequate resuscitation and anticoagulation.

3. Eclampsia

Background

See discussion of PET in Chapter 31.

INCIDENCE – Approximately 1 in 1000, with up to one third of these occurring in the puerperium.

MAIN COMPLICATIONS – There is a risk of cerebrovascular accident with hypertension, pulmonary oedema with overzealous fluid administration, and DIC.

Treatment Options

Treatment requires resuscitation (ABC) followed by problem-specific management. Adequate ventilation will require intubation. Circulation should be maintained, and shock treated.

PROBLEM-SPECIFIC – If fit is still persisting, stop initial episode with Diazepam. Commence prophylactic therapy with magnesium sulphate to prevent recurrent seizures. In the presence of significant hypertension, antihypertensives should be given, e.g. labetolol or hydralazine.

4. Myocardial Infarction

Background

INCIDENCE – Less than 1 in 10 000 pregnancies. Mortality rate is up to 45%, and usually death, where it occurs, is immediate.

MAIN COMPLICATIONS – Arrhythmias are very common. Left ventricular dysfunction can give rise to congestive heart failure. 10% of sufferers develop cardiogenic shock with a high immediate mortality.

Treatment Options

Treatment requires resuscitation followed by problem-specific management. Adequate ventilation will require intubation. Circulation should be maintained, and shock should be treated.

PROBLEM-SPECIFIC – Cardiopulmonary resuscitation should be commenced and senior cardiological assistance summoned. Vasopressor, antiarrhythmic and anticoagulant therapy may be required at the direction of the cardiologist.

5. Complications of Regional Anaesthesia

Background

INCIDENCE – Approximately 1 in 1000 epidurals, though actual collapse is much rarer.

AETIOLOGY – Inadvertent intravascular injection or an

excess dose of local anaesthetic agent is the usual cause. During pregnancy there is an increased blood flow in the vessels around the cord. These are distended and reduce the amount of space in the epidural space, thus increasing the risk of inadvertent cannulation. The increased pressure changes during contractions and pushing increase the dispersion of any agent in the space.

MAIN COMPLICATIONS – Paralysis by the local anaesthetic of the respiratory muscles, leading to collapse.

Treatment Options

Treatment requires resuscitation (ABC) followed by problem-specific management. Adequate ventilation will require intubation. Circulation should be maintained, and shock should be treated.

PROBLEM-SPECIFIC – Anticonvulsant therapy should be administered, if required. Prompt treatment should avoid prolonged hypoxia and acidosis, in which case the outlook for full recovery is excellent.

Prevention

Skilled management of all regional anaesthetic techniques is essential. Establishment should be by experienced anaesthetists. Attention must be paid to the dosages, and careful top-up technique, and careful observations during and after top-ups are required.

6. Major Obstetric Haemorrhage

This is discussed in detail in Chapters 30 and 43, and therefore only uterine rupture and incidental abdominal haemorrhage will be discussed here.

Differential Diagnosis

- Abruption
- Placenta praevia
- Disseminated intravascular coagulation
- Uterine rupture
- Postpartum haemorrhage
- Incidental intra-abdominal haemorrhage.

Uterine Rupture

INCIDENCE – This is a rare complication. It is more common in women with previous caesarean section (especially classical incision), hysterotomy, myomectomy, and after oxytocin infusion where there has been a previous caesarean section. It may follow oxytocin in fusion in parous women where there is cephalopelvic disproportion. Forceps delivery, especially rotational, may cause it.

CLINICAL ASSESSMENT – Complete uterine rupture may present with bleeding per vaginam, but the bleeding may be into the broad ligament and thus be rather occult. For the woman who shows signs compatible with blood loss greater than visible blood loss, a high index of suspicion should be maintained, particularly in women in higher-risk groups. An ultrasound scan may show a collection of blood in the broad ligament, but this is not an easy diagnosis to make immediately postpartum. Management is for general resuscitative measures or by examination under anaesthesia, proceeding to laparotomy. At laparotomy, depending upon the site and nature of the rupture, it may be possible to repair the rupture, or hysterectomy may be indicated.

Incidental Intra-abdominal Haemorrhage

INCIDENCE – Very rarely, spontaneous haemorrhage can occur intra-abdominally from rupture of splenic artery, adrenal artery or ovarian artery.

AETIOLOGY – The aetiology of these spontaneous vessel ruptures is unknown.

TREATMENT – Surgical assistance at laparotomy is essential in these cases.

GOLDEN POINTS

1. Rapid accurate management is required to reduce maternal morbidity and mortality to a minimum.

2. Resuscitate first.

3. Get the history from the midwife/partner.

4. Treatment requires resuscitation followed by problem-specific management.

45 Postnatal depression

CLINICAL SIGNIFICANCE

There is a spectrum of recognised postnatal depressive disorders ranging from the essentially benign postnatal blues through postnatal depression to the severely incapacitating puerperal psychosis. It is not clear whether these are variants of the same underlying condition or essentially separate conditions. Most research has been into psychosocial aspects of these disorders, and there is little knowledge of their biological background. All three conditions share certain similar underlying features, suggesting a biological cause. There is no correlation between these conditions and mode of delivery, nor any correlation with psychosocial factors including social class, race, or life events. However, there is a persistent link between postnatal depressive illnesses and poor support from the woman's partner and the family. There is no effective way of screening for women at risk, and diagnosis is not easy. The diagnosis is a major concern, as only 15% of affected women receive treatment for postnatal depression.

DIFFERENTIAL DIAGNOSIS

1. *Postnatal blues*

2. *Postnatal depression*

3. *Puerperal psychosis*

CLINICAL ASSESSMENT

Clinical assessment in these sensitive conditions can be difficult. It is important to establish the type of depression, and in many cases consultation with the psychiatry department is required.

Rapid Emergency Assessment

It is important to exclude puerperal psychosis because there is a risk of both self-harm and harm to the baby unless effective treatment is rapidly instituted.

Relevant History

Presenting Complaint

MAIN COMPLAINT – Postnatal blues are characterised by transient symptoms lasting for up to 3 days, with the onset typically on the third day (the third-day blues) but certainly within 10 days postpartum.

Postnatal depression is commonly underdiagnosed and it is associated with mood swings, changes in cognitive function and a decreased ability to bond with the baby. It characteristically presents after 2 weeks postpartum.

Puerperal psychosis presents similarly to any other psychosis. Psychosis occurs more frequently in the first 3 months postpartum than at any other time in a woman's life. The disorders are usually affective in nature. Rejection of the child, and obsessive behaviour, are common.

COMMONLY ASSOCIATED SYMPTOMS – Other symptoms include anxiety, tiredness, insomnia, mood lability.

Gynaecological History

There appears to be an association between women

suffering from premenstrual syndrome, particularly where there are psychological rather than physical manifestations, and an increased risk of postnatal blues.

Obstetric History

Each condition is likely to recur in subsequent pregnancies. In puerperal psychosis 15–20% of affected women will have had a previous psychotic episode either during or outside pregnancy.

Medical History

PSYCHIATRIC HISTORY – There is no significant relationship between a history of psychiatric disorders and postnatal blues. There is a strong association between a history of psychiatric illness, particularly a previous affective disorder, and postnatal depression; the risk may be up to 30%. Similarly, in puerperal psychosis, 15–20% of affected women will have had a previous psychotic episode. Up to 40% of women with puerperal psychosis will suffer a recurrence when not pregnant.

Drug History

Postnatal blues appears to have been less common in the past when oestradiol was given to decrease lactation.

Social History

In postnatal blues there is no relationship to social class, race, age or life events. The condition is less common and less severe where there is a strong relationship with the partner and appropriate support from the family. There is a family history of psychosis in 10% of women with puerperal psychosis.

Relevant Clinical Examination

There are no significant features on examination.

Relevant Investigations

There are no specific diagnostic tests for any of the conditions.

DETAILS OF INDIVIDUAL CONDITIONS

1. Postnatal Blues

Background

INCIDENCE – Postnatal blues are very common: rates vary between studies, but up to 70% of women are affected.

AETIOLOGY – The aetiology is unknown but the timing of onset does suggest a hormonal cause. The sudden drop in progesterone immediately after delivery has been implicated.

MAIN COMPLICATIONS – Postnatal blues describes a transient experience of weepiness, mood instability and anxiety.

Should it persist beyond 2 weeks then there is an increased risk of postnatal depression.

PREVENTION – There are no screening or prophylactic measures that have been shown to work effectively.

Treatment Options

CONSERVATIVE AND REASSURANCE – The condition is essentially self-limiting, and no specific therapy other than reassurance and support from the family is required.

Follow-up

SHORT TERM – The treatment is supportive, and therefore follow-up in the community can be helpful. Some support groups, including the National Childbirth Trust (NCT), offer postnatal support. Medical follow-up is rarely required.

2. Postnatal Depression

Background

DEFINITION – The definition of postnatal depression is vague: it can be similar to postnatal blues but with a longer duration and exaggerated symptoms. Up to 60% of women are still affected after 6 months and 40% at 1 year; legally, the consequences of postnatal depression are recognised for up to a year after delivery. The chronicity of the condition increases the stress on relationships with the partner, and family and behavioural problems are common in the children of affected women.

INCIDENCE – Prospective studies have suggested an incidence of up to 17%. From the number of diagnoses made, this would suggest that only 10–15% of affected women are actually receiving treatment.

AETIOLOGY – As with the other postnatal disorders, this is thought to be multifactorial, including psychosocial and biological factors. An unsatisfactory 'birth experience' can be a factor.

MAIN COMPLICATIONS – The woman can experience a sense of ambivalence towards her infant as well as the previously described symptoms of tearfulness and anxiety. Suicide and injury to the baby are extremely rare unless there is a history of previous psychiatric disorder.

PREVENTION – There are no recognised preventative measures, but women at increased risk are those with a previous history and recognised social and domestic stresses during this pregnancy. Progesterone therapy has been advocated as a prophylactic measure, but there is no satisfactory evidence of its efficacy.

Treatment Options

CONSERVATIVE AND REASSURANCE – Relief from total childcare responsibility may help, as can access to other mothers with babies – see 'Self-help groups'.

Table 45.1   Postnatal depressive illnesses

	Blues	Depression	Psychosis
Onset	2–3 days postnatally	>2 weeks postnatally	Variable
Symptoms	Tearfulness, anxiety	Depression	Psychotic symptoms
Duration	<2 weeks	Up to 1 year	Variable
Risks	Few	Recurrence	Suicide and infant injury
Treatment	Supportive	Antidepressants	+ antipsychotics
	Home/community	Home/community	Inpatient

MEDICAL – Underlying medical disorders, particularly hypothyroidism, should be excluded.

Traditionally, the treatment has been antidepressant therapy, and help may be required from psychiatrist colleagues. Progesterone therapy has been used, and success is claimed by its proponents, although scientific studies are lacking.

Following up on the apparent decreased incidence where oestrogen was used for lactation suppression, a recent randomised, double-blind, placebo-controlled trial has shown significant improvement in women receiving 200 mcg of oestradiol daily, during both the 6 month trial period and 3 month post-trial follow-up period.

OVERVIEW – Postnatal depression can be severely debilitating. It characteristically has a long time course and requires continued empathy. Antidepressant medication is often required. Table 45.1 compares postnatal depression with postnatal blues and puerperal psychosis.

Information for Patients

PROGNOSIS – There is no direct relation to parity, but the condition recurs in up to 50% of subsequent pregnancies.
SELF-HELP GROUPS – As for postnatal blues.

3. Puerperal Psychosis

Background

DEFINITION – Postpartum psychosis is a major affective disorder with symptoms ranging from mania to severe depression.
INCIDENCE – Fortunately, this severe condition is rare (about one per thousand births). It develops most commonly within the first 2 weeks after delivery.
AETIOLOGY – Is unknown. Possible biological causes are recognised but hard evidence is lacking, being mainly circumstantial, e.g. the occurrence of psychiatric disorders at times of significant hormonal change (e.g. premenstrually and perimenopausally) and the temporal relationship to pregnancy.

A number of studies have been undertaken looking at the relationship with oestradiol, progesterone, thyroid, hormone, prolactin and pituitary gonadatrophin levels. There is no relationship to plasma levels but there is an increasing view that oestrogen levels may be important.

MAIN COMPLICATIONS –
Maternal: The main maternal complications are psychiatric, including hallucinations, mania and irritability and depression. There is also an increased risk of self harm.
Neonatal: Unlike the other postnatal depressive problems, there is a significant risk of the mother injuring the baby as well as herself.

PREVENTION – As with the other postnatal psychiatric disorders, there are no effective preventative measures, but a high index of suspicion should be maintained with women at increased risk, particularly those with a previous history.

Treatment Options

MEDICAL – For severe puerperal psychosis, inpatient psychiatric care is required. Both antidepressants and neuroleptics are used under psychiatric supervision. Electroconvulsive therapy (ECT) is occasionally needed where medication fails.

If possible, the mother should not be separated from the baby. Specialist mother and baby units exist to provide adequate supervision for postpartum psychosis in particular.

The role of oestrogen in this condition is also being considered. In one long-term study, 40 women were followed over a period of 18 years. There were no recurrences in subsequent pregnancies in a group where a 20% recurrence rate was expected with oestrogen.
OVERVIEW – Postpartum psychosis is potentially a very dangerous complication of the puerperium because there is a risk of injury both to the mother and the baby. There is often a history of previous psychiatric illness, and intensive inpatient psychiatric care is warranted.

Information for Patients

PROGNOSIS – There is a 20% risk of recurrence in a subsequent pregnancy.

Follow-up

SHORT TERM – Postpartum psychosis can been managed on an outpatient basis in selected women, with appropriate psychiatric follow-up.

LONG TERM – Long-term psychiatric follow-up may be required.

GOLDEN POINTS

1. Postnatal blues is extremely common and is usually transient, rarely requiring more than reassurance and empathy.

2. Postnatal depression persists after the first 2 weeks of the puerperium and may require anti-depressant medication.

3. Self-help groups such as the NCT can provide valuable local support for mothers with both postnatal blues and postnatal depression.

4. Puerperal psychosis is a potentially dangerous complication with a risk of injury to both the mother and the baby.

5. There is a significant association between puerperal psychosis and previous psychiatric episodes.

6. Inpatient psychiatric care and treatment with antidepressants is required for puerperal psychosis.

46 Painful breasts

CLINICAL SIGNIFICANCE

Breast problems are rare antenatally, but common after delivery. Although more common in breast-feeding women, occurring in around 30% on discharge home and persisting in 12% beyond 8 weeks, they are by no means rare in women who bottle feed (20% in hospital, falling to 8% after discharge home).

Breast feeding has significant potential benefits for both baby and mother; babies who are breast fed are less likely to suffer from diarrhoea or ear infections in early life. However, breast-feeding rates are low in the United Kingdom (40% in England and Wales and only 30% in Scotland at 6 weeks) compared with the rest of Europe. Mastitis and breast engorgement are commonly quoted reasons for stopping breast feeding, even in well-motivated mothers. Therefore prevention and treatment of these common conditions may increase the breast-feeding rates as well as reducing unnecessary pain and distress for mothers.

CLINICAL ASSESSMENT

Engorgement is common, causing an uncomfortable distension and heaviness. It rarely causes pyrexia, and if pyrexia is present, associated with redness and heat, mastitis is likely. If not promptly treated with antibiotics, abscess formation can occur with fluctuation. This requires surgical drainage. Malignant disease is very rare, but in cases occurring during pregnancy and the puerperium it can follow a very rapid course.

Relevant History

Presenting Complaint

MAIN COMPLAINT – Pain is the one symptom common to all. The pain may be diffuse over both breasts with engorgement, or specific to one quadrant or point with mastitis and abscesses respectively.

COMMONLY ASSOCIATED SYMPTOMS – Puerperal fever associated with breast feeding. Although pyrexia is more common with infection, e.g. mastitis or an abscess, it can also occur in simple engorgement. The fever associated with mastitis (and abscess formation) often produces malaise and flu-like symptoms.

Obstetric History

PREVIOUS BREAST FEEDING – There is little research into recurrences of breast problems, but, where a woman has had any breast problems in a previous pregnancy, particular attention should be paid to correct breast-feeding technique if that is what the woman wishes; or, if she is determined not to breast feed, then serious consideration should be given to active suppression of lactation.

Medical History

MEDICAL CONDITIONS – Diabetes mellitus predisposes to infection, and therefore both mastitis and breast abscesses are more common.

Relevant Clinical Examination

General Features

Pyrexia is common to all the conditions, though it is characteristically worse in mastitis and breast abscesses.

Breasts

In the presence of engorgement the breasts are enlarged, firm and may well be tender. Often the superficial veins are very prominent. There is usually distension of the axillary tail, which should not be mistaken for enlarged lymph glands. There is no localised heat or redness and no induration. There should be no pyrexia. The white count is raised at this stage of pregnancy anyway, and, if there is any doubt, the differential count looking at the neutrophilia may help.

In addition to engorgement, which is common, mastitis is usually associated with painful breasts, which are red with increased temperature. In addition to the engorged axillary tails, there may well be discreet glands palpable in the axillae. Induration may well be present.

When mastitis leads to abscess formation the induration becomes fluctuant with pointing. At this stage antibiotic treatment is contraindicated and the best therapy is surgical drainage.

Where there is the slightest suspicion that there may be malignancies, a breast surgeon should be consulted straight away. The presence of ulceration of the skin is highly suspicious.

Relevant Investigations

Biochemistry

It may be appropriate to undertake a blood glucose in the presence of an abscess to exclude diabetes.

Microbiology

A swab of any discharge or abscess contents may be useful. Microbiological investigation of a milk sample can also be useful in cases of mastitis.

DETAILS OF INDIVIDUAL CONDITIONS

1. Engorgement

Background

INCIDENCE – Prevalence rates vary between studies, but it is commonly quoted as occurring in between 50% and 70% of all cases.

AETIOLOGY – Essentially, the aetiology is unknown, but the timing of onset does suggest a hormonal cause.

MAIN COMPLICATIONS – The main complications of engorgement are pain, subsequent infection and ceasing breast feeding.

PREVENTION – Prevention is far better than cure with these conditions. The majority of problems can be prevented by correct breast-feeding technique with unrestricted feeding by a well-positioned baby not sucking on the nipple. Cracked nipples due to poor technique are the usual cause of infection. Much attention has been paid to inverted nipples antenatally, but there is as yet no consensus on the best form of management of this condition.

Treatment Options

CONSERVATIVE AND REASSURANCE – Treatment for engorgement is based on a firm support bra/binder and continuing breast feeding.

There is also debate about the best form of treatment for engorgement. Some authorities recommend expression to alleviate the painful distension, whilst others suggest that this can perpetuate the problem. In general, intermittent expression seems appropriate to make the patient comfortable.

MEDICAL – Where engorgement is severe or when appropriate to suppress lactation (e.g. following a stillbirth or neonatal death) bromocriptine can be used, usually in a dose of 2.5 mg b.d. for 10 days. Oestrogen is best avoided at this stage because of the increased risk of thromboembolism, but its role in the treatment of postnatal depression is currently being evaluated. Diuretics and fluid restriction have little role. Symptomatic relief is provided by analgesics.

OVERVIEW – Engorgement is a common problem in the puerperium for both breast-feeding and non-breast-feeding mothers. With adequate care and support the complications can be minimised and, one hopes breast feeding is encouraged wherever possible.

2. Mastitis and Abscess Formation

Background

DEFINITION – Mastitis is a non-specific term employed to describe puerperal breast infection.

INCIDENCE – Up to 2.5% of women develop mastitis in the puerperium – more commonly, breast-feeding mothers. Approximately 5% of these women will develop an abscess.

AETIOLOGY – Nipple trauma, exacerbated by incorrect positioning of the baby, allows pathogenic bacteria to start a cellulitis. The most commonly implicated bacteria are Staphylococcus aureus, S. epidermidis and Escherichia coli. The infection involves the interlobar cellular tissue and therefore usually presents in one discrete quadrant.

Milk stasis increases the risk further by supplying a fertile medium for bacterial growth. Milk stasis has been implicated as a major risk factor for abscess formation in particular.

MAIN COMPLICATIONS –
Maternal: The main maternal complications are as for breast engorgement.
Neonate: Stopping breast feeding.

Treatment Options

CONSERVATIVE AND REASSURANCE – Treatment for engorgement is based on a firm support bra/binder and continuing breast feeding.

MEDICAL – When mastitis is present, prompt antibiotic therapy is required. A sample of milk can be sent for culture and sensitivities, the treatment being commenced with a broad-spectrum antibiotic in the meantime. Where abscess formation is suspected, it is probably better to avoid antibiotic therapy and to arrange surgical drainage, as it is possible to cause a sterile abscess which causes more long-term problems if antibiotics are given at this late stage.

SURGICAL – The management of abscess formation is surgical drainage followed by antibiotics.

OVERVIEW – Breast engorgement, mastitis and abscess formation are all related, if not constituting a direct continuum. Prevention is better than cure; good feeding technique and support may prevent infection and also maintain feeding rates by removing a major cause of stopping feeding.

Information for Patients

PROGNOSIS – The prognosis is generally good. Most women can be treated with simple supportive measures; only a minority will require antibiotics or further treatment. It is important to emphasise that continuation of breast feeding is both beneficial to the infant and part of the treatment.

SELF-HELP GROUPS – The National Childbirth Trust (NCT) and the La Leche group both provide support for breast-feeding mothers in particular.

Follow-up

SHORT TERM – Support is essential, and regular follow-up by the community midwifery teams or self-help groups can be invaluable.

GOLDEN POINTS

1. Painful breasts are one of the commonest causes for stopping breast feeding.

2. Prevention is far better than cure: good support and adequate technique may reduce the incidence of mastitis and breast abscesses.

3. Unless there is pus discharging from the nipple, feeding should be continued as part of the treatment, as milk stasis exacerbates the problem.

4. Antibiotics should be used for mastitis

5. Surgical drainage is required for abscesses.

47 Swollen legs in the puerperium

CLINICAL SIGNIFICANCE

Swollen legs are very common in late pregnancy and the early puerperium, particularly so in hot weather, and especially in obese women and those with pre-eclampsia. The causes of swollen legs vary from the common, and benign, oedema through to the potentially life-threatening thromboembolic disease; therefore it is important to carefully assess the legs in order to exclude deep vein thrombosis (DVT).

Because of the poor reliability of clinical signs in establishing the diagnosis, patients with suspected DVT should be referred urgently for investigations to confirm the diagnosis.

DIFFERENTIAL DIAGNOSIS

1. *Oedema*

2. *Superficial thrombophlebitis*

3. *Deep vein thrombosis*

CLINICAL ASSESSMENT

A careful history will determine the onset of the swelling and whether it is unilateral or bilateral. Other features sought include any pain or tenderness.

Rapid Emergency Assessment

It is important to exclude thromboembolic disease quickly because there is an increased risk of pulmonary embolus with an associated increase in maternal mortality.

Relevant History

Presenting Complaint

MAIN COMPLAINT – The main complaint is obviously swelling. Uncomplicated oedema is usually bilateral. Superficial thrombophlebitis can occur in women with varicose veins, and this can lead to increased swelling of the leg which is usually unilateral. Deep vein thrombosis is usually unilateral but rarely can be bilateral if it is a high thrombus.

COMMONLY ASSOCIATED SYMPTOMS – The other main complaint is pain. All swollen legs may be painful; however, superficial pain, particularly over inflamed varicose veins, is suggestive of thrombophlebitis, and a deeper dull pain is more suggestive of DVT.

Severe DVTs may also present with night cramps and, rarely, cyanosis of the affected leg.

Gynaecological History

Heritable thrombophilias, i.e. antiphospholipid antibody syndrome and anti-factor V Leiden, predispose to miscarriage as well as DVT.

Obstetric History

INDEX PREGNANCY – Swollen ankles complicate many pregnancies, but ankle oedema is more common in conditions like PET or multiple pregnancy. DVTs are more common after caesarean section and prolonged immobility.

OBSTETRIC HISTORY – A previous history of DVT and/or stillbirth – in the presence of thrombophilias – increases the risk of future DVT.

Medical History

A previous history of superficial thrombophlebitis or thromboembolic phenomena is important. A small number of women will be known to be at increased risk of DVT because of a previous episode or a known abnormality of clotting factors.

Drug History

A previous history of DVT on the oral contraceptive pill may suggest a predisposition, and women should be investigated for heritable thrombophilias after pregnancy.

Social History

AGE – Thromboembolic phenomena are more common with increasing age, particularly after 35 years of age.

BODY-MASS INDEX – Obesity increases the risk of DVT and also, indirectly, the risk of superficial thrombophlebitis by exacerbating varicose veins.

SMOKING – There is also an increased risk of thrombo-embolic disease with smoking.

Relevant Clinical Examination

General
Low-grade pyrexia is common in the presence of DVTs.

Legs
In order to check the symmetry, the circumference of both legs should be measured 10-cm above the upper pole and 10 cm below the lower pole of the patella. A difference of more than 1.5 cm in either of these measurements between right and left legs is significant.

The abdomen and both lower limbs should be examined, looking for the level of oedema. If the patient has been lying down then sacral oedema would support oedema as a cause for the swollen legs.

Looking at the legs, one should determine whether there is unilateral or bilateral swelling; bilateral swelling is usually benign, though a high pelvic vein thrombosis can rarely also cause bilateral swelling.

Homan's sign is unreliable as an indicator of DVT.

Tenderness
Superficial thrombophlebitis can be excruciatingly tender, particularly over varicosities. Patients often complain that they cannot bear anything next to their skin, it is so tender. DVTs are characteristically less tender, though the tenderness increases on deep palpation.

Colour
Local redness over varicose veins suggests superficial thrombophlebitis.

Relevant Investigations

No specific investigations are required for oedema and superficial thrombophlebitis, but, where there is any suspicion of DVT, further investigation is required. It is no longer acceptable simply to place a hand-held Doppler instrument over the femoral vein below the middle ligament and to listen for an increased flow on compression of the leg veins.

Venogram
The gold standard investigation for DVT is still the veno-gram, though Doppler ultrasound is increasingly being used.

Doppler Duplex
Duplex and colour doppler is non-invasive and very useful for proximal (pelvic/femoral) venous thromboses though it is less sensitive for calf vein thromboses. Doppler is the investigation of choice in pregnant women, as there is no radiation risk.

DETAILS OF INDIVIDUAL CONDITIONS

1. Superficial Thrombophlebitis

Background
DEFINITION – Superficial thrombophlebitis is an inflammation of the superficial leg veins.

INCIDENCE – Superficial thrombophlebitis can complicate up to 1% of pregnancies.

MAIN COMPLICATIONS – There is no increased mortality associated with superficial thrombophlebitis, as there is no excess risk of clot extension or pulmonary embolisation.

PREVENTION – There are no adequate preventative measures for simple oedema or superficial thrombophlebitis.

Treatment Options
CONSERVATIVE AND REASSURANCE – Superficial thrombophlebitis responds to administration of non-steroidal anti-inflammatory agents, and local applications can be comforting. The local application of a mixture of glycerol and ichthamol paste was popular for many years. It is uncertain whether it actually helped, but the combination of the messy application and its potent smell have at the very least a potent placebo effect.

OVERVIEW – Superficial thrombophlebitis is a postnatal complication which can cause significant discomfort but does not increase maternal risk otherwise. Local treatment only is required.

Information for Patients
PROGNOSIS – Superficial thrombophlebitis usually resolves spontaneously, and there are very few implications for the future.

2. Thromboembolic Disease

Background
INCIDENCE – The incidence of DVT is approximately 0.5%.

AETIOLOGY – The increased stasis in the veins and in the venous blood flow during pregnancy predisposes to thrombophlebitis in varicose veins and also to DVT (Figure 47.1). There is a 40% reduction in the flow through the common femoral vein in late pregnancy, and the effects are greater on the left leg than the right.

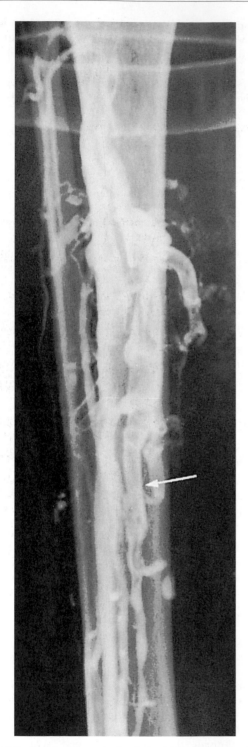

Fig 47.1 *Venogram demonstrating deep vein thrombosis. Reproduced from D. Sutton,* Radiology and Imaging for Medical Students, *7th edn, 1998, Churchill Livingstone.*

During pregnancy there is increased production in the liver of clotting factors I, VII, VIII, IX and X.

MAIN COMPLICATIONS – There is a 13% mortality from untreated pulmonary embolus and there is a risk of pulmonary embolus after DVTs, though the exact risk is unclear. Pulmonary embolus from calf veins is rare, though the risk of haemodynamically significant pulmonary emboli increases with popliteal and femoral venous thromboses, probably because they are larger.

There is also a risk of long-term venous insufficiency after venous thrombosis, as the clot can damage the deep veins and the valves therein. This manifests as varicose veins, as the blood travels in superficial vessels, and occasionally as swollen legs and venous ulceration.

PREVENTION – Prophylaxis is essential. Risk factors have been identified and those women at high risk should be offered prophylaxis. The best prophylactic measure to reduce the risk of DVT is early mobilisation following delivery, especially if this is by caesarean section. There is no proof that the use of antiembolic stockings or prophylactic heparin as a matter of course for operative deliveries offer any advantage. However, for women at increased risk of thromboembolism, serious consideration should be given to heparin therapy. Low-molecular-weight heparin is easy to use and appears to offer good protection against DVT in at-risk women. It is safe in pregnancy and does not appear to increase the risk of PPH.

Aspirin is increasingly being used as prophylaxis for women who have suffered a DVT in the past with no other risk factors.

Treatment Options

MEDICAL – In the presence of DVT, prompt anticoagulation is required with an initial bolus of 5–10 000 units of heparin followed by an infusion at a rate advised by the haematologist. Women can be changed to warfarin for home management or subcutaneous heparin. Treatment should be continued for 6 weeks postnatally. Warfarin is no longer commonly used antenatally, as there is a risk of fetal abnormality. However, there are no contraindications to its use postnatally. There is increasing interest in the use of low-molecular-weight heparins (Clexane, Fragmin) which only need once-per-day administration and appear to be at least as effective as heparin infusions.

OVERVIEW – Pregnancy itself is a risk factor for DVT, and the risk is increased by caesarean section, previous thromboembolic disease, etc. Women at high risk should be offered prophylaxis against DVT. There should be a low threshold for suspicion of thromboembolic disease, and investigation should be performed early where it is

Table 47.1   Swollen legs

	Oedema	Superficial thrombophlebitis	DVT
Swelling	Bilateral	Unilateral	Usually unilateral
Pain	Uncomfortable	Very tender over varicosities	Painful to deep palpation
Pyrexia	No	No	+/−
Treatment	Supportive	NSAIDs and compression	Heparin

suspected. Table 47.1 compares oedema, superficial thrombophlebitis and DVT.

Information for Patients

PROGNOSIS – The prognosis after DVT is generally good, though there is an increased risk of thromboembolic disease in future pregnancies and chronic venous insufficiency afterwards. Because of the increased recurrence risk, women should be seen early in any future pregnancy and prophylaxis commenced.

Follow-up

SHORT TERM – Women diagnosed with a DVT antenatally should be followed regularly and low-molecular-weight heparin administered once per day. The heparin can be stopped in labour and recommended for 6 weeks postpartum.

LONG TERM – Long-term follow-up is rarely required.

GOLDEN POINTS

1. Swollen legs are common in late pregnancy and the early puerperium.

2. Oedema is the most common cause of bilaterally swollen legs.

3. Superficial thrombophlebitis is usually self-limiting and presents little risk to the mother.

4. Thromboembolic disease is a major cause of maternal mortality.

5. Clinical signs are unreliable; women should be investigated by either venogram or Doppler where venous thrombosis is suspected.

6. Heparin is the drug of choice for both prophylaxis and treatment of venous thrombosis.

7. Risk assessment and prophylaxis for high-risk women should be mandatory.

Appendix

How to pass final MB

Table 1	Essay plan skeleton	
Opening paragraph:	Definition of condition Significance (mini-conclusion)	
Body:	Aetiology (causes) Incidence	
Complications:	**Obstetric**	**Gynaecological**
	1st Trimester	Pre-op assessment
	2nd Trimester	Anaesthetic
	3rd Trimester	Thromboembolic risk
	Intrapartum Postpartum Neonatal	
Management:	Always start with RESUSCITATION	
Treatment:	Condition specific	
Follow-up:		
Mini-conclusion:	Same as above but different wording	

FINAL MBBS – CLINICAL AND VIVA

Clinical

Almost all of the patients will be obstetric and don't be surprised if they seem absolutely normal; they probably are.

Remember how boring listening to 30 histories/day is. Concentrate on succinct summary, beginning and end which includes all the salient information.

Use obstetric language: e.g. pre-eclampsia, not a bit of blood pressure; antepartum haemorrhage rather than 'had a bleed'.

Sample Summary

'I'd like to introduce Mrs Wotssit who is a 30-year-old woman who is 34 weeks gestation in her second pregnancy who has been admitted to hospital after a painless antepartum haemorrhage'.

- Presenting Complaint – if any!
- History of current pregnancy:

- 1st Trimester: Pain and bleeding, hyperemesis
- 2nd Trimester: Booking visit; Down's risk and USS
- 3rd Trimester: Fetal history is kicking?
  Any other problems
- Previous O&G history
  - Antenatal
  - Intrapartum including induction and delivery?
  - Postnatal
- Family/genetic history

Examination
(NB: You can only fail by hurting/ignoring the patient)

- Inspection
  - Scars (LSCS) and linea nigra. Symphyseal–fundal height
- Palpation
  - Where is it? Use jargon. If all else fails, guess longitudinal lie, cephalic presentation, 3/5 palpable
- Auscultation
  - Over ant. shoulder

Table 2	Examination subjects
Likely subjects	**Think about**
Normal pregnancy	Get all basics, including Down's risk
Multiple pregnancy	Infertility Rx, exaggerated Sx of pregnancy
Placenta praevia	Bleeding, management? PP free
Previous LSCS	Recurring indication? Labour?
Mild PET	Booking BP, proteinuria? IUGR?
Small for dates	Differential Dx – baby, liquor, dates
Large for dates	Differential Dx – baby, liquor, dates

Viva

Practise likely topics in groups. Make certain you have at least seen the instruments below. You will instantly treble your chance of failure by reading a CTG upside down!

Practise viva topics as a question: 'Tell me about...'
  Try to use the same framework for each answer:

* definition/explanation
* clinical significance
* management, which includes diagnosis/indication, treatment and/or potential complications.

Remember – You will all pass!

Table 3   Likely viva table toys!

Obstetrics	Gynaecology
Forceps/ventouse	Ring pessary
Fetal scalp electrode	Uterine sound
Amnihook	Pipelle biopsy
CTG	IUCD/OCP
	Smear spatula/cytobrush
	Simms speculum

Table 4   Some suggested topics (not an exhaustive list)

Atrophic vaginitis	Antepartum haemorrhage	Anti-D
Blighted ovum	Augmentation of labour	Incontinence
CA 125	Cephalopelvic disproportion	CTG
Chlamydia	Diabetes in pregnancy	Endometriosis
Eclampsia	External cephalic version	TCRE
Fibroids (O&G)	Breech presentation	HRT
Hysteroscopy	Induction of labour	LLETZ
LHRH analogues	Prolapse	NTD
Ovarian cysts	Postcoital bleeding	PMB
PPH	Twin pregnancy	PET

Index